Chronobiology and Cardiovascular Diseases

Editor

ROBERTO MANFREDINI

HEART FAILURE CLINICS

www.heartfailure.theclinics.com

Consulting Editor
EDUARDO BOSSONE

Founding Editor
JAGAT NARULA

October 2017 • Volume 13 • Number 4

ELSEVIER

1600 John F. Kennedy Boulevard • Suite 1800 • Philadelphia, Pennsylvania, 19103-2899

http://www.theclinics.com

HEART FAILURE CLINICS Volume 13, Number 4
October 2017 ISSN 1551-7136, ISBN-13: 978-0-323-54666-9

Editor: Stacy Eastman
Developmental Editor: Alison Swety

Heart Failure Clinics (ISSN 1551-7136) is published quarterly by Elsevier Inc., 360 Park Avenue South, New York, NY 10010-1710. Months of publication are January, April, July, and October. Business and editorial offices: 1600 John F. Kennedy Boulevard, Suite 1800, Philadelphia, PA 19103-2899. Periodicals postage paid at New York, NY, and additional mailing offices. Subscription prices are USD 247.00 per year for US individuals, USD 448.00 per year for US institutions, USD 100.00 per year for US students and residents, USD 288.00 per year for Canadian individuals, USD 519.00 per year for Canadian institutions, USD 309.00 per year for international individuals, USD 519.00 per year for international institutions, and USD 100.00 per year for Canadian and foreign students/residents. To receive student and resident rate, orders must be accompanied by name of affiliated institution, date of term, and the *signature* of program/residency coordinator on institution letterhead. Orders will be billed at individual rate until proof of status is received. Foreign air speed delivery is included in all *Clinics* subscription prices. All prices are subject to change without notice. **POSTMASTER:** Send address changes to *Heart Failure Clinics*, Elsevier Health Sciences Division, Subscription Customer Service, 3251 Riverport Lane, Maryland Heights, MO 63043. **Customer Service: 1-800-654-2452 (US and Canada). From outside of the US and Canada, call 314-447-8871. Fax: 314-447-8029. For print support, E-mail: JournalsCustomerService-usa@elsevier.com. For online support, E-mail: JournalsOnlineSupport-usa@elsevier.com.**

Reprints. For copies of 100 or more of articles in this publication, please contact the Commercial Reprints Department, Elsevier Inc., 360 Park Avenue South, New York, NY 10010-1710. Tel.: 212-633-3874; Fax: 212-633-3820; E-mail: reprints@elsevier.com.

Heart Failure Clinics is covered in *MEDLINE/PubMed (Index Medicus).*

Contributors

CONSULTING EDITOR

**EDUARDO BOSSONE, MD, PhD, FCCP,
FESC, FACC**
Director, "Cava de' Tirreni" Cardiology Unit,
Heart Department, Scuola Medica Salernitana,
University Hospital, Lauro (AV), Salerno, Italy

EDITOR

ROBERTO MANFREDINI, MD, FRSPH
Full Professor, Internal Medicine, Head, Clinica
Medica Unit, Director, Department of Medical
Sciences, School of Medicine, Pharmacy and
Prevention, University of Ferrara, Ferrara, Italy

AUTHORS

WALTER AGENO, MD
Department of Medicine and Surgery,
Research Center on Thromboembolic
Diseases and Antithrombotic Therapies,
University of Insubria, Varese, Italy

DIANA E. AYALA, MD, MPH, PhD
Bioengineering & Chronobiology Laboratories,
Atlantic Research Center for Information and
Communication Technologies (AtlantTIC), E.I.
Telecomunicación, University of Vigo,
Pontevedra, Vigo, Spain

STEFANIA BASILI, MD
Associate Professor, Internal Medicine,
Department of Internal Medicine and Medical
Specialties, Sapienza University of Rome,
Rome, Italy

SRAVYA BHATIA, BS
Duke University School of Medicine, Duke
University Medical Center Greenspace,
Durham, North Carolina, USA

SUBIR BHATIA, MD
Department of Internal Medicine, Mayo Clinic,
Rochester, Minnesota, USA

**EDUARDO BOSSONE, MD, PhD, FCCP,
FESC, FACC**
Director, "Cava de' Tirreni" Cardiology
Unit, Heart Department, Scuola Medica
Salernitana, University Hospital, Lauro (AV),
Salerno, Italy

ROSARIA CAPPADONA, MW
Director of Teaching Activities, Department of
Morphology, Surgery and Experimental
Medicine, School of Medicine, Pharmacy and
Prevention, University of Ferrara, Ferrara, Italy

JUAN J. CRESPO, MD, PhD
Bioengineering & Chronobiology
Laboratories, Atlantic Research Center for
Information and Communication Technologies
(AtlantTIC), E.I. Telecomunicación, University
of Vigo, Centro de Salud de Bembrive,
Estructura de Gestión Integrada de Vigo,
Servicio Galego de Saúde (SERGAS), Vigo,
Spain

AFREDO DE GIORGI, MD
Department of Medical Sciences, University of
Ferrara, University Hospital St Anna, Ferrara,
Italy

FRANCESCO DENTALI, MD
Department of Medicine and Surgery, Research Center on Thromboembolic Diseases and Antithrombotic Therapies, University of Insubria, Varese, Italy

ABHISHEK DESHMUKH, MD
Division of Cardiovascular Diseases, Mayo Clinic, Rochester, Minnesota, USA

GEORGE DIBU, MD
Division of Cardiovascular Medicine, University of Florida, Gainesville, Florida, USA

AUSTIN DUONG, BSc, MBS
Department of Biomedical Sciences, Centre for Cardiovascular Investigations, University of Guelph, Guelph, Ontario, Canada

KIM A. EAGLE, MD, MACC
Division of Cardiology, Albion Walter Hewlett Professor of Internal Medicine, Professor of Health Management and Policy, University of Michigan School of Public Health, Director of the Frankel Cardiovascular Center, Domino's Farms, University of Michigan, Ann Arbor, Michigan, USA

FABIO FABBIAN, MD
Department of Medical Sciences, University of Ferrara, University Hospital St Anna, Ferrara, Italy

CHIARA FANTONI, MD
Department of Medicine and Surgery, Research Center on Thromboembolic Diseases and Antithrombotic Therapies, University of Insubria, Varese, Italy

UGO FEDELI, MD
Epidemiological Department, Veneto Region, Padova, Italy

JOSÉ R. FERNÁNDEZ, PhD
Bioengineering & Chronobiology Laboratories, Atlantic Research Center for Information and Communication Technologies (AtlantTIC), E.I. Telecomunicación, University of Vigo, Pontevedra, Vigo, Spain

MASSIMO GALLERANI, MD
Department of Internal Medicine, Hospital of Ferrara, Azienda Ospedaliero-Universitaria, Ferrara, Italy

RAMÓN C. HERMIDA, PhD, FASH
Director, Bioengineering & Chronobiology Laboratories, Atlantic Research Center for Information and Communication Technologies (AtlantTIC), E.I. Telecomunicación, University of Vigo, Pontevedra, Vigo, Spain

NIKI KATSIKI, MD, MSc, PhD, FRSPH
Second Propaedeutic Department of Internal Medicine, Hippokration University Hospital, Medical School, Aristotle University of Thessaloniki, Thessaloniki, Greece

LORRIE KIRSHENBAUM, PhD
Department of Physiology and Pathophysiology, Institute of Cardiovascular Sciences, St Boniface Hospital Research Centre, College of Medicine, Faculty of Health Sciences, University of Manitoba, Winnipeg, Manitoba, Canada

BJÖRN LEMMER, Prof.em., Dr.med., Dr.h.c.
Medical Faculty Mannheim, Institute of Experimental and Clinical Pharmacology and Toxicology, Ruprecht-Karls-University of Heidelberg, Mannheim, Germany

ELISA MAIETTI, CStat
Department of Medical Sciences, University of Ferrara, Center for Clinical Epidemiology, Ferrara, Italy

ROBERTO MANFREDINI, MD, FRSPH
Full Professor, Internal Medicine, Head, Clinica Medica Unit, Director, Department of Medical Sciences, School of Medicine, Pharmacy and Prevention, University of Ferrara, Ferrara, Italy

TAMI A. MARTINO, PhD
Department of Biomedical Sciences, Centre for Cardiovascular Investigations, University of Guelph, Guelph, Ontario, Canada

GIANLUIGI MAZZOCCOLI, MD
Chronobiology Unit, Division of Internal Medicine, Department of Medical Sciences, IRCCS "Casa Sollievo della Sofferenza," San Giovanni Rotondo, Foggia, Italy

JENNIFER MEARS, BS
Division of Cardiovascular Diseases, Mayo Clinic, Rochester, Minnesota, USA

PRIYA MISTRY, BSc
Department of Biomedical Sciences, Centre for
Cardiovascular Investigations, University of
Guelph, Guelph, Ontario, Canada

ARTEMIO MOJÓN, PhD
Bioengineering & Chronobiology Laboratories,
Atlantic Research Center for Information and
Communication Technologies (AtlantTIC), E.I.
Telecomunicación, University of Vigo,
Pontevedra, Vigo, Spain

MARCO PALA, MD
Department of Internal Medicine, Hospital of
Ferrara, Azienda Ospedaliero-Universitaria,
Ferrara, Italy

REED E. PYERITZ, MD, PhD, FACP, FACMG
Department of Medicine, William Smilow
Professor of Medicine and Professor of
Genetics, Senior Fellow, Leonard Davis
Institute of Health Economics, Smilow Center
for Translational Research, Perelman School of
Medicine, University of Pennsylvania,
Philadelphia, Pennsylvania, USA

MARÍA T. RÍOS, MD, PhD
Bioengineering & Chronobiology Laboratories,
Atlantic Research Center for Information and
Communication Technologies (AtlantTIC), E.I.
Telecomunicación, University of Vigo, and
Centro de Salud de A Doblada, Estructura de
Gestión Integrada de Vigo, Servicio Galego de
Saúde (SERGAS), Vigo, Spain

RAFFAELLA SALMI, MD
Head, Second Internal Medicine Unit, Azienda
Ospedaliera-Universitaria 'S.Anna' Ferrara,
Italy

ANUSHA SHANBHAG, MD
Department of Internal Medicine, University of
Arkansas for Medical Sciences, Little Rock,
Arkansas, USA

HASAN K. SIDDIQI, MD, MSCR
Fellow, Cardiovascular Medicine, Brigham and
Women's Hospital, Boston, Massachusetts,
USA

FULVIA SIGNANI, PsyD
Psychologist, Azienda Sanitaria Locale,
Ferrara, Italy

MICHAEL H. SMOLENSKY, PhD
Department of Biomedical Engineering,
Cockrell School of Engineering,
The University of Texas at Austin, Austin,
Texas, USA

ROBERTO TARQUINI, MD
Department of Clinical and Experimental
Medicine, Inter-institutional Department for
Continuity of Care of Empoli, School of
Medicine, University of Florence, Florence,
Italy

Contents

> The molecular clockwork drives rhythmic oscillations of signaling pathways managing intermediate metabolism; the circadian timing system synchronizes behavioral cycles and anabolic/catabolic processes with environmental cues, mainly represented by light/darkness alternation. Metabolic pathways, bile acid synthesis, and autophagic and immune/inflammatory processes are driven by the biological clock. Proper timing of hormone secretion, metabolism, bile acid turnover, autophagy, and inflammation with behavioral cycles is necessary to avoid dysmetabolism. Disruption of the biological clock and mistiming of body rhythmicity with respect to environmental cues provoke loss of internal synchronization and metabolic derangements, causing liver steatosis, obesity, metabolic syndrome, and diabetes mellitus.

> Circadian rhythms are fundamentally important for cardiovascular health, including heart rate, blood pressure, and molecular gene and protein responses. Rhythms also play a direct role in the pathophysiology of heart disease, such as in the timing of onset and severity of myocardial infarction, sudden cardiac death, ventricular arrhythmias, and stroke. Importantly, a flurry of new studies reveals translational applications for circadian biology to clinical medicine, and especially cardiology. Circadian medicine is a promising new approach that targets the heart's daily physiologic and molecular rhythms to benefit the treatment of patients with cardiovascular disease.

> The authors performed a MEDLINE search to identify reports, published during the past 20 years, focused on circadian variation of acute myocardial infarction (AMI) and prevalence, and the ratios between the number of events per hour during the morning and the other hours of the day were calculated. Despite the optimization of interventional and medical therapy of AMI since the first reports of circadian patterns in AMI occurrence, it was found that such a pattern still exists and that AMI happens most frequently in the morning hours.

> Seasonal variation for ischemic heart disease and heart failure is known. The interplay of environmental, biological, and physiologic changes is fascinating. This article highlights the seasonal periodicity of ischemic heart disease and heart failure and examines some of the potential reasons for these unique observations.

In recent years, several studies have consistently described the chronobiologic aspects of many cardiovascular diseases. Several studies have also assessed the circadian and circannual patterns of occurrence and mortality of deep vein thrombosis and pulmonary embolism, but the results have been less univocal. Different mechanisms have been proposed to explain these possible patterns, including oscillation of coagulation proteins, the role of meteorologic parameters, and air pollution. This article summarizes the available evidence on chronobiologic aspects of venous thromboembolism and discusses the casual mechanism.

Acute aortic syndromes are highly morbid conditions that require prompt diagnosis and management. Aortic dissections have rhythmic patterns, with notable peaks at certain points in every 24 hours as well as weekly and seasonal variations. Several retrospective studies have assessed the chronobiology of acute aortic dissections and there seems to be a winter seasonal peak and morning daily peak in incidence. Although the pathophysiology of this chronobiology is unclear, there are several environmental and physiologic possibilities. This article reviews the major studies examining the chronobiology of acute aortic dissection, and summarizes some theories on the pathophysiology of this phenomenon.

The occurrence of cardiovascular events shows a different distribution during the week, with many studies reporting a Monday peak, possibly related to the role of stress associated with commencing weekly activities. Furthermore, a higher mortality has been observed among patients hospitalized for cardiovascular and other disorders on weekends, a phenomenon known as "weekend effect." Such effect may be explained by a higher level of disease severity among patients admitted over the weekend, and/or by a poorer quality of care associated with shortage of staff, lower experience of personnel, and limited availability of therapeutic and diagnostic procedures.

Women are often excluded/underrepresented in clinical trials; sometimes, the number of men/women participants or separate analysis by sex are not reported. A robust body of evidence demonstrated that several life-threatening acute cardiovascular diseases, for example, acute myocardial infarction, sudden cardiac death, cardiac arrest, rupture or dissection of aortic aneurysms, and stroke, exhibit a circadian periodicity with a morning peak. An analysis of 20 years of chronobiologic studies (44% of them, accounting for 85% of total cases, with separate analysis by sex) confirmed that morning hours are a critical time of onset of acute cardiovascular diseases in men and women.

Signal Transduction and Chronopharmacology of Regulation of Circadian Cardiovascular Rhythms in Animal Models of Human Hypertension

Björn Lemmer

Inbred strains of rats can be used as models of human hypertension to evaluate mechanisms of regulation of the circadian rhythms underlying hypertension. Blood pressure and heart rate rhythms in rodents are endogenous (circadian). Studies have been performed in rats on the turnover of norepinephrine, on processes of signal transduction in the beta-adrenoceptor–adenylate cyclase–cyclic AMP–phosphodiesterase system and in the renin-angiotensin-aldosterone system, and on circadian rhythms in blood pressure and heart rate using radiotelemetry. The findings allowed a better understanding of the circadian phase–dependent kinetics and effects of cardiovascular active drugs (chronopharmacology) used in humans.

Bedtime Blood Pressure Chronotherapy Significantly Improves Hypertension Management

Ramón C. Hermida, Diana E. Ayala, José R. Fernández, Artemio Mojón, Juan J. Crespo, María T. Ríos, and Michael H. Smolensky

Consistent evidence of numerous studies substantiates the asleep blood pressure (BP) mean derived from ambulatory BP monitoring (ABPM) is both an independent and a stronger predictor of cardiovascular disease risk than are daytime clinic BP measurements or the ABPM-determined awake or 24-hour BP means. Hence, cost-effective adequate control of sleep-time BP is of marked clinical relevance. Ingestion time, according to circadian rhythms, of hypertension medications of 6 different classes and their combinations, significantly improves BP control, particularly sleep-time BP, and reduces adverse effects.

Bedtime Chronotherapy with Conventional Hypertension Medications to Target Increased Asleep Blood Pressure Results in Markedly Better *Chrono*prevention of Cardiovascular and Other Risks than Customary On-awakening Therapy

Michael H. Smolensky, Ramón C. Hermida, Diana E. Ayala, Artemio Mojón, and José R. Fernández

The bases for bedtime hypertension chronotherapy (BHCT) as superior chronoprevention against cardiovascular disease (CVD) are (1) correlation between blood pressure (BP) and various risks is greater for ambulatory BP monitoring (ABPM) than office BP measurements (OBPM); (2) asleep BP mean is a better predictor of CVD risk than ABPM awake and 24-hour means and OBPM; and (3) targeting of asleep BP by BHCT with one or more conventional medications versus usual on-awakening therapy better reduces major and total CVD events. BHCT offers the most cost-effective chronoprevention against adverse CVD outcomes in regular and vulnerable patients with renal, diabetic, and resistant hypertension.

HEART FAILURE CLINICS

ISSUE OF RELATED INTEREST

Medical Clinics, July 2015 (Vol. 99, Issue 4)
Management of Cardiovascular Disease
Deborah L. Wolbrette, *Editor*
Available at: http://www.medical.theclinics.com

THE CLINICS ARE AVAILABLE ONLINE!
Access your subscription at:
www.theclinics.com

Erratum

An error was made in two contributor addresses for the article, "Cardiac Resynchronization Therapy in Older Adults with Heart Failure," in the July 2017 issue of *Heart Failure Clinics* (Volume 13, Issue 3). The correct address for George E. Taffet, MD is Department of Geriatrics and Cardiovascular Medicine, Baylor College of Medicine, 1200 Binz Street, Suite 1470, Houston, TX, 77004, USA. The correct address for Ali Ahmed, MD, MPH is Department of Medicine, George Washington University, 2150 Pennsylvania Avenue, NW, Suite 8-416, Washington, DC 20037, USA. The online version of the article has been corrected.

Heart Failure Clin 13 (2017) xi
http://dx.doi.org/10.1016/j.hfc.2017.08.003
1551-7136/17/© 2017 Elsevier Inc. All rights reserved.

Preface
A Journey into the Science of Cardiovascular Chronobiology

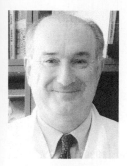 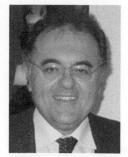

Roberto Manfredini,
MD, FRSPH
Editor

Eduardo Bossone, MD,
PhD, FESC, FACC
Consulting Editor

A lot of water has flowed under the bridge since, near twenty-four centuries ago, Androsthenes of Thasos described in a small clay board the first example of a circadian rhythm. It is not certain if he was an admiral of the Alexander's fleet or, more likely, a scientist, a naturalist, a geographer who accepted the invitation of his friend Nearchus, the trierarch of Alexander's fleet, to join the military expedition as a unique opportunity to discover new worlds. Androsthenes discovered that plants, and not only animals, are capable of movement. In fact, the leaves of *Tamarindus indica* opened and closed accordingly with sunlight.[1] However, only in the twentieth century did some landmark studies, such as the discovery of circadian clock mutants in *Drosophila melanogaster*[2] and the "forward genetics" approach to identify the *Clock* gene,[3] open up a new amazing world for scientists.

From this moment, an incredible explosion of studies was published with the MeSH term "circadian rhythm" with 42,470 articles published between 1990 and 2015 out of 64,847 overall (**Fig. 1**); that means more than 30 articles every week. A great interest has involved not only researchers of basic sciences but also many clinicians as well. After the milestone article on the circadian variation in the occurrence of myocardial infarction,[4] hundreds of studies and robust meta-analyses have identified the temporal frames in which the risk of onset of cardiovascular diseases (CVD) is highest, the time of the day, the day of week, and the season.[5–9] The final objective is to try to prevent the onset of unfavorable CVDs by using appropriate medications at appropriate times (chronotherapy).[10]

In this issue, some prestigious worldwide experts will introduce you to the fascinating world of the genetics and molecular biology of body clocks, and their influence on the heart and cardiovascular system.[11] Again, the available evidence on the link existing between biological rhythms and CVDs, such as ischemic heart disease, heart failure, aortic syndromes, and venous thromboembolism, will be accurately reviewed,[11–16] with particular attention to possible differences by gender.[17] Finally, last but not least, the more recent opportunities offered by chronotherapy will be reviewed, with particular attention to arterial hypertension, one of the leading risk factors for CVDs.[18–20]

We are deeply proud of the opportunity to introduce our readers to this interesting, amazing, and fascinating way of approaching cardiovascular medicine.

Heart Failure Clin 13 (2017) xiii–xv
http://dx.doi.org/10.1016/j.hfc.2017.06.001
1551-7136/17/© 2017 Published by Elsevier Inc.

heartfailure.theclinics.com

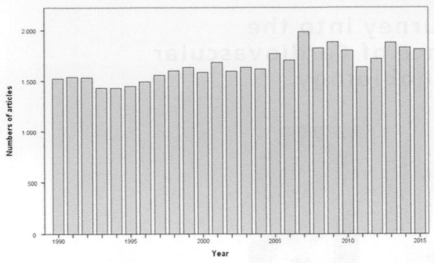

Fig. 1. PubMed search of published papers with the MeSH term "circadian rhythm," years 1990 to 2015.

Roberto Manfredini, MD, FRSPH
Department of Medical Sciences
School of Medicine, Pharmacy and Prevention
University of Ferrara Via L. Ariosto 35
44121 Ferrara, Italy

Eduardo Bossone, MD, PhD, FESC, FACC
'Cava de' Tirreni and Amalfi Coast'
Division of Cardiology
Heart Department
University Hospital
Salerno, Italy

E-mail addresses:
roberto.manfredini@unife.it (R. Manfredini)
ebossone@hotmail.com (E. Bossone)

REFERENCES

1. Bretzl H. Botanische Forschungen des Alexander-zuges. Leipzig: B.G. Teubner; 1903. p. 120–32.
2. Konopka RJ, Benzer S. Clock mutants of Drosophila melanogaster. Proc Natl Acad Sci U S A 1971;68: 2112–6.
3. Takahashi JS, Pinto LH, Vitaterna MH. Forward and reverse genetic approaches to behavior in mouse. Science 1994;264:1724–33.
4. Muller JE, Stone PH, Turi ZG, et al. Circadian variation in the frequency of onset of acute myocardial infarction. N Engl J Med 1985;313:1315–22.
5. Cohen MC, Rohtla KM, Lavery CE, et al. Meta-analysis of the morning excess of acute myocardial infarction and sudden cardiac death. Am J Cardiol 1997;79:1512–6.
6. Elliott WJ. Circadian variation in the timing of stroke onset: a meta-analysis. Stroke 1998;29:992–6.
7. Dentali F, Ageno W, Rancan E, et al. Seasonal and monthly variability in the incidence of venous thromboembolism. A systematic review and a meta-analysis of the literature. Thromb Haemost 2011; 106:439–47.
8. Witte DR, Grobbee DR, Bots ML, et al. A meta-analysis of excess cardiac mortality on Monday. Eur J Epidemiol 2005;20:401–6.
9. Vitale J, Manfredini R, Gallerani M, et al. Chronobiology of acute aortic rupture or dissection: a systematic review and a meta-analysis of the literature. Chronobiol Int 2015;32:385–94.
10. Manfredini R, Gallerani M, Salmi R, et al. Circadian rhythms and the heart: implications for chronotherapy of cardiovascular diseases. Clin Pharmacol Ther 1994;56:244–7.
11. Tarquini R, Mazzoccoli G. Clock genes, metabolism and cardiovascular risk. Heart Fail Clin 2017;13(4): 645–55.
12. Mistry P, Duong A, Kirshenbaum L, et al. Cardiac clocks and preclinical translation. Heart Fail Clin 2017;13(4):657–72.
13. Fabbian F, Bathia S, De Giorgi, et al. Circadian periodicity of ischemic heart disease. Heart Fail Clin 2017;13(4):673–80.
14. Gallerani M, Pala M, Fedeli U. Circaseptan periodicity of cardiovascular diseases. Heart Fail Clin 2017;13(4):703–19.
15. Siddiqi HK, Bossone E, Pyeritz RE, et al. Chronobiology of acute aortic syndromes. Heart Fail Clin 2017;13(4):697–701.
16. Fantoni C, Dentali F, Ageno W. Chronobiologic aspects of venous thromboembolism. Heart Fail Clin 2017;13(4):691–6.
17. Manfredini R, Salmi R, Cappadona R, et al. Sex and circadian periodicity of cardiovascular diseases. Are

women sufficiently represented in chronobiological studies? Heart Fail Clin 2017;13(4):719–38.

18. Lemmer B. Signal transduction and chronopharmacology of regulation of circadian cardiovascular rhythms in animal models of human hypertension. Heart Fail Clin 2017;13(4):739–57.

19. Hermida RC, Ayala DE, Fernandez JR, et al. Bedtime blood pressure chronotherapy significantly improves hypertension management. Heart Fail Clin 2017;13(4):759–73.

20. Smolensky MH, Hermida RH, Ayala DE, et al. Bedtime chronotherapy with conventional medications to target elevated asleep pressure results in markedly better chronoprevention of cardiovascular and other risk than customary on-awakening therapy. Heart Fail Clin 2017;13(4):775–92.

Clock Genes, Metabolism, and Cardiovascular Risk

Roberto Tarquini, MD[a,b], Gianluigi Mazzoccoli, MD[c,*]

KEYWORDS

• Clock • Gene • Circadian • Rhythm • Metabolism • Cardiovascular

KEY POINTS

• The biological clock rules periodic adjustments of biochemical processes controlling lipid and glucose metabolism, and the circadian timing system coordinates behavioral cycles and metabolic pathways with environmental cues.
• Metabolism, bile acid signaling, autophagy, and immunity/inflammation are driven by the clock gene machinery, which in turn is modulated by gut microbiota. Appropriate synchronization of these processes with behavioral cycles is required to thwart metabolism alteration.
• Derangements of the molecular clockwork or misalignment of the circadian timing system with respect to environmental cues causes chronodisruption and dysmetabolism, leading to cardio-metabolic disease.

INTRODUCTION

The continued existence of living beings on planet Earth is taunted, especially in the wild, by environmental challenges as well as changes of ecological niches and life conditions, such as temperature swinging, food availability, and predation risk, which in turn impact processes and activities crucial for individual and species survival, such as feeding, mating, and hunting, among others. Survival advantage is warranted by proper physiologic and behavioral modifications anticipating periodic and predictable variations of the environment and cycling in a huge frequency range.[1] The periodicity interval may span from the hourly variations of

heart rate to the monthly and seasonal fluctuations of hormone secretion and even to the circa-decennial rhythm of oscillation of umbilical cord blood parameters.[2,3] The most frequent and explored biological rhythms are hallmarked by a 24-hour period of oscillation resonating with the daily transition from darkness to solar illumination dictated by Earth's rotation on its axis. This potent environmental cue is perceived by the retina via melanopsin-containing ganglion cells and transferred to the suprachiasmatic nuclei (SCN) of the hypothalamus through the glutamatergic fibers of the retino-hypothalamic tract. In mammals, 24-hour rhythmicity is driven by the circadian timing system, a hierarchical multilevel organization

Conflict of Interest Statement: The authors declare that there are no conflicts of interest with respect to the authorship and/or publication of this article.
Financial Support: The study was supported by the 5 × 1000 voluntary contribution and by a grant (G. Mazzoccoli) through Division of Internal Medicine and Chronobiology Unit (RC1203ME46, RC1302ME31, RC1403ME50, RC1504ME53, and RC1603ME43), IRCCS Scientific Institute and Regional General Hospital "Casa Sollievo della Sofferenza", Opera di Padre Pio da Pietrelcina, San Giovanni Rotondo (F.G.), Italy.
[a] Department of Clinical and Experimental Medicine, School of Medicine, University of Florence, Viale Gaetano Pieraccini, 6, 50139, Florence, Italy; [b] Inter-institutional Department for Continuity of Care of Empoli, School of Medicine, University of Florence, Viale Gaetano Pieraccini, 6, 50139 Florence, Italy; [c] Chronobiology Unit, Division of Internal Medicine, Department of Medical Sciences, IRCCS "Casa Sollievo della Sofferenza", Cappuccini Avenue, San Giovanni Rotondo, Foggia 71013, Italy
* Corresponding author.
E-mail address: g.mazzoccoli@operapadrepio.it

Heart Failure Clin 13 (2017) 645–655
http://dx.doi.org/10.1016/j.hfc.2017.05.001
1551-7136/17/© 2017 Elsevier Inc. All rights reserved.

composed of the SCN, composed of approximately 15,000 to 20,000 neurons in rodents ad 80,000 to 100,000 neurons in humans, working as the principal oscillator synchronizing self-sustained oscillators in the peripheral tissues by means of neural fibers of the autonomic nervous system or by humoral factors (melatonin, cortisol).[4,5] Anatomic links connect the SCN to other brain regions, such as arcuate nucleus, ventromedial, dorsomedial, and lateral hypothalamic nuclei, controlling appetite, energy expenditure, and behavioral activity.[6,7] Environmental lighting is the prevailing entraining factor for SCN and sequentially for other brain areas and peripheral tissues, anyway alternative cues can overcome SCN control on peripheral clocks. In particular, feeding time is capable of disengaging peripheral oscillators and central oscillators; if experimental animals are fed only during the subjective day, when nocturnal animals usually are not active (restricted feeding), central and peripheral clocks tick in opposite phases.[8,9]

THE MOLECULAR CLOCKWORK

Neurons in SCN and interplaying brain areas as well as each cell in nearly all peripheral tissues harbor endowed biological clocks ticking through transcriptional-translational feedback loops (TTFLs) operated by a set of so-called clock genes and their coded proteins and revolving rhythmically with a roughly 24-hour period.[10–12] The positive limb of the TTFL in mammals, such as rodents and humans, is operated by the Period-Arnt-Single-minded and basic helix-loop-helix (PAS-bHLH) proteins circadian locomotor output cycles kaput (CLOCK), and its paralog neuronal PAS domain protein 2 (NPAS2), and by brain and muscle aryl-hydrocarbon receptor nuclear translocatorlike/aryl-hydrocarbon receptor nuclear translocatorlike (BMAL1/ARNTL1) or its homolog BMAL2/ARNTL2.[13] These transcription factors heterodimerize and bind to canonical E-box (5'-CACGTG-3') cis-regulatory enhancer sequences of their target genes Period (Per1-3) and Cryptochrome (Cry 1-2). The negative limb of the TTFL is operated by PER and CRY proteins, which in turn dimerize and form a repressor complex that translocates back to the nucleus and hinders CLOCK or NPAS2/BMAL1-2 transcriptional activity.[14,15] In Drosophila melanogaster as well as in other flies and insects, a cog of the molecular clockwork is represented by Timeless, which in mammals is conserved and collaborates with TIMELESS interacting protein in biological processes comprising embryonic development, cell cycle progression, DNA replication, and DNA damage response.[16]

SIRTUINS AND THE BIOLOGICAL CLOCK

The oscillation amplitude of numerous clock genes depends on the activity of SIRT1, a type III nicotinamide (NAM) adenine dinucleotide (NAD$^+$)-dependent histone/protein deacetylase, which rhythmically deacetylates BMAL1, histone H3, and PER2, decreasing PER2 stability in a circadian manner.[17,18] SIRT1 cofactor is de novo and cyclically synthesized from tryptophan through NAM phosphoribosyltransferase (NAMPT), the rate-limiting enzyme in the NAD$^+$ salvage pathway, whose expression is driven directly by BMAL1 with 24-hour periodicity and in the circulating form is defined as visfatin/pre-B-cell colony–enhancing factor.[19–22] High NAD+ and low adenosine triphosphate levels specify low-energy status in the cell, and high adenosine monophosphate (AMP) triggers AMP-activated kinase (AMPK), which activates NAMPT and modulates the NAD+/NADH balance,[23,24] working as a nutrient sensor prompted to reestablish energy balance in case of exercise, fasting, or hypoxia.[25,26] SIRT1 activity is obstructed through protein-protein interaction by deleted in breast cancer–1 (DBC1), which controls SIRT1 activity in metabolically active tissues, especially in the liver.[27] DBC1 was shown in animal models fed a high-calorie diet to bind SIRT1 and impede its deacetylase activity, whereas in animals starved or fed a low-calorie diet, DBC1 remains unbound and SIRT1 activity bolsters.[28] Experiments performed in vitro using cultured cells synchronized using different protocols show mitochondrial respiratory activity oscillation depends on BMAL1 levels and takes place independently from the cell type tested, the protocol of synchronization used, and the carbon source in the medium. Fluctuation in cellular NAD+ content and clock-genes–dependent expression of NAMPT and Sirtuins 1/3 dictate the rhythmic respiratory activity and is related to the acetylation/deacetylation cycle of a single subunit of the mitochondrial respiratory chain complex I, suggesting a molecular interplay between cellular bioenergetics and the molecular clockwork operated by a dedicated interlocked transcriptional-enzymatic feedback loop.[29,30]

POSTTRANSLATIONAL AND EPIGENETIC MODIFICATIONS

The functioning of the molecular clockwork crucially depends on posttranslational modification of the circadian proteins, comprising phosphorylation, acetylation, sumoylation, and ubiquitination, which modulates their transcriptional activity and intracellular localization.[31,32]

Mainly, casein kinases 1-δ and 1-ε (CK1δ and CK1ε) target Bmal1 as well as the PER and CRY proteins, tagging the latter for polyubiquitination by the E3 ubiquitin ligase complex β-transducin repeat containing protein 1 and SCF/Fbxl3 ubiquitin ligase complex (Skp1, Cullin1, F-box, and leucine-rich repeat protein 3), respectively.[33,34] The AKT-GSK3β system phosphorylates BMAL1,[35] and AMPK targets the CRY proteins tagging them for degradation through the 26S proteasome via the SCF/Fbxl3 ubiquitin ligase complex.[36] Another layer of regulation of the biological clock depends on cyclic epigenetic modifications. CLOCK is a histone acetyltransferase (HAT) and prompts protein acetylation and chromatin remodeling holding up gene transcription. Clock joins to E-boxes in the company of cyclic adenosine monophosphate (cAMP) response element–binding protein (CBP)/p300 and acetylates histones H3 and H4 and BMAL1, particularly the following: (1) the transcriptional coactivators and HAT p300/CBP, PCAF, and ACTR associate with CLOCK and NPAS2 to regulate trigger clock gene expression; (2) Cry2-mediated hindrance of NPAS2:BMAL1 transcriptional activity is surmounted by p300 overexpression; (3) p300 shows a 24-hour periodic association with NPAS2 in the vasculature heralding target genes expression climax; (4) a rhythm in core histone H3 acetylation on the mPer1 promoter in vivo correlates with mRNAs cyclical expression.[37–39] Besides, 24-hour rhythms of gene transcription at the level of the whole genome are driven by cycles of histone methylation catalyzed by methyltransferase MLL3 with alternation of activating (H3K4me3) and inhibitory (H3K9me3) chromatin marks[40] and cycles of histone lysine demethylation driven by the histone lysine demethylase JARID1a, which stimulates CLOCK-BMAL1 heterodimer transcriptional activity.[41]

AN AUXILIARY LOOP IN THE MOLECULAR CLOCKWORK

The oscillation of the starting cog of the TTFL-positive limb depends on the cycling of the reverse transcript of the erythroblastosis gene (REV-ERB) α/β and the retinoic acid–related (RAR) orphan receptor (ROR) α, β/δ, γ, whose expression is driven by the molecular clockwork and hard-wires an additional regulatory loop controlling BMAL1 expression. REV-ERBα/β, not capable of engaging coactivators and trigger target gene transcription, binds ROR-specific response elements (RORE) in Bmal1, Clock, and Cry1 promoters, impeding binding and activation of transcription by RORα.[42–44] RORα cooperates with the transcriptional coactivator peroxisome proliferator-activated receptor (PPAR)γ coactivator-1α (PGC-1α), which engages chromatin-remodeling complexes to the proximal Bmal1 promoter and prompts Bmal1 transcription. Conversely, REV-ERBα cooperates with histone deacetylase 3 (HDAC3) and nuclear receptor corepressor 1 (NCOR1), operates as an HDAC3 activating subunit and induces repression of transcription.[45] As a result, the 24-hour rhythm of the RORα/PGC-1α activator complex and REV-ERBα/NCOR1-HDAC3 repressor complex recruitment manages the 24-hour rhythmicity of Bmal1 expression. Experiments performed in mouse models showed that HDAC3 binds to the liver genome with circadian periodicity and drives the expression of gene-enriching pathways involved in lipid metabolism, whose alteration induces in vivo hepatic steatosis.[46] Heme is a physiologic ligand of REV-ERBα/β, binds to the ligand-binding domain with a 1:1 stoichiometry, and enhances thermal stability of these nuclear receptors. Heme synthesis is catalyzed by the rate-limiting enzyme delta-aminolevulinate synthase 1, whose expression is driven by the molecular clockwork; its binding to REV-ERBs induces corepressor NCOR1 recruitment, with repression of target genes (Bmal1 included), whereas heme dissociation prompts the expression of target genes according to modifications in intracellular redox balance.[47,48] REV-ERBs are also highly responsive to the redox state and gases. The addition of nitric oxide pulls out transcription repression induced by heme-bound REV-ERBs.[49] In addition, a thiol-disulfide redox switch modulates heme and REV-ERBβ interaction; the reduced dithiol state of REV-ERBβ binds heme 5-fold more tightly than the oxidized disulfide state. However, changes in the iron redox state do not impact heme binding to the ligand binding domain.[50] Moreover, heme influences BMAL1-NPAS2 transcription activity in vitro through a NPAS2 heme-binding motif via inhibition of DNA binding in response to carbon monoxide.[51]

THE CLOCK-CONTROLLED GENES

The molecular clockwork drives the expression of so-called clock-controlled genes, some in common among the different peripheral tissues and others specific to particular tissues and defined output genes, which manage biological processes at the cell level and physiologic functions at the tissue and organ level.[52] Principally, CLOCK:BMAL1 heterodimer drives the expression of the proline- and acidic amino acid–rich domain basic leucine zipper transcription factors albumin gene D-site binding protein (DBP), thyrotroph embryonic factor, and hepatic leukemia factor (HLF); these sequentially drive the transcription of thousands of genes.[53] In turn, DBP triggers *Per1* transcription feeding back on the molecular clockwork,[54] whereas REV-ERBs bind to RORE and trigger the expression of the nuclear factor interleukin 3 regulated protein (defined adenoviral E4 protein–binding protein, [E4BP4] as well), which fluctuates in antiphase regarding DBP, in order that these transcription factors manage the expression of downstream genes peaking in an opposite phase.[55] Another cog of the machinery is represented by the bHLH transcription factors differentially expressed in chondrocytes protein 1 (DEC1) and 2 (DEC2), which manage transcriptional repression/regulation of multiple circadian genes and feed back to the molecular clockwork.[56,57]

THE BIOLOGICAL CLOCK AND THE NUCLEAR RECEPTORS

The clock gene machinery drives rhythmic oscillations of several biological processes whose output feeds back in the biological clock (**Fig. 1**). A crucial role in this interplay is played by the nuclear receptors, ligand-dependent transcription factors capable of binding lipophilic ligands and interact directly with promoters of specific DNA sequences to modulate target gene expression. The intracellular level of several nuclear receptors oscillate with circadian rhythmicity in several metabolically active tissues, such as liver, muscle, and adipose tissue and in particular include constitutive androstane receptor (CAR); estrogen-related receptor (ERR) α, β, and γ; farnesoid receptor (FXR) α and β; glucocorticoid receptor (GR); Nur-related protein 1; PPAR α, δ/β, and γ; RAR α, β, and γ; retinoid X receptors (RXR) α, β, and γ; small heterodimeric partner (SHP); and thyroid hormone receptor α.[58,59] The rhythmic assembly of metabolites capable of binding nuclear receptors and the interplay among molecular clockworks and signaling pathways activated on ligand binding to nuclear receptors sustain the circadian regulation of metabolism. The biological clock drives the oscillation of nuclear receptors as well as their ligands; sequentially, the nuclear receptors gauge the metabolic status and feed back in the clock gene machinery binding to response elements on definite clock genes, specifying transcriptional networks that convey time-related and feeding-related cues to the metabolic pathways.[60] For instance, oxysterols and bile acids are produced with 24-hour periodicity, bind liver X receptor (LXR) and FXR, respectively, and in turn oxysterols binding LXRs trigger, whereas bile acids binding FXRs hinder the expression of *Cyp7a1*, which encodes CYP7A1, the rate-limiting enzyme in bile acid synthesis whose expression oscillates with circadian rhythmicity driven by the alternate binding of LXR and FXR on response elements at the gene promoter level.[61,62]

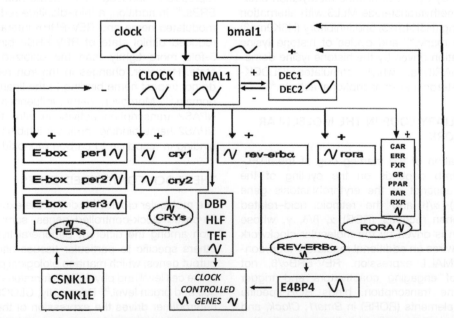

Fig. 1. The functioning of the clock gene machinery. Plus signs indicate activation; minus signs indicate inhibition; arrow-ended continuous lines indicate molecular interaction. CAR, constitutive androstane receptor; ERR, estrogen-related receptor; FXR, farnesoid receptor; GR, glucocorticoid receptor; RXR, retinoid X receptors.

THE MOLECULAR CLOCKWORK AND INTERMEDIATE METABOLISM

The biological clock drives the expression of many genes enriching the metabolic pathways that manage intermediate metabolism and coordinates the enzymatic cascades implicated in lipid and glucose metabolism.[63]

Lipid Metabolism

The circulating levels of lipids and the activity of enzymes catalyzing their synthesis and lysis, such as 3-hydroxy-3-methylglutaryl coenzyme A (HMG-CoA) reductase, fatty acid synthase, fatty acyl-CoA synthetase 1, as well as the carriers involved in their transport, such as apolipoprotein A-IV and C-III, fatty acid transport protein 1, or the receptors mediating their turnover, such as low-density lipoprotein receptor, oscillate with circadian rhythmicity in mammals.[63] The 24-hour cycle of Cyp7a1 expression is additionally controlled by REV-ERBα, DBP/E4BP4, and DEC2, which manage correct ruling of the circadian pattern, working through Rev-ROR response elements, DBP/E4BP4-binding elements, and E-boxes, respectively.[64] RORα is capable of binding cholesterol and its metabolites, for example, 7-oxygenated sterol, with transcriptional activity modulation,[65] and triggers the expression of apoC-III, a very low-density lipoprotein component,[66] whose transcription is thwarted by REV-ERBα.[67] On its side, REV-ERBα drives sterol regulatory element binding protein (SREBP) activity controlling the 24-hour rhythm of oscillation of the insulin-induced gene (INSIG) 2, which encodes an enzyme that seizes at the level of the endoplasmic reticulum membranes, the SREB-cleavage activating protein–INSIG-SREBP complex, which gauges cholesterol accessibility; in addition, driving the rhythmic nuclear accrual of SREBP, REV-ERBα also drives the time-related expression of Hmgcr, encoding HMG-CoA reductase, the rate-limiting enzyme of the mevalonate pathway, involved in the biosynthesis of cholesterol and other isoprenoids.[68] Besides, REV-ERBα manages bile acid metabolism via fluctuations of oxysterol synthesis and LXR activity and interplays with FXR to regulate SHP, hinders the expression of SHP and E4BP4 expression and triggers the expression of Cyp7a1 in the liver.[69] REV-ERBα manages lipid metabolism also through epigenetic changes brought on via HDAC3-NCOR1 complex recruitment at the level of genes involved in lipid metabolism, causing chromatin remodeling and histone modification: during the activity/feeding time, small REV-ERBα levels decrease HDAC3 binding to the liver genome and allow lipid buildup; however, during the resting/fasting time, high REV-ERBα levels augment HDAC3 recruitment to liver metabolic genes, hampering lipid biosynthesis.[46]

Glucose Metabolism

Glucose levels must be accurately gauged to provide a vital energy supply for cells in the different tissues of the organism and the equilibrium between glycogen anabolism and catabolism in metabolically active tissues helps to maintain roughly stable concentrations in the peripheral blood during the 24-hour day. On food intake, increasing plasma glucose levels prompts insulin secretion by Langerhans islets β cells in the pancreas, insulin signaling pathway triggering, glucose uptake, and polymerization into glycogen stores. However, glycogenolysis and/or gluconeogenesis in the liver during fasting generates glucose and the increase of GLUT2 expression induces GLUT2-mediated transport of glucose in the peripheral blood. Circadian changes ruled by central and peripheral biological oscillators drive the transcription of genes encoding enzymes and carriers implicated in glucose metabolism, comprising glycogen synthase 2 (GYS2), glycogen phosphorylase, phosphoenolpyruvate carboxykinase (PEPCK), glucokinase, glucose-6-phosphatase (GLC-6-Pase), and the glucose transporter GLUT2, among the others.[70,71] The biological clock drives glucose metabolism and in particular CRY1 and CRY2 control gluconeogenesis in the liver decreasing cAMP signaling in response to G protein–coupled receptor activation,[72] CLOCK drives glycogen synthesis in the liver triggering Gys2 transcription,[73] KLF10, a transcription factor encoded by a clock-controlled gene, hinders hepatic glucose production decreasing Pepck expression.[74] Glucocorticoids control glucose homeostasis and circadian rhythmicity modulating the expression of core clock genes, specifically Per1 and Per2, through binding via GRs to glucocorticoid response elements in their promoters.[75,76] GR levels oscillate with 24-hour periodicity in metabolically active tissues, in particular in white and brown adipose tissue, linking time-related and feeding-related cues to manage synchronicity between metabolic adjustments and clock gene machinery as well as activity and feeding.[76] Furthermore, Rev-erbα inhibits gluconeogenic gene expression in the liver and modulates hepatic glucose production in response to heme,[77] whereas RORα induces the expression of GLC-6-Pase and adjusts glycogen metabolism in the liver.[78] Specifically, the SWI/SNF chromatin-remodeling complex subunit

BAF60a, expressed in mouse liver with circadian rhythmicity, is bound at ROR response elements on the proximal *Bmal1* and *G6Pc* promoters, prompts their transcription through coactivation of RORα, and impacts the harmonized regulation of circadian clock, glucose metabolism, and energy homeostasis in the liver.[79] Moreover, experiments performed in primary hepatocytes showed that PGC-1α physically interacts with CK1δ and is phosphorylated at multiple sites within its arginine/serine-rich domain and sequentially degraded through the proteasome system, with the decrease of transcription of genes enriching pathways involved in hepatic gluconeogenesis and glucose secretion.[80]

THE BIOLOGICAL CLOCK AND DERANGED METABOLISM

The several cogs of the biological clock manage signaling pathways and biochemical reactions crucially involved in metabolic regulation and alteration of the molecular clockwork severely impacts lipid and glucose homeostasis. A comprehensive revision of the scientific literature regarding the role played by the altered functioning of the molecular clockwork in the derangement of lipid metabolism and in particular in liver steatosis, the most important anatomopathological manifestation of metabolic syndrome, is provided by a previous review article.[81] Regarding the role played by the molecular clockwork in glucose metabolism, its crucial involvement is corroborated by the reduced rhythmicity of clock genes expression found in peripheral leukocytes of patients affected by type 2 diabetes[82] and by the increased risk of impaired fasting glucose and type 2 diabetes highlighted by genome-wide association studies in subjects carrying a *Cry2* variant allele.[83,84] Accordingly, experiments performed in mouse models showed that *Clock* and *Bmal1* mutation induces disrupted glucose homeostasis.[85] $Clock^{\Delta19/\Delta19}$ and pancreas-specific $Bmal1^{-/-}$ mutant mice are hallmarked by altered glucose tolerance, decreased insulin secretion, and reduced size and proliferation of pancreatic islets deteriorating in the course of time.[86,87] Furthermore, Langerhans islets β cells harbor a self-sustained and autonomous molecular clockwork,[88] and disruption of the biological clock induced altered transcription of genes enriching pathways involved in insulin secretion (GNAQ, ATP1A1, ATP5G2, KCNJ11) as well as granule maturation and release (VAMP3, STX6, SLC30A8) and caused altered circadian pattern of basal insulin secretion by human islet cells synchronized in vitro.[89] Besides, mice with specific *Bmal1* disruption in the liver are hallmarked by deranged hepatocyte molecular clockwork; GLUT2 expression is stably low; these animal models show undue glucose clearance, altered rhythmic patterns of hepatic glucose regulatory genes expression, and hypoglycemia expression during the fasting/resting phase of the nychthemeral period.[90]

THE CLOCK GENE MACHINERY, LIVER STEATOSIS, AND CARDIOVASCULAR DISEASE

The altered functioning of the biological clock is critically involved in the pathogenesis of nonalcoholic fatty liver disease (NAFLD), which is associated with increased risk of cardiovascular disease.[91] NAFLD is the most frequent hepatic pathology in the Western world[92] and in one-fifth of all cases may progress to chronic hepatic inflammation (nonalcoholic steatohepatitis [NASH]) associated with cirrhosis, portal hypertension, and hepatocellular carcinoma.[93] Diseases related to dysmetabolism represent public health problems and pose a huge economic and social burden on national health systems worldwide. Obesity, a distinctive metabolic syndrome trait, augments the risk for diabetes and cardiovascular diseases; NAFLD is considered the hepatic manifestation of metabolic syndrome.[94] Impressive modifications occurred throughout the previous decades in dietary macronutrient intake, such as overconsumption of energy-dense foods, particularly high-fat and high-sugar diets, which, in addition to reduced physical activity, determine energy imbalance leading to obesity and impacted metabolic diseases prevalence.[95] Nutrient-sensing information is exchanged among organs to preserve systemic energy homeostasis, and the liver plays a key role in the integration and processing of signals derived from other tissues, such as intestine, pancreas, and adipose tissue. Interorgan communication is conveyed by humoral factors, such as insulin, adipocytokines, and glucocorticoids; by the autonomic nervous system[96]; and by dietary signals, such as fatty acids, glucose, and other metabolites: these factors are sensed by nuclear receptors that consecutively control nutrient signaling pathways. Bile acids, chiefly identified as important detergents necessary for lipid absorption in the intestine, are able to turn on nuclear receptor signaling pathways and come out as crucial metabolism regulators.[60] In the past decade, an everincreasing bulk of evidence has highlighted a critical role played by the intestine in molecular regulation of diet-related diseases that exceeds its function in nutrient digestion and extraction to maintain body metabolic homeostasis. The intestine secretes enteroendocrine hormones as well, and the harbored gut microbial flora is ever more regarded as an essential player in the modulation of metabolic processes. Consequently, innovative preventive and therapeutic approaches, for instance, drugs targeting nuclear receptors, bile acid signaling, or gut microbiota modulation, are investigated in addition to conventional strategies, including diet and physical activity, which have been ineffective in diminishing metabolic disease prevalence.[97]

THE BIOLOGICAL CLOCK AT THE CROSSROAD OF AUTOPHAGY, GUT MICROBIOTA, INFLAMMATION, BILE ACID SIGNALING, AND INTERMEDIATE METABOLISM

Multifaceted interactions occur among metabolic pathways of lipids, glucose, bile acids and autophagy, inflammation, and their regulation by the biological clock in response to nutrients, bile acids, hormones, nuclear receptors, or gut microbiota.[98–103] This interplay is supported by strong evidence: (1) the metabolic derangements underlying NAFLD and the progression from NAFLD to NASH hint of a key role played by nutrients and bile acids acting as ligands of nuclear receptors, which manage the metabolic pathways, and as signaling molecules in metabolism and inflammation. Bile acids influence macrophage function, energy homeostasis, and gastrointestinal insulinotropic hormones secretion and are metabolized by the gut microbiota, which may change the bile acids binding capacity of their receptors and influence the intestinal immune system and the metabolic processes[104–109]; (2) NLRP6 and NLRP3 inflammasomes negatively regulate NAFLD to NASH progression through changes of the gut microbiota configuration and entry of Toll-like receptor (TLR) 4 and TLR9 agonists into the portal circulation, with modulation of hepatic tumor-necrosis factor (TNF)-α expression driving NASH progression, and TLR7 impacts NAFLD pathogenesis as well[110,111]; (3) recent studies have pinpointed the role played by autophagy in NAFLD pathogenesis, suggesting the therapeutic potential of its regulation.[112] Remarkably, hepatic metabolic pathways and bile acid synthesis as well as autophagic and immune/inflammatory processes are driven by the biological clock. Besides, gut microbiota impact the biological clock[113]; appropriate timing of circadian patterns of hormone secretion, metabolism, bile acid turnover, autophagy, and inflammation with behavioral cycles is necessary to avoid hepatic dysfunction and metabolic disorders.[114–123] Furthermore, experiments performed in aryl hydrocarbon receptor (AHR, a xenobiotic receptor for exogenous toxicants) liver-specific and inducible transgenic mice fed an obesogenic diet showed that AHR signaling pathway activation worsens liver steatosis and in contradiction avoids obesity and systemic insulin resistance interplaying with the biological clock.[124,125] Interestingly, fibroblast growth factor 21, which interacting with β-Klotho coordinates a change to oxidative metabolism during fasting and starvation and has been involved as a mediator joining nutrition, growth, reproduction, and longevity,[126] was recognized as a direct AHR target in the liver and as the inducer of the systemic metabolic benefits in addition to liver steatosis observed in AHR transgenic mice.[124,125]

SUMMARY

The biological clock controls the molecular signaling pathways involved in metabolism regulation; the circadian timing system drives sleep/wake, rest/activity, and fasting/feeding rhythmicity, harmonizing behavioral cycles with energy flux and expenditure and synchronizing the timing of anabolic/catabolic processes with environmental cues, predominantly light/dark alternation and temperature fluctuations. The cogs of the molecular clockwork drive the periodic oscillation of biochemical processes; the nuclear receptors sense nutrient levels and the cellular redox state, guiding the recruitment of coactivators, corepressors, HATs, and HDACs to DNA sequences. These molecular events prompt chromatin remodeling and histone modifications and trigger rhythms of epigenetic modification, transcriptional activity, and gene expression, coordinating metabolic pathways with nychthemeral rhythmicity of behavior. Alteration of the biological clock as well as misalignment of body 24-hour rhythmicity with respect to environmental cues lead to chronodisruption with internal synchronization failure and metabolic derangements, ultimately causing liver steatosis, obesity, metabolic syndrome, and diabetes mellitus, with increased risk of cardiovascular diseases.

REFERENCES

1. Dunlap JC. Molecular bases for circadian clocks. Cell 1999;96(2):271–90.
2. Mazzoccoli G, Miscio G, Fontana A, et al. Time related variations in stem cell harvesting of umbilical cord blood. Sci Rep 2016;6:21404.
3. Scholkmann F, Miscio G, Tarquini R, et al. The circadecadal rhythm of oscillation of umbilical cord blood parameters correlates with geomagnetic activity - an analysis of long-term measurements (1999-2011). Chronobiol Int 2016;33(9):1136–47.

4. Albrecht U. Timing to perfection: the biology of central and peripheral circadian clocks. Neuron 2012;74(2):246–60.

5. Nagoshi E, Saini C, Bauer C, et al. Circadian gene expression in individual fibroblasts: cell-autonomous and self-sustained oscillators pass time to daughter cells. Cell 2004;119:693–705.

6. Kalsbeek A, Palm IF, La Fleur SE, et al. SCN outputs and the hypothalamic balance of life. J Biol Rhythms 2006;21(6):458–69.

7. Luo AH, Aston-Jones G. Circuit projection from suprachiasmatic nucleus to ventral tegmental area: a novel circadian output pathway. Eur J Neurosci 2009;29(4):748–60.

8. Damiola F, Le Minh N, Preitner N, et al. Restricted feeding uncouples circadian oscillators in peripheral tissues from the central pacemaker in the suprachiasmatic nucleus. Genes Dev 2000;14:2950–61.

9. Stokkan KA, Yamazaki S, Tei H, et al. Entrainment of the circadian clock in the liver by feeding. Science 2001;291:490–3.

10. Mazzoccoli G, Francavilla M, Pazienza V, et al. Differential patterns in the periodicity and dynamics of clock gene expression in mouse liver and stomach. Chronobiol Int 2012;29(10):1300–11.

11. Mazzoccoli G, Francavilla M, Giuliani F, et al. Clock gene expression in mouse kidney and testis: analysis of periodical and dynamical patterns. J Biol Regul Homeost Agents 2012;26(2):303–11.

12. Bonny O, Vinciguerra M, Gumtz ML, et al. Molecular bases of circadian rhythmicity in renal physiology and pathology. Nephrol Dial Transplant 2013;28(10):2421–31.

13. Mazzoccoli G, Rubino R, Tiberio C, et al. Clock gene expression in human and mouse hepatic models shows similar periodicity but different dynamics of variation. Chronobiol Int 2016;33(2):181–90.

14. Ko CH, Takahashi JS. Molecular components of the mammalian circadian clock. Hum Mol Genet 2006;15(Spec No. 2):R271–7.

15. Lowrey PL, Takahashi JS. Genetics of circadian rhythms in mammalian model organisms. Adv Genet 2011;74:175–230.

16. Mazzoccoli G, Laukkanen MO, Vinciguerra M, et al. A timeless link between circadian patterns and disease. Trends Mol Med 2016;22(1):68–81.

17. Nakahata Y, Kaluzova M, Grimaldi B, et al. The NAD+-dependent deacetylase SIRT1 modulates CLOCK-mediated chromatin remodeling and circadian control. Cell 2008;134(2):329–40.

18. Asher G, Gatfield D, Stratmann M, et al. SIRT1 regulates circadian clock gene expression through PER2 deacetylation. Cell 2008;134(2):317–28.

19. Nakahata Y, Sahar S, Astarita G, et al. Circadian control of the NAD+ salvage pathway by CLOCK-SIRT1. Science 2009;324:654–7.

20. Ramsey K, Yoshino J, Brace CS, et al. Circadian clock feedback cycle through NAMPT-mediated NAD+ biosynthesis. Science 2009;324:651–4.

21. Sahar S, Nin V, Barbosa MT, et al. Altered behavioral and metabolic circadian rhythms in mice with disrupted NAD+ oscillation. Aging (Albany NY) 2011;3(8):794–802.

22. Benedict C, Shostak A, Lange T, et al. Diurnal rhythm of circulating nicotinamide phosphoribosyltransferase (Nampt/visfatin/PBEF): impact of sleep loss and relation to glucose metabolism. J Clin Endocrinol Metab 2012;97(2):E218–22.

23. Fulco M, Sartorelli V. Comparing and contrasting the roles of AMPK and SIRT1 in metabolic tissues. Cell Cycle 2008;7:3669–79.

24. Cantó C, Auwerx J. PGC-1alpha, SIRT1 and AMPK, an energy sensing network that controls energy expenditure. Curr Opin Lipidol 2009;20:98–105.

25. Kahn BB, Alquier T, Carling D, et al. AMP-activated protein kinase: ancient energy gauge provides clues to modern understanding of metabolism. Cell Metab 2005;1(1):15–25.

26. Long YC, Zierath JR. AMP-activated protein kinase signaling in metabolic regulation. J Clin Invest 2006;116(7):1776–83.

27. Kim JE, Chen J, Lou Z. DBC1 is a negative regulator of SIRT1. Nature 2008;451(7178):583–6.

28. Escande C, Chini CC, Nin V, et al. Deleted in breast cancer-1 regulates SIRT1 activity and contributes to high-fat diet-induced liver steatosis in mice. J Clin Invest 2010;120(2):545–58.

29. Cela O, Scrima R, Pazienza V, et al. Clock genes-dependent acetylation of complex I sets rhythmic activity of mitochondrial OxPhos. Biochim Biophys Acta 2016;1863(4):596–606.

30. Scrima R, Cela O, Merla G, et al. Clock-genes and mitochondrial respiratory activity: evidence of a reciprocal interplay. Biochim Biophys Acta 2016;1857(8):1344–51.

31. Lee J, Lee Y, Lee MJ, et al. Dual modification of BMAL1 by SUMO2/3 and ubiquitin promotes circadian activation of the CLOCK/BMAL1 complex. Mol Cell Biol 2008;28(19):6056–65.

32. Eide EJ, Vielhaber EL, Hinz WA, et al. The circadian regulatory proteins BMAL1 and cryptochromes are substrates of casein kinase Iε. J Biol Chem 2002;277:17248–54.

33. Agostino PV, Harrington ME, Ralph MR, et al. Casein kinase-1-epsilon (CK1epsilon) and circadian photic responses in hamsters. Chronobiol Int 2009;26:126–33.

34. Sahar S, Zocchi L, Kinoshita C, et al. Regulation of BMAL1 protein stability and circadian function by GSK3beta-mediated phosphorylation. PLoS One 2010;5(1):e8561.

35. Lamia KA, Sachdeva UM, Ditacchio L, et al. AMPK regulates the circadian clock by cryptochrome

phosphorylation and degradation. Science 2009; 326:437–40.

36. Cardone L, Hirayama J, Giordano F, et al. Circadian clock control by SUMOylation of BMAL1. Science 2005;309(5739):1390–4.

37. Curtis AM, Seo SB, Westgate EJ, et al. Histone acetyltransferase-dependent chromatin remodeling and the vascular clock. J Biol Chem 2004; 279(8):7091–7.

38. Doi M, Hirayama J, Sassone-Corsi P. Circadian regulator CLOCK is a histone acetyltransferase. Cell 2006;125:497–508.

39. Hirayama J, Sahar S, Grimaldi B, et al. CLOCK-mediated acetylation of BMAL1 controls circadian function. Nature 2007;450:1086–90.

40. Valekunja UK, Edgar RS, Oklejewicz M, et al. Histone methyltransferase MLL3 contributes to genome-scale circadian transcription. Proc Natl Acad Sci U S A 2013;110(4):1554–9.

41. Di Tacchio L, Le HD, Vollmers C, et al. Histone lysine demethylase JARID1a activates CLOCK-BMAL1 and influences the circadian clock. Science 2011;333(6051):1881–5.

42. Preitner N, Damiola F, Lopez-Molina L, et al. The orphan nuclear receptor REV-ERBalpha controls circadian transcription within the positive limb of the mammalian circadian oscillator. Cell 2002; 110:251–60.

43. Burris TP. Nuclear hormone receptors for heme: REV-ERBalpha and REV-ERBbeta are ligand-regulated components of the mammalian clock. Mol Endocrinol 2008;22(7):1509–20.

44. Mazzoccoli G, Cai Y, Liu S, et al. REV-ERBalpha and the clock gene machinery in mouse peripheral tissues: a possible role as a synchronizing hinge. J Biol Regul Homeost Agents 2012;26(2):265–76.

45. Alenghat T, Meyers K, Mullican SE, et al. Nuclear receptor corepressor and histone deacetylase 3 govern circadian metabolic physiology. Nature 2008;456:997–1000.

46. Feng D, Liu T, Sun Z, et al. A circadian rhythm orchestrated by histone deacetylase 3 controls hepatic lipid metabolism. Science 2011;331(6022): 1315–9.

47. Kaasik K, Lee CC. Reciprocal regulation of haem biosynthesis and the circadian clock in mammals. Nature 2004;430(6998):467–71.

48. Raghuram S, Stayrook KR, Huang P, et al. Identification of heme as the ligand for the orphan nuclear receptors REV-ERBalpha and REV-ERBbeta. Nat Struct Mol Biol 2007;14(12):1207–13.

49. Pardee KI, Xu X, Reinking J, et al. The structural basis of gas-responsive transcription by the human nuclear hormone receptor REV-ERBbeta. PLoS Biol 2009;7(2):e43.

50. Gupta N, Ragsdale SW. Thiol-disulfide redox dependence of heme binding and heme ligand switching in nuclear hormone receptor rev-erb {beta}. J Biol Chem 2011;286(6):4392–403.

51. Gilles-Gonzalez MA, Gonzalez G. Signal transduction by heme-containing PAS-domain proteins. J Appl Physiol (1985) 2004;96(2):774–83.

52. Bozek K, Relógio A, Kielbasa SM, et al. Regulation of clock-controlled genes in mammals. PLoS One 2009;4(3):e4882.

53. Gachon F, Olela FF, Schaad O, et al. The circadian PAR-domain basic leucine zipper transcription factors DBP, TEF, and HLF modulate basal and inducible xenobiotic detoxification. Cell Metabol 2006;4:25–36.

54. Yamaguchi S, Mitsui S, Yan L, et al. Role of DBP in the circadian oscillatory mechanism. Mol Cell Biol 2000;20(13):4773–81.

55. Mitsui S, Yamaguchi S, Matsuo T, et al. Antagonistic role of E4BP4 and PAR proteins in the circadian oscillatory mechanism. Genes Dev 2001; 15(8):995–1006.

56. Miyazaki K, Kawamoto T, Tanimoto K, et al. Identification of functional hypoxia response elements in the promoter region of the DEC1 and DEC2 genes. J Biol Chem 2002;277(49):47014–21.

57. Noshiro M, Kawamoto T, Furukawa M, et al. Rhythmic expression of DEC1 and DEC2 in peripheral tissues: DEC2 is a potent suppressor for hepatic cytochrome P450s opposing DBP. Genes Cells 2004;9:317–29.

58. Bookout AL, Jeong Y, Downes M, et al. Anatomical profiling of nuclear receptor expression reveals a hierarchical transcriptional network. Cell 2006; 126:789–99.

59. Yang X, Downes M, Yu RT, et al. Nuclear receptor expression links the circadian clock to metabolism. Cell 2006;126:801–10.

60. Yang X. A wheel of time: the circadian clock, nuclear receptors, and physiology. Genes Dev 2010;24(8):741–7.

61. Galman C, Angelin B, Rudling M. Bile acid synthesis in humans has a rapid diurnal variation that is asynchronous with cholesterol synthesis. Gastroenterology 2005;129:1445–53.

62. Moore JT, Goodwin B, Willson TM, et al. Nuclear receptor regulation of genes involved in bile acid metabolism. Crit Rev Eukaryot Gene Expr 2002; 12:119–35.

63. Mazzoccoli G, Pazienza V, Vinciguerra M. Clock genes and clock controlled genes in the regulation of metabolic rhythms. Chronobiol Int 2012;29(3): 227–51.

64. Lavery DJ, Schibler U. Circadian transcription of the cholesterol 7alpha hydroxylase gene may involve the liver-enriched bZIP protein DBP. Genes Dev 1993;7:1871–84.

65. Wang Y, Kumar N, Solt LA, et al. Modulation of ROR {alpha} and ROR{gamma} activity by 7-oxygenated sterol ligands. J Biol Chem 2009;285:5013–25.

66. Raspé E, Duez H, Gervois P, et al. Transcriptional regulation of apolipoprotein C-III gene expression by the orphan nuclear receptor RORalpha. J Biol Chem 2001;276(4):2865–71.

67. Raspé E, Duez H, Mansen A, et al. Identification of Rev-erbalpha as a physiological repressor of apoC-III gene transcription. J Lipid Res 2002;43:2172–9.

68. Le Martelot G, Claudel T, Gatfield D, et al. REV-ERBalpha participates in circadian SREBP signaling and bile acid homeostasis. PLoS Biol 2009;7(9):e1000181.

69. Duez H, van der Veen JN, Duhem C, et al. Regulation of bile acid synthesis by the nuclear receptor Rev-erbα. Gastroenterology 2008;135:689–98.

70. Gachon F, Nagoshi E, Brown SA, et al. The mammalian circadian timing system: from gene expression to physiology. Chromosoma 2004;113:103–12.

71. Gatfield D, Schibler U. Circadian glucose homeostasis requires compensatory interference between brain and liver clocks. Proc Natl Acad Sci U S A 2008;105(39):14753–4.

72. Zhang EE, Liu Y, Dentin R, et al. Cryptochrome mediates circadian regulation of cAMP signaling and hepatic gluconeogenesis. Nat Med 2010;16(10):1152–6.

73. Doi R, Oishi K, Ishida N. CLOCK regulates circadian rhythms of hepatic glycogen synthesis through transcriptional activation of Gys2. J Biol Chem 2010;285(29):22114–21.

74. Guillaumond F, Gréchez-Cassiau A, Subramaniam M, et al. Kruppel-like factor KLF10 is a link between the circadian clock and metabolism in liver. Mol Cell Biol 2010;30(12):3059–70.

75. Yamamoto T, Nakahata Y, Tanaka M, et al. Acute physical stress elevates mouse period1 mRNA expression in mouse peripheral tissues via a glucocorticoid- responsive element. J Biol Chem 2005;280:42036–43.

76. So AY, Bernal TU, Pillsbury ML, et al. Glucocorticoid regulation of the circadian clock modulates glucose homeostasis. Proc Natl Acad Sci U S A 2009;106(41):17582–7.

77. Yin L, Wu N, Curtin JC, et al. Rev-erbalpha, a heme sensor that coordinates metabolic and circadian pathways. Science 2007;318:1786–9.

78. Chauvet C, Vanhoutteghem A, Duhem C, et al. Control of gene expression by the retinoic acid-related orphan receptor alpha in HepG2 human hepatoma cells. PLoS One 2011;6(7):e22545.

79. Tao W, Chen S, Shi G, et al. SWItch/sucrose nonfermentable (SWI/SNF) complex subunit BAF60a integrates hepatic circadian clock and energy metabolism. Hepatology 2011;54(4):1410–20.

80. Li S, Chen XW, Yu L, et al. Circadian metabolic regulation through crosstalk between casein kinase 1δ and transcriptional coactivator PGC-1α. Mol Endocrinol 2011;25(12):2084–93.

81. Mazzoccoli G, Vinciguerra M, Oben J, et al. Nonalcoholic fatty liver disease: the role of nuclear receptors and circadian rhythmicity. Liver Int 2014;34(8):1133–52.

82. Ando H, Takamura T, Matsuzawa-Nagata N, et al. Clock gene expression in peripheral leucocytes of patients with type 2 diabetes. Diabetologia 2009;52(2):329–35.

83. Dupuis J, Langenberg C, Prokopenko I, et al. New genetic loci implicated in fasting glucose homeostasis and their impact on type 2 diabetes risk. Nat Genet 2010;42(2):105–16.

84. Liu C, Li H, Qi L, et al. Variants in GLIS3 and CRY2 are associated with type 2 diabetes and impaired fasting glucose in Chinese Hans. PLoS One 2011;6(6):e21464.

85. Rudic R, McNamara P, Curtis AM, et al. BMAL1 and CLOCK, two essential components of the circadian clock, are involved in glucose homeostasis. PLoS Biol 2004;2:e377.

86. Marcheva B, Ramsey KM, Buhr ED, et al. Disruption of the clock components CLOCK and BMAL1 leads to hypoinsulinaemia and diabetes. Nature 2010;466(7306):627–31.

87. Sadacca LA, Lamia KA, deLemos AS, et al. An intrinsic circadian clock of the pancreas is required for normal insulin release and glucose homeostasis in mice. Diabetologia 2011;54(1):120–4.

88. Pulimeno P, Mannic T, Sage D, et al. Autonomous and self-sustained circadian oscillators displayed in human islet cells. Diabetologia 2013;56(3):497–507.

89. Saini C, Petrenko V, Pulimeno P, et al. A functional circadian clock is required for proper insulin secretion by human pancreatic islet cells. Diabetes Obes Metab 2016;18(4):355–65.

90. Lamia KA, Storch KF, Weitz CJ. Physiological significance of a peripheral tissue circadian clock. Proc Natl Acad Sci U S A 2008;105(39):15172–7.

91. Targher G, Day CP, Bonora E. Risk of cardiovascular disease in patients with nonalcoholic fatty liver disease. N Engl J Med 2010;363:1341–50.

92. Williams CD, Stengel J, Asike MI, et al. Prevalence of nonalcoholic fatty liver disease and nonalcoholic steatohepatitis among a largely middle-aged population utilizing ultrasound and liver biopsy: a prospective study. Gastroenterology 2011;140(1):124–31.

93. Bugianesi E, Leone N, Vanni E, et al. Expanding the natural history of nonalcoholic steatohepatitis: from cryptogenic cirrhosis to hepatocellular carcinoma. Gastroenterology 2002;123(1):134–40.

94. Podrini C, Borghesan M, Greco A, et al. Redox homeostasis and epigenetics in non-alcoholic fatty liver disease (NALFD). Curr Pharm Des 2013;19(15):2737–46.

95. Mazzoccoli G, Longhitano C, Vinciguerra M. Cardio-hepatic metabolic derangements and valproic acid. Curr Clin Pharmacol 2014;9(2):165–70.

96. Rotman Y, Sanyal AJ. Current and upcoming pharmacotherapy for non-alcoholic fatty liver disease. Gut 2017;66(1):180–90.

97. Sayin SI, Wahlström A, Felin J, et al. Gut microbiota regulates bile acid metabolism by reducing the levels of tauro-beta-muricholic acid, a naturally occurring FXR antagonist. Cell Metab 2013;17(2):225–35.

98. Tremaroli V, Backhed F. Functional interactions between the gut microbiota and host metabolism. Nature 2012;489:242–9.

99. Cermakian N, Lange T, Golombek D, et al. Crosstalk between the circadian clock circuitry and the immune system. Chronobiol Int 2013;30(7):870–88.

100. Vinciguerra M, Borghesan M, Pazienza V, et al. The transcriptional regulators, the circadian clock and the immune system. J Biol Regul Homeost Agents 2013;27(1):9–22.

101. Mazzoccoli G, Sothern RB, Greco G, et al. Time-related dynamics of variation in core clock gene expression levels in tissues relevant to the immune system. Int J Immunopathol Pharmacol 2011;24(4):869–79.

102. Ma D, Panda S, Lin JD. Temporal orchestration of circadian autophagy rhythm by C/EBPβ. EMBO J 2011;30(22):4642–51.

103. Muegge BD, Kuczynski J, Knights D, et al. Diet drives convergence in gut microbiome functions across mammalian phylogeny and within humans. Science 2011;332:970–4.

104. Chu H, Khosravi A, Kusumawardhani IP, et al. Gene-microbiota interactions contribute to the pathogenesis of inflammatory bowel disease. Science 2016;352(6289):1116–20.

105. Kim KH, Lee MS. Autophagy-a key player in cellular and body metabolism. Nat Rev Endocrinol 2014;10(6):322–37.

106. Lee JM, Wagner M, Xiao R, et al. Nutrient-sensing nuclear receptors coordinate autophagy. Nature 2014;516(7529):112–5.

107. Seok S, Fu T, Choi SE, et al. Transcriptional regulation of autophagy by an FXR-CREB axis. Nature 2014;516(7529):108–11.

108. Madrigal-Matute J, Cuervo AM. Regulation of liver metabolism by autophagy. Gastroenterology 2016;150(2):328–39.

109. Zhang X, Han J, Man K, et al. CXC chemokine receptor 3 promotes steatohepatitis in mice through mediating inflammatory cytokines, macrophages and autophagy. J Hepatol 2016;64(1):160–70.

110. Bieghs V, Trautwein C. Innate immune signaling and gut-liver interactions in non-alcoholic fatty liver disease. Hepatobiliary Surg Nutr 2014;3(6):377–85.

111. Kim S, Park S, Kim B, et al. Toll-like receptor 7 affects the pathogenesis of non-alcoholic fatty liver disease. Sci Rep 2016;6:27849.

112. Lin CW, Zhang H, Li M, et al. Pharmacological promotion of autophagy alleviates steatosis and injury in alcoholic and non-alcoholic fatty liver conditions in mice. J Hepatol 2013;58(5):993–9.

113. Mukherji A, Kobiita A, Ye T, et al. Homeostasis in intestinal epithelium is orchestrated by the circadian clock and microbiota cues transduced by TLRs. Cell 2013;153(4):812–27.

114. Clemente JC, Ursell LK, Parfrey LW, et al. The impact of the gut microbiota on human health: an integrative view. Cell 2012;148(6):1258–70.

115. Li F, Jiang C, Krausz KW, et al. Microbiome remodelling leads to inhibition of intestinal farnesoid X receptor signalling and decreased obesity. Nat Commun 2013;4:2384.

116. Tevy MF, Giebultowicz J, Pincus Z, et al. Aging signaling pathways and circadian clock-dependent metabolic derangements. Trends Endocrinol Metab 2013;24(5):229–37.

117. Vinciguerra M, Tevy MF, Mazzoccoli G. A ticking clock links metabolic pathways and organ systems function in health and disease. Clin Exp Med 2014;14(2):133–40.

118. Jones ML, Tomaro-Duchesneau C, Prakash S. The gut microbiome, probiotics, bile acids axis, and human health. Trends Microbiol 2014;22(6):306–8.

119. Joyce SA, MacSharry J, Casey PG, et al. Regulation of host weight gain and lipid metabolism by bacterial bile acid modification in the gut. Proc Natl Acad Sci U S A 2014;111(20):7421–6.

120. Ridlon JM, Kang DJ, Hylemon PB, et al. Bile acids and the gut microbiome. Curr Opin Gastroenterol 2014;30(3):332–8.

121. Fiorucci S, Distrutti E. Bile acid-activated receptors, intestinal microbiota, and the treatment of metabolic disorders. Trends Mol Med 2015;21(11):702–14.

122. Flynn CR, Albaugh VL, Cai S, et al. Bile diversion to the distal small intestine has comparable metabolic benefits to bariatric surgery. Nat Commun 2015;6:7715.

123. Jiang C, Xie C, Li F, et al. Intestinal farnesoid X receptor signaling promotes nonalcoholic fatty liver disease. J Clin Invest 2015;125(1):386–402.

124. Lu P, Yan J, Liu K, et al. Activation of aryl hydrocarbon receptor dissociates fatty liver from insulin resistance by inducing fibroblast growth factor 21. Hepatology 2015;61:1908–19.

125. Vinciguerra M, Mazzoccoli G. Aryl hydrocarbon receptor-fibroblast growth factor 21 dissociation of fatty liver from insulin resistance: a timely matter? Hepatology 2016;63(4):1396–7.

126. Bookout AL, de Groot MH, Owen BM, et al. FGF21 regulates metabolism and circadian behavior by acting on the nervous system. Nat Med 2013;19(9):1147–52.

Cardiac Clocks and Preclinical Translation

Priya Mistry, BSc[a], Austin Duong, BSc, MBS[a], Lorrie Kirshenbaum, PhD[b],
Tami A. Martino, PhD[a],*

KEYWORDS

- Circadian • Clocks • Cardiovascular • Heart disease • Circadian rhythm

KEY POINTS

- Circadian rhythms play a crucial role in cardiovascular health.
- Disturbing rhythms causes heart disease and worsens outcomes.
- Translational application of circadian biology to clinical medicine shows enormous potential for directly benefiting patients with cardiovascular disease.

INTRODUCTION

Circadian rhythms are important for healthy cardiovascular physiology. Staying in synchrony with the earth's 24-hour day and night (diurnal) cycle provides benefits to the daily functioning of our cardiovascular system. Conversely, desynchrony with the external environment, for example, through jet lag, shift work, or sleep disorders, has profound adverse effects on our cardiovascular system. Importantly, this has led a flurry of recent investigations with a translational focus, specifically on how circadian biology can be applied to benefit treatment of heart disease. For example, time-of-day therapy (chronotherapy) with angiotensin-converting enzyme inhibitors (ACEi) benefits treatment in experimental murine models of heart disease. Moreover, clinical cardiology benefits from chronotherapy and recent successes include evening administration of antihypertensives for nondippers, aspirin at night to reduce morning risk of myocardial infarction (MI), nocturnal hemodialysis, and nocturnal continuous positive airway pressure (CPAP) for patients with obstructive sleep apnea (OSA). Evidence is also emerging that short-term circadian and sleep disruption, as occurs in intensive care units (ICUs), may hamper recovery after MI. Maintaining the diurnal environment and patients biological rhythms is a promising nonpharmaceutic approach to reduce scar expansion and improve outcomes after MI. Finally, recent studies give rise to 3 new frontiers for translational research: (1) applications to benefit cardiovascular disease in the aging population; (2) new understanding of circadian mitophagy in regulating cardiac bioenergetics; and (3) links between the circadian clock mechanism and cognitive impairment or depression in heart disease. Recognizing the fundamental role that the circadian mechanism plays in cardiovascular health and disease is leading to new translational applications for clinical cardiology.

CIRCADIAN RHYTHMS IN THE CARDIOVASCULAR SYSTEM

This section provides an overview of the molecular circadian mechanism, and its role in regulating

Disclosures: None.
This work is supported by a grant from the Canadian Institutes of Health Research (CIHR, to T.A. Martino) and the Heart and Stroke Foundation of Canada (HSFC, to T.A. Martino).
[a] Department of Biomedical Sciences, Centre for Cardiovascular Investigations, University of Guelph, Guelph, Ontario N1G2W1, Canada; [b] Department of Physiology and Pathophysiology, Institute of Cardiovascular Sciences, St Boniface Hospital Research Centre, College of Medicine, Faculty of Health Sciences, University of Manitoba, Winnipeg, Manitoba R2H 2A6, Canada
* Corresponding author. Department of Biomedical Sciences, Centre for Cardiovascular Investigations, OVC, University of Guelph, Guelph, Ontario N1G2W1, Canada.
E-mail address: tmartino@uoguelph.ca

Heart Failure Clin 13 (2017) 657–672
http://dx.doi.org/10.1016/j.hfc.2017.05.002
1551-7136/17/© 2017 The Author(s). Published by Elsevier Inc. This is an open access article under the CC BY-NC-ND license (http://creativecommons.org/licenses/by-nc-nd/4.0/).

healthy cardiovascular physiology as well as in the in the timing of onset of adverse cardiovascular events.

Overview of the Circadian Mechanism in the Heart

Molecular circadian clocks are present in all our cells, including cardiomyocytes.[1–4] This mechanism enables us to entrain to environmental cues and anticipate the differing physiology demands of our everyday events, including those of the cardiovascular system. The circadian mechanism at a most basic level is a transcriptional-translational loop that cycles once every 24 hours to keep cellular time, and it is illustrated in **Fig. 1** (there are excellent reviews[5,6]). Briefly, the positive arm (see **Fig. 1**, *green*) consists of a heterodimeric pairing of CLOCK and BMAL1 proteins, which bind to promoter E-boxes to induce expression of the repressors PERIOD and CRYPTOCHROME. In the negative arm (see **Fig. 1**, *purple*), the repressors PER and CRY are phosphorylated by CASEIN KINASE, leading to inhibition of their transcription. In addition to regulating 24-hour diurnal clock cycles, this mechanism also controls diurnal patterns of tissue-specific output genes, those which regulate cardiac structure and function on a daily basis.[7,8] Collectively, transcription of approximately 10% of the genes[1,2,8–11] and translation of approximately 10% of the proteins[12,13] in the heart, as well as vasculature[8,14,15] and other tissues,[16,17] are under circadian control.

Circadian Rhythms and Healthy Cardiovascular Physiology

The output of the circadian mechanism is observed as diurnal physiologic rhythms, many crucial to the cardiovascular system. For example, there is daily cyclic variation in heart rate (HR), which is highest in the day and lowest during the night.[18] Blood pressure (BP) also displays a daily rhythm that is highest in the morning, falls progressively throughout the day and early evening, and then reaches a nadir around 3:00 AM.[19] Diurnal rhythms in BP are considered especially important for cardiovascular health, because clinically, humans with 24-hour BP profiles that do not follow the normal diurnal pattern are at a higher risk of heart disease. That is, most people have a nocturnal dip in BP of approximately 10% as compared with the daytime.[19] However, hypertensive nondippers (patients who do not experience the anticipated drop in BP at night),[20] or patients without hypertension but still a diminished nocturnal decline in BP,[21] exhibit an increased risk of heart disease. These diurnal rhythms in HR and BP parallel the sympathetic and parasympathetic biases of our autonomic nervous system,[22,23] and they are endogenously generated.[24–26]

Circadian Rhythms in the Timing of Onset of Adverse Cardiovascular Events

Rhythms are important not only for healthy cardiovascular physiology but also for the timing of onset

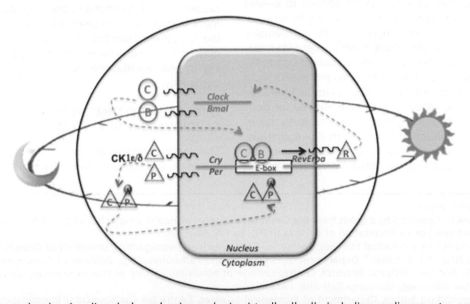

Fig. 1. The molecular circadian clock mechanism cycles in virtually all cells, including cardiomyocytes, and plays a direct role in regulating the daily output of thousands of genes, proteins, and metabolites. These in turn play key roles in regulating the structure and function of the healthy heart and contribute to cardiac remodeling and the pathophysiology of heart disease.

of acute cardiovascular events. These events do not occur randomly throughout the day. A classic example, reported by Muller and colleagues (**Table 1**) in the *New England Journal of Medicine*, is that acute MI is most likely to occur between approximately 6:00 AM and noon, as compared with any other time of day or night. In the years following this important initial observation by Muller and colleagues, there have been many subsequent epidemiologic reports on the diurnal timing of acute cardiovascular events. In this article, the authors have summarized the literature on the timing of onset of MI (see **Table 1**), time of day and severity of MI (**Table 2**), timing of onset of sudden cardiac death (**Table 3**), timing of onset of ventricular arrhythmias (**Table 4**), and timing of onset of stroke (**Table 5**). In addition, clinical and experimental studies indicate that severity of MI varies by time of day of onset,[27–29] and this is due in part to the triggering of different immune and genetic responses in the daytime as compared with nighttime.[30]

TRANSLATING CIRCADIAN RHYTHMS FOR THE TREATMENT OF HEART DISEASE

This section describes direct applications of circadian biology to clinical medicine.

Chronotherapy Benefits Treatment of Heart Disease, Basic Research

There is remarkable circadian rhythmicity in healthy cardiovascular physiology, and in the timing of onset of acute cardiovascular events, as noted above. Moreover, a growing body of evidence from basic animal research studies suggests that this can lead directly to translational applications, such as timing of therapy (chronotherapy) to benefit the treatment of cardiac hypertrophy. In earlier studies, the authors' group demonstrated that chronotherapy with ACEi benefits cardiac remodeling in mice.[31] They chose ACEi for the study because they are commonly prescribed to patients with hypertension or after MI. The authors showed improved efficacy if ACEi were given at sleep time; in their murine model of pressure overload–induced cardiac hypertrophy (Trans Aortic Constriction [TAC] model). In contrast, wake time treatment did not differ from placebo. A key reason ACEi chronotherapy works is because of rhythms in the renin-angiotensin system (RAS), the target of this drug class. If mice are given ACEi when RAS is high, then it is much more effective than given when RAS is low. It has subsequently been reported that chronotherapy could improve efficacy for a wide variety of drugs. Many of the world's best-selling medications

target the products of rhythmic genes; many of these drugs have short half-lives, and they may well benefit from timed dosage.[32]

Chronotherapy and Clinical Applications for Treatment of Heart Disease

There is also a growing clinical appreciation that timing of therapy can be applied to several different cardiovascular therapies.[3,33–37] Recent successes include the following: (1) Nocturnal BP: BP has a circadian rhythm that is high in the day and dips down by approximately 10% at night.[19] This dipper profile is important for cardiovascular health, and hypertensive non-dippers have significantly increased heart size as compared with hypertensive dippers or normotensive dippers.[20] Manfredini and Fabbian[38] have compiled a vast array of clinical reports and reviews supporting the notion that evening administration of antihypertensive drugs helps to maintain the dipper profile and can reduce cardiovascular risk. (2) Aspirin at night: Aspirin taken at night time, as compared with on awakening, may reduce the morning peak in platelet reactivity and thus may reduce cardiovascular risk.[39] (3) Nocturnal hemodialysis: Cardiovascular disease is a significant cause of death in patients with end-stage renal disease.[40] Intriguingly, nocturnal hemodialysis, as compared with conventional daytime therapy, is accompanied by regression of left ventricular cardiac hypertrophy.[41] (4) OSA: OSA is a common sleep disorder with cardiovascular consequences, and it is treated during nighttime by CPAP therapy. Nocturnal CPAP therapy attenuates some of the adverse effects of OSA on the cardiovascular system (reviews[42–46]). The authors created a blog of recent clinical studies and reviews, which highlight chronotherapy for cardiovascular and other clinical conditions (http://chronobioapp.blogspot.ca).[37] In summary, timing of drug therapy matters, and administration of therapies timed with the body's physiologic and molecular rhythms can benefit patients with heart disease.

Rhythms in the Intensive Care Unit

Modern hospitals, and especially intensive and coronary care units, still use multi-bed rooms. Contemporary medicine seems to ignore the importance of undisturbed diurnal rhythms, even in the critically ill. Although the ICU benefits patient management, inadvertent noise, lighting, and frequent patient-staff interactions conspire to disturb sleep and circadian rhythms in acutely ill patients.[47,48] Recently, the authors investigated the consequences of rhythm disturbance on heart disease, using the experimental murine model of

Table 1
Timing of onset of myocardial infarction

	Cases (N)	Main Finding	Criteria
Pell & D'Alonzo,[77] 1963	902	Diurnal variation, with decreased incidence from midnight to 6:00 AM	Clinical history, ECG, laboratory findings, autopsy reports
Muller et al,[78] 1985	847	Frequency of onset of MI peaks from 6:00 AM to noon	CK-MB levels
Thompson et al,[79] 1985	1099	Onset of chest pain peaks at 7:00 AM and at midnight	MI pain >30 min, CPK levels, Minnesota code ECG
Rocco et al,[80] 1987	32	Frequency of ischemic episodes peaks between 6:00 AM and noon	Ambulatory ECG
Nademanee et al,[81] 1987	77	Transient ischemic episodes have a peak incidence between 8:00 AM and 3:00 PM	Holter monitoring, angiography, positive exercise test, chest pain
Hjalmarson et al,[82] 1989	4796	AMI symptom onset is most frequent from 6:00 AM to noon; reduced 6:00 PM to midnight	Chest pain, ECG, CK
Willich et al,[83] 1989	1741	Incidence of MI is increased between 6:00 AM and noon	Clinical symptoms, CK-MB levels, ECG
Hausmann et al,[84] 1990	97	Ischemic episodes predominate between 6:00 AM and noon	Ambulatory ECG, chronic stable angina pectoris, exercise stress test, angiography
Goldberg et al,[85] 1990	137	Onset of AMI symptoms increases in the first hour after awakening	Chest pain >30 min, CK levels, ECG
Ridker et al,[86] 1990	211	Onset of MI has a primary peak between 4:00 AM and 10:00 AM and a secondary smaller peak in the evening. Patients taking aspirin have a reduced morning peak	Self-reports of symptom onset, physician reviews of hospital charts
Thompson et al,[87] 1992	792	Onset of chest pain peaks from 11:30 PM to 12:30 AM and from 6:30 AM to 8:30 AM	Ischemic pain >30 min, CPK levels, Minnesota code ECG
Tofler et al,[88] 1992	3339	Higher frequency of onset of MI between 6:00 AM and noon. Patients taking beta-blockers have a reduced incidence of morning MI	Chest discomfort >30 min, ECG
Hansen et al,[89] 1992	6763	Symptom onset of AMI increased between 6:00 AM and noon, and between 6:00 PM and midnight	Central chest pain, lung edema, syncope, shock, ECG, aspartate aminotransferase levels, autopsy reports
ISIS-2 (Second International Study of Infarct Survival)[90]	12,163	MI peaks 8:00 AM to 11:00 AM and has a steady trough at night	ISIS-2 trial MI onset of symptoms
Behar et al,[91] 1993	1818	Frequency of onset of symptoms shows a predominant peak between 6:00 AM and noon	Angina pain, ECG, cardiac enzymes (CK, glutamic oxaloacetic transaminase, lactate dehydrogenase)

(continued on next page)

Table 1
(continued)

	Cases (N)	Main Finding	Criteria
Peters et al,[92] 1993	2439	Onset of MI symptoms is highest in the first hour of awakening with a secondary peak 11–12 h later	Ambulatory ECG Holter monitoring
Kono et al,[93] 1996	608	Onset of AMI and resistance to thrombolysis peaks in the early morning and in the late evening	Chest pain >30 min, ECG, cardiac enzymes
Spielberg et al,[94] 1996	1901	MI occurs more frequently from 7:00 AM to 10:00 AM	Chest pain, ECG, enzymes, autopsy
Cannon et al,[95] 1997	1472	Onset of pain is increased between 6:00 AM and noon	Chest pain, ECG, coronary artery disease
Sayer et al,[96] 1997	1182	Onset of AMI symptoms peak at 9:00 AM	Chest pain, ECG, CK, no diabetes, South Asian, beta-blockers, aspirin, female gender, smokers, or history of MI
Zhou et al,[97] 1998	428	AMI occurrence peaks between 1:00 AM and 7:00 AM, and troughs between 1:00 PM and 7:00 PM	Symptoms, ECG, serum enzymes
Kinjo et al,[98] 2001	1252	Onset of AMI peaks 8:00 AM to noon, and 8:00 PM.to midnight	Chest pain or tightness >30 min, ECG, CK
Yamasaki et al,[99] 2002	725	AMI incidence peaks 6:00 AM to noon; secondary, late afternoon peak	Chest pain, ECG, serum myocardial enzymes
Rana et al,[100] 2003	3068	AMI symptom onset peaks in the morning	CK levels, CK-MB levels, identifiable onset of symptoms, nondiabetic patients
Manfredini et al,[101] 2004	442	MI occurs more frequently between 6:00 AM and noon.	Patient history, clinical signs, myocardial enzymes, ECG, autopsy.
López Messa et al,[102] 2004	54,249	AMI symptom onset peaks at 10:07 AM and troughs at 4:46 AM	Troponin, CK-MB, symptoms, ECG, angioplasty, pathology
Tanaka et al,[103] 2004	174	AMI onset more common from 6:00 AM to noon	Chest pain >30 min, ECG, CK levels
Lopez et al,[104] 2005	340	MI predominates in British Caucasians, Indo-Asians from midnight and noon; predominates in Mediterranean Caucasians from noon to midnight	ECG, biochemical markers of myocardial damage, eligibility for thrombolytic therapy
D'Negri et al,[105] 2006	1063	MI incidence peaks 8:00 AM to noon and 3:00 PM to 10:00 PM; nadir is 3:00 AM to 7:00 AM	Chest pain >30 min, ECG, CPK levels
Sari et al,[106] 2009	476	Frequency of onset of acute STEMI peaks noon to 6:00 PM; troughs midnight to 6:00 AM	Chest pain >30 min, ECG, CK-MB levels
Holmes et al,[107] 2010	2143	STEMI symptom onset increased from 8:00 AM to 3:00 PM	Onset of symptoms, arrival at hospital, time to therapy

(continued on next page)

Table 1
(continued)

	Cases (N)	Main Finding	Criteria
Celik et al,[108] 2011	465	Frequency of onset of acute anterior MI peaks during the day and troughs at night. Acute inferior MI peaks midnight to noon and troughs between noon to midnight	ECG, echocardiography, low-density lipoprotein cholesterol levels
Fournier et al,[109] 2012	353	Frequency of MI onset is higher between 8:00 AM and 3:00 PM	Time of symptom onset, CK levels
Mogabgab et al,[110] 2012	35,492	Symptom onset of STEMI is more frequent early in the day	Clinical evidence of STEMI, ECG
Chan et al,[111] 2012	505	Incidence of AMI peaks between midnight and 6:00 AM	Troponin, CK-MB, symptoms, ECG
Ammirati et al,[112] 2013	1099	STEMI incidence is increased from 6:00 AM to noon	Symptom onset, ECG
Kanth et al,[113] 2013	519	STEMI peaks at 11:30 AM	ECG, troponin, CK, patients not using beta-blockers, no diabetes
Wieringa et al,[114] 2014	6970	Onset of STEMI symptoms peak at 9:00 AM	Chest pain, ECG
Rallidis et al,[115] 2015	256	Symptom onset of AMI is more frequent from 6:00 AM to noon; lower from midnight to 6:00 AM	Chest pain >30 min, ECG, myocardial injury markers
Seneviratna et al,[116] 2015	6710	Peak incidence of STEMI symptom onset from 6:00 AM to noon	Chest pain >30 min, ECG, biomarkers
Mahmoud et al,[117] 2015	6799	MI symptom onset has lower incidence during the night and a peak in the morning	CK levels

Abbreviations: AMI, acute myocardial infarction; CK, creatine kinase; CK-MB, Creatine Linase, Muscle and Brain; CPK, creatine phosphokinase; ECG, electrocardiography.

MI. They showed that short-term disruption of diurnal rhythms, for just the few days after MI, worsened long-term outcomes (increased scar expansion and left ventricular dilation and decreased % ejection fraction) as compared with mice housed in a normal diurnal environment after MI.[49] The short-term diurnal disruption had a profound adverse effect on outcome because the circadian rhythms of the immune system were disturbed. Normally there is coordinated removal of dead tissue through an early inflammatory phase, followed by remodeling of the myocardium, and scar maturation.[50] However, when rhythms were disturbed, this early inflammatory response was altered. As a result, this led to a domino-like triggered a domino-like effect, whereby aberrant early remodeling set an inappropriate stage for the subsequent healing phases and ultimately worsened outcome. Maintaining the diurnal environment and patients' biological rhythms is a promising nonpharmaceutic approach to improve outcomes.[33,35] This translational application, as well as chronocardiology, is the subject of recent cardiology news, in the high-impact journal *Circulation* published by the American Heart Association.[51]

NEW FRONTIERS IN CARDIAC CLOCKS AND PRECLINICAL TRANSLATION

Circadian medicine already shows enormous promise by targeting the heart's daily physiologic and molecular rhythms. In addition, there are exciting new frontiers for investigation, and these too show significant potential for translational application for the treatment of heart disease. These new frontiers are described in later discussion.

Table 2
Time of day and severity of myocardial infarction

	Cases (N)	Main Finding	Criteria
Hansen et al,[118] 1993	6763	AMI onset between 6:00 AM and noon predicts a greater infarct size	Aspartate aminotransferase levels
Suarez-Barrientos et al,[29] 2011	811	Infarct size is largest with STEMI onset between 6:00 AM and noon	CK levels, troponin I levels
Fournier et al,[109] 2012	353	Infarct size higher in patients with onset midnight to 6:00 AM	CK levels
Arroyo Ucar et al,[119] 2012	108	Larger infarct size with AMI between midnight and noon	Troponin I levels
Reiter et al,[28] 2012	165	Greater injury with 1:00 AM ischemia and 5:00 AM reperfusion. Greatest decrease in cardiac function with infarction at 1:00 AM	CK levels, cardiac MRI
Wieringa et al,[114] 2014	6970	Ischemic time is longest and infarct size is larger with STEMI onset between midnight and 6:00 AM	CK levels, myocardial-band of CK levels, myocardial blush grade
Seneviratna et al,[116] 2015	6710	Symptom onset midnight to 6:00 AM associated with larger mean infarct size; 6:00 AM to noon with smaller mean infarct size	CK levels
Mahmoud et al,[117] 2015	6799	Infarct size is largest with STEMI symptom onset at 3:00 AM and smallest with onset at 11:00 AM	CK levels
Fournier et al,[120] 2015	6223	STEMI symptom onset at 11:00 PM presents with highest peak CK values; CK lower in patients with symptom onset at 11:00 AM	CK levels
Ari et al,[121] 2016	252	Largest infarct size and poor left ventricular function associates with infarcts occurring 6:00 AM to noon	Myocardial-band of CK, echocardiography

Circadian Rhythms and Cardiovascular Aging

The prevalence and incidence of cardiovascular disease increase with aging and frequently progress toward heart failure (HF).[52,53] HF is a common cause for hospitalization in patients older than 65 years of age and is a considerable economic burden, and more than 50% of patients die within 5 years of diagnosis. Total costs are projected to double over the next 2 decades because of increasing prevalence of HF associated with aging.[54,55] The authors recently identified a direct role for the circadian mechanism factor *Clock* in the pathophysiology of cardiac aging, using a murine model.[56] Disturbing *Clock* in circadian mutant mice (*Clock*$^{\Delta 19/\Delta 19}$) leads to an age-dependent increase in heart size, cardiomyocyte hypertrophy, interstitial fibrosis, and maladaptive cardiac remodeling leading to HF (increased left ventricular dimensions, reduced % ejection fraction, and % fractional shortening).[56] Cardiomyocyte-specific mutation of *Clock* can cause hypertrophy and fibrosis,[57] and moreover, disruption in the vasculature in *Clock*$^{\Delta 19/\Delta 19}$ mice contributes to reduced myogenic responsiveness and leads to decreased cardiac contractility.[56] Mechanistically, Clock is a key mediator in the PTEN-AKT signal pathways, and thus, it plays a crucial role in cardiac growth and renewal. Intriguingly, pharmacologic targeting of the circadian mechanism may provide a new opportunity

Table 3
Timing of onset of sudden cardiac death

	Cases (N)	Main Finding	Criteria
Muller et al,[122] 1987	2203	SCD primary peak 7:00 AM to 11:00 AM, secondary peak 5:00 PM to 6:00 PM	Mortality records
Willich et al,[123] 1987	429	Incidence of SCD peaks 7:00 AM to 9:00 AM	Mortality records
Peters et al,[124] 1989	101	SCD peaks in the midmorning. Beta-blockers prevent or blunt this	Mortality records from the Beta Blocker Heart Attack Trial
Willich et al,[125] 1992	84	Likelihood of SCD increased during the initial 3-h after awakening	Death certificates
Levine et al,[126] 1992	1019	Frequency of cardiac arrest increases 6:00 AM to noon	City of Houston Emergency Medical Services reports
Aronow et al,[127] 1993	362	Frequency of SCD increased 6:00 AM to noon	Long-term care data
Arntz et al,[128] 1993	703	Occurrence of SCD primary peak 6:00 AM to noon; secondary peak 3:00 PM to 7:00 PM	Automated external defibrillator tape recordings
Moser et al,[129] 1994	72	SCD more frequent 6:00 AM to noon	Ahmansen-UCLA Cardiomyopathy Center death certificates

Abbreviation: SCD, sudden cardiac death.

Table 4
Timing of onset of ventricular arrhythmias

	Cases (N)	Episodes	Main Finding	Criteria
Lucente et al,[130] 1988	94	157	VT frequency peaks 11:00 AM to 1:00 PM; secondary peak 4:00 PM to 6:00 PM	Holter monitoring of AMI patients
Twidale et al,[131] 1989	68		Peak incidence 10:00 AM to noon, reduced 11:00 PM to 1:00 AM	Electrocardiography
Lanza et al,[132] 1990	38		Highest frequency of ventricular premature complexes during wake	Holter, physical examination, chest radiograph, echocardiography
Zehender et al,[133] 1992	129		Ventricular arrhythmias peak early morning to late afternoon	Holter monitoring
Siegel et al,[134] 1992	199		Higher prevalence 6:00 AM to noon	Holter monitoring
Valkama et al,[135] 1992	34	1314	Occurrence of VT episodes peaks 6:00 AM	Ambulatory electrocardiography
Arntz et al,[128] 1993	294	294	Peak 6:00 AM to noon	Defibrillator tape recordings
Lampert et al,[136] 1994	32	2558	Peaks 6:00 AM to noon; secondary later in day	ICD
Wood et al,[137] 1995	43	830	Peaks noon to 5:00 PM	ICD
Tofler et al,[138] 1995	483	1217	VT peaks 9:00 AM to noon, nadir at night	ICD
Englund et al,[139] 1999	310	1061	Ventricular arrhythmias have a morning peak and a less pronounced afternoon peak	ICD

Abbreviations: ICD, implantable cardioverter defibrillators; VT, ventricular tachycardia.

Table 5
Timing of onset of stroke

	Cases (N)	Main Finding	Criteria
Marshall,[140] 1977	554	Cerebral infarction strokes more common midnight to 6:00 AM	Retrospective stroke records
Tsementzis et al,[141] 1985	557	Subarachnoid hemorrhage, intracerebral hemorrhage, and thromboembolic cerebral infarction peak incidence 10:00 AM to noon	Prospective CT scans, cerebrospinal fluid, angiography, postmortem, Allen test
Van der Windt et al,[142] 1988	59	Cerebral infarction occurs mostly between 6:00 AM and 6:00 PM	Retrospective reports of cerebral infarction, CT scans
Marler et al,[143] 1989	1167	Ischemic strokes predominate in awake patients 10:00 AM to noon	Angiography, CT scans, Doppler ultrasound
Pasqualetti et al,[144] 1990	667	Maximum incidence of stroke occurs 2:00 AM to 8:00 AM	Spinal lumbar puncture, CT scans
Argentino et al,[145] 1990	426	The frequency of onset of hemispheric stroke is higher from 6:00 AM to noon	CT scans
Marsh et al,[146] 1990	151	Most acute ischemic strokes occur between 6:00 AM and noon	Stroke registry, clinical presentation, diagnoses
Ricci et al,[147] 1992	368	Cerebral infarction, primary intracerebral hemorrhage, and subarachnoid hemorrhage more common 6:00 AM to noon	CT scans, Allen test, lumbar puncture, clinical profile
Wroe et al,[148] 1992	554	Onset of stroke in wake time more frequent 6:00 AM to noon	CT scans, postmortem examination, Guy's Hospital diagnostics
Sloan et al,[149] 1992	480	Intracerebral hemorrhage peaks 10:00 AM to noon. Subarachnoid hemorrhage in hypertensives peaks in mid-to-late morning	Stroke Data Bank
Gallerani et al,[150] 1993	897	Most strokes occur between 7:00 AM and noon	CT scans, angiography, autopsy reports
Kelly-Hayes et al,[151] 1995	401	Strokes most frequent 8:00 AM to noon.	Framingham Study Cohort
Lago et al,[152] 1998	914	Stroke peaks 6:00 AM to noon	CT scans
Chaturvedi et al,[153] 1999	1272	Atherothromboembolic and cardioembolic stroke peak 6:00 AM to noon. Small-vessel/lacunar stroke peaks noon to 6:00 PM	CT scans, MRI, vascular imaging, echocardiography
Raj et al,[154] 2015	367	Rate of occurrence of stroke is highest 6:00 AM to noon hours and lowest 6:00 PM to midnight	Observational study, clinical diagnosis, radiological diagnosis

Abbreviation: CT, computerized tomographic.

for treating heart disease. The therapeutic implications may be particularly relevant for individuals subjected to circadian rhythms disruption, such as shift workers and individuals with sleep disorders in the aging population.

Circadian Rhythms and Mitophagy

The circadian mechanism component Rev-erb-a is key regulator of mitochondrial content and oxidative function in skeletal muscle, exerting control in part by repressing genes that trigger mitophagy.[58] This notion, combined with a recent flurry of mechanistic studies suggesting that mitochondrial quality is important for the heart and that dysregulation of quality control mechanisms such as mitophagy can contribute to cardiomyocyte pathophysiology,[59] suggests a role for circadian rhythms in mitophagy in heart disease. It is currently known that the PINK1-Parkin pathway plays an essential role in eliminating damaged mitochondria by mitophagy. Under basal conditions the E3-ligase Parkin is retained in the cytoplasm but rapidly translocates to damaged mitochondria in a manner dependent upon PINK1.[60,61] Activation of parkin results in the ubiquitination of several proteins on the outer mitochondrial membrane, which targets ubiquitinated mitochondria for autophagic removal.[62] Notably, defects in autophagy have been associated with contractile dysfunction and HF.[63–66] For example, autophagy increases in cardiac myocytes following ischemia-reperfusion injury. In fact, activation of autophagy upon early phases of reperfusion is critical for removing damaged organelles, including mitochondria and averting proteotoxic stress. This mechanism is largely substantiated by studies in which delayed autophagy exacerbated reperfusion injury, resulting in cardiac-increased cell death and cardiac dysfunction.[67,68] Because mitochondria are highly dynamic organelles and continually undergoing fission and fusion, future investigations examining the role of the circadian mechanism on mitophagy in the heart are warranted.

Circadian Rhythms and Depression in Patients with Heart Disease

Depression is common in patients with coronary heart disease, and the comorbidity complicates treatment and worsens prognosis.[69,70] Moreover, cognitive impairment, depression, or brain changes have all been frequently reported as coincidental in patients with HF.[71–73] Although there is a complex interplay between pathophysiologic factors that can contribute to these mental health conditions in patients with heart disease, a role for the circadian mechanism may also be warranted. In support of this notion, several studies suggest that disruption of the circadian clock system plays a role in mood disorders, including depression and bipolar disorder.[74,75] Moreover, it has been shown experimentally that disruption of circadian rhythms in mice lowers dendritic length and decreases the complexity of neurons in the prelimbic frontal cortex, a brain region important for emotional control.[76] The authors also showed that this diurnal disruption worsens heart disease, using a model

of pressure overload–induced cardiac hypertrophy in mice.[8] Further understanding of the links between circadian rhythms and neuropathophysiology could lead to new approaches to improve the quality of life and improve outcomes for patients with heart disease.

SUMMARY

Recent epidemiologic, experimental, and clinical studies demonstrate the profound importance of circadian rhythms for healthy cardiovascular physiology. Disturbing rhythms is etiologically associated with heart disease and worse outcomes. Rhythm disturbance is common in contemporary society, for example, frequent jet travel between time zones, 24/7 shift work, or sleep disorders. Importantly, these discoveries have led to an exciting new opportunity, that is, translating circadian biology to clinical medicine. Recent successes include optimizing the timing of cardiovascular medications to improve drug efficacy and maintaining circadian rhythms and sleep to benefit outcomes after MI. Upcoming areas for preclinical translation include targeting the circadian mechanism to reduce cardiac aging, targeting circadian-driven bioenergetics to improve heart function, and examining the complex interplay between neurophysiology and heart disease to improve outcomes for patients with heart disease.

REFERENCES

1. Martino T, Arab S, Straume M, et al. Day/night rhythms in gene expression of the normal murine heart. J Mol Med (Berl) 2004;82(4):256–64.
2. Storch KF, Lipan O, Leykin I, et al. Extensive and divergent circadian gene expression in liver and heart. Nature 2002;417(6884):78–83.
3. Martino TA, Young ME. Influence of the cardiomyocyte circadian clock on cardiac physiology and pathophysiology. J Biol Rhythms 2015;30(3): 183–205.
4. Young ME, Razeghi P, Taegtmeyer H. Clock genes in the heart - characterization and attenuation with hypertrophy. Circ Res 2001;88(11):1142–50.
5. Reppert SM, Weaver DR. Coordination of circadian timing in mammals. Nature 2002;418(6901): 935–41.
6. Roenneberg T, Merrow M. Circadian clocks - the fall and rise of physiology. Nat Rev Mol Cell Biol 2005;6(12):965–71.
7. Martino TA, Oudit GY, Herzenberg AM, et al. Circadian rhythm disorganization produces profound cardiovascular and renal disease in hamsters. Am J Physiol Regul Integr Comp Physiol 2008; 294(5):R1675–83.

8. Martino TA, Tata N, Belsham DD, et al. Disturbed diurnal rhythm alters gene expression and exacerbates cardiovascular disease with rescue by resynchronization. Hypertension 2007;49(5):1104–13.

9. Bray MS, Shaw CA, Moore MW, et al. Disruption of the circadian clock within the cardiomyocyte influences myocardial contractile function, metabolism, and gene expression. Am J Physiol Heart Circ Physiol 2008;294(2):H1036–47.

10. Young ME, Brewer RA, Peliciari-Garcia RA, et al. Cardiomyocyte-specific BMAL1 plays critical roles in metabolism, signaling, and maintenance of contractile function of the heart. J Biol Rhythms 2014; 29(4):257–76.

11. Tsimakouridze EV, Straume M, Podobed PS, et al. Chronomics of pressure overload-induced cardiac hypertrophy in mice reveals altered day/night gene expression and biomarkers of heart disease. Chronobiol Int 2012;29(7):810–21.

12. Podobed P, Pyle WG, Ackloo S, et al. The day/night proteome in the murine heart. Am J Physiol Regul Integr Comp Physiol 2014;307(2):R121–37.

13. Podobed PS, Alibhai FJ, Chow CW, et al. Circadian regulation of myocardial sarcomeric Titin-cap (Tcap, telethonin): identification of cardiac clock-controlled genes using open access bioinformatics data. PLoS One 2014;9(8):e104907.

14. Chalmers JA, Martino TA, Tata N, et al. Vascular circadian rhythms in a mouse vascular smooth muscle cell line (Movas-1). Am J Physiol Regul Integr Comp Physiol 2008;295(5):R1529–38.

15. Rudic RD, McNamara P, Reilly D, et al. Bioinformatic analysis of circadian gene oscillation in mouse aorta. Circulation 2005;112(17):2716–24.

16. Chalmers JA, Lin SY, Martino TA, et al. Diurnal profiling of neuroendocrine genes in murine heart, and shift in proopiomelanocortin gene expression with pressure-overload cardiac hypertrophy. J Mol Endocrinol 2008;41(3):117–24.

17. Martino TA, Tata N, Bjarnason GA, et al. Diurnal protein expression in blood revealed by high throughput mass spectrometry proteomics and implications for translational medicine and body time of day. Am J Physiol Regul Integr Comp Physiol 2007;293(3):R1430–7.

18. Clarke JM, Hamer J, Shelton JR, et al. The rhythm of the normal human heart. Lancet 1976;1(7984): 508–12.

19. Millar-Craig MW, Bishop CN, Raftery EB. Circadian variation of blood-pressure. Lancet 1978;1(8068): 795–7.

20. Verdecchia P, Schillaci G, Guerrieri M, et al. Circadian blood pressure changes and left ventricular hypertrophy in essential hypertension. Circulation 1990;81(2):528–36.

21. Ohkubo T, Hozawa A, Yamaguchi J, et al. Prognostic significance of the nocturnal decline in blood pressure in individuals with and without high 24-h blood pressure: the Ohasama study. J Hypertens 2002;20(11):2183–9.

22. Furlan R, Guzzetti S, Crivellaro W, et al. Continuous 24-hour assessment of the neural regulation of systemic arterial pressure and RR variabilities in ambulant subjects. Circulation 1990;81(2):537–47.

23. Richards AM, Nicholls MG, Espiner EA, et al. Diurnal patterns of blood pressure, heart rate and vasoactive hormones in normal man. Clin Exp Hypertens A 1986;8(2):153–66.

24. Scheer FA, van Doornen LJ, Buijs RM. Light and diurnal cycle affect human heart rate: possible role for the circadian pacemaker. J Biol Rhythms 1999;14(3):202–12.

25. Shea SA, Hilton MF, Hu K, et al. Existence of an endogenous circadian blood pressure rhythm in humans that peaks in the evening. Circ Res 2011; 108(8):980–4.

26. Hu K, Ivanov P, Hilton MF, et al. Endogenous circadian rhythm in an index of cardiac vulnerability independent of changes in behavior. Proc Natl Acad Sci U S A 2004;101(52):18223–7.

27. Durgan DJ, Pulinilkunnil T, Villegas-Montoya C, et al. Short communication: ischemia/reperfusion tolerance is time-of-day-dependent: mediation by the cardiomyocyte circadian clock. Circ Res 2010;106(3):546–50.

28. Reiter R, Swingen C, Moore L, et al. Circadian dependence of infarct size and left ventricular function after ST elevation myocardial infarction. Circ Res 2012;110(1):105–10.

29. Suarez-Barrientos A, Lopez-Romero P, Vivas D, et al. Circadian variations of infarct size in acute myocardial infarction. Heart 2011;97(12):970–6.

30. Bennardo M, Alibhai F, Tsimakouridze E, et al. Day-night dependence of gene expression and inflammatory responses in the remodeling murine heart post-myocardial infarction. Am J Physiol Regul Integr Comp Physiol 2016;311(6): R1243–54.

31. Martino TA, Tata N, Simpson JA, et al. The primary benefits of angiotensin-converting enzyme inhibition on cardiac remodeling occur during sleep time in murine pressure overload hypertrophy. J Am Coll Cardiol 2011;57(20):2020–8.

32. Zhang R, Lahens NF, Ballance HI, et al. A circadian gene expression atlas in mammals: implications for biology and medicine. Proc Natl Acad Sci U S A 2014;111(45):16219–24.

33. Alibhai FJ, Tsimakouridze EV, Reitz CJ, et al. Consequences of circadian and sleep disturbances for the cardiovascular system. Can J Cardiol 2015;31(7):860–72.

34. Martino TA, Sole MJ. Molecular time: an often overlooked dimension to cardiovascular disease. Circ Res 2009;105(11):1047–61.

35. Reitz CJ, Martino TA. Disruption of circadian rhythms and sleep on critical illness and the impact on cardiovascular events. Curr Pharm Des 2015; 21(24):3505–11.

36. Sole MJ, Martino TA. Diurnal physiology: core principles with application to the pathogenesis, diagnosis, prevention, and treatment of myocardial hypertrophy and failure. J Appl Physiol (1985) 2009;107(4):1318–27.

37. Tsimakouridze EV, Alibhai FJ, Martino TA. Therapeutic applications of circadian rhythms for the cardiovascular system. Front Pharmacol 2015;6:77.

38. Manfredini R, Fabbian F. A pill at bedtime, and your heart is fine? Bedtime hypertension chronotherapy: an opportune and advantageous inexpensive treatment strategy. Sleep Med Rev 2017;33:1–3.

39. Bonten TN, Saris A, van Oostrom MJ, et al. Effect of aspirin intake at bedtime versus on awakening on circadian rhythm of platelet reactivity. A randomised cross-over trial. Thromb Haemost 2014; 112(6):1209–18.

40. Harnett JD, Kent GM, Barre PE, et al. Risk factors for the development of left ventricular hypertrophy in a prospectively followed cohort of dialysis patients. J Am Soc Nephrol 1994;4(7):1486–90.

41. Chan CT, Floras JS, Miller JA, et al. Regression of left ventricular hypertrophy after conversion to nocturnal hemodialysis. Kidney Int 2002;61(6): 2235–9.

42. Bradley TD, Floras JS. Obstructive sleep apnoea and its cardiovascular consequences. Lancet 2009;373(9657):82–93.

43. Somers VK, White DP, Amin R, et al. Sleep apnea and cardiovascular disease: an American Heart Association/American College of Cardiology Foundation Scientific Statement from the American Heart Association Council for High Blood Pressure Research Professional Education Committee, Council on Clinical Cardiology, Stroke Council, and Council on Cardiovascular Nursing. J Am Coll Cardiol 2008;52(8):686–717.

44. floras JS. Sleep apnea and cardiovascular risk. J Cardiol 2014;63(1):3–8.

45. Ayas NT, Hirsch AA, Laher I, et al. New frontiers in obstructive sleep apnoea. Clin Sci (Lond) 2014; 127(4):209–16.

46. Marin JM, Carrizo SJ, Vicente E, et al. Long-term cardiovascular outcomes in men with obstructive sleep apnoea-hypopnoea with or without treatment with continuous positive airway pressure: an observational study. Lancet 2005;365(9464):1046–53.

47. Buxton OM, Ellenbogen JM, Wang W, et al. Sleep disruption due to hospital noises: a prospective evaluation. Ann Intern Med 2012;157(3):170–9.

48. Drouot X, Cabello B, d'Ortho MP, et al. Sleep in the intensive care unit. Sleep Med Rev 2008;12(5): 391–403.

49. Alibhai FJ, Tsimakouridze EV, Chinnappareddy N, et al. Short-term disruption of diurnal rhythms after murine myocardial infarction adversely affects long-term myocardial structure and function. Circ Res 2014;114(11):1713–22.

50. Frangogiannis NG. Regulation of the inflammatory response in cardiac repair. Circ Res 2012;110(1): 159–73.

51. Kuehn BM. The heart's circadian rhythms point to potential treatment strategies. Circulation 2016; 134(23):1907–8.

52. Strait JB, Lakatta EG. Aging-associated cardiovascular changes and their relationship to heart failure. Heart Fail Clin 2012;8(1):143–64.

53. Thomas S, Rich MW. Epidemiology, pathophysiology, and prognosis of heart failure in the elderly. Heart Fail Clin 2007;3(4):381–7.

54. Yancy CW, Jessup M, Bozkurt B, et al. 2013 ACCF/AHA guideline for the management of heart failure: executive summary: a report of the American College of Cardiology Foundation/American Heart Association Task Force on practice guidelines. Circulation 2013;128(16):1810–52.

55. Mozaffarian D, Benjamin EJ, Go AS, et al. Heart disease and stroke statistics–2015 update: a report from the American Heart Association. Circulation 2015;131(4):e29–322.

56. Alibhai FJ, LaMarre J, Reitz CJ, et al. Disrupting the key circadian regulatory CLOCK leads to age-dependent cardiovascular disease. J Mol Cell Cardiol 2017;105:24–37.

57. Durgan DJ, Tsai JY, Grenett MH, et al. Evidence suggesting that the cardiomyocyte circadian clock modulates responsiveness of the heart to hypertrophic stimuli in mice. Chronobiol Int 2011;28(3):187–203.

58. Woldt E, Sebti Y, Solt LA, et al. Rev-erb-alpha modulates skeletal muscle oxidative capacity by regulating mitochondrial biogenesis and autophagy. Nat Med 2013;19(8):1039–46.

59. Yamaguchi O, Murakawa T, Nishida K, et al. Receptor-mediated mitophagy. J Mol Cell Cardiol 2016;95:50–6.

60. Gong G, Song M, Csordas G, et al. Parkin-mediated mitophagy directs perinatal cardiac metabolic maturation in mice. Science 2015;350(6265): aad2459.

61. Jimenez RE, Kubli DA, Gustafsson AB. Autophagy and mitophagy in the myocardium: therapeutic potential and concerns. Br J Pharmacol 2014;171(8): 1907–16.

62. Chen Y, Dorn GW 2nd. PINK1-phosphorylated mitofusin 2 is a Parkin receptor for culling damaged mitochondria. Science 2013;340(6131):471–5.

63. Bhandari P, Song M, Chen Y, et al. Mitochondrial contagion induced by Parkin deficiency in Drosophila hearts and its containment by suppressing mitofusin. Circ Res 2014;114(2):257–65.

64. Dhingra R, Margulets V, Chowdhury SR, et al. Bnip3 mediates doxorubicin-induced cardiac myocyte necrosis and mortality through changes in mitochondrial signaling. Proc Natl Acad Sci U S A 2014;111(51):E5537–44.

65. Sadoshima J. The role of autophagy during ischemia/reperfusion. Autophagy 2008;4(4):402–3.

66. Rothermel BA, Hill JA. Autophagy in load-induced heart disease. Circ Res 2008;103(12):1363–9.

67. Matsui Y, Kyoi S, Takagi H, et al. Molecular mechanisms and physiological significance of autophagy during myocardial ischemia and reperfusion. Autophagy 2008;4(4):409–15.

68. Matsui Y, Takagi H, Qu X, et al. Distinct roles of autophagy in the heart during ischemia and reperfusion: roles of AMP-activated protein kinase and Beclin 1 in mediating autophagy. Circ Res 2007; 100(6):914–22.

69. Shapiro PA. Management of depression after myocardial infarction. Curr Cardiol Rep 2015; 17(10):80.

70. Hance M, Carney RM, Freedland KE, et al. Depression in patients with coronary heart disease. A 12-month follow-up. Gen Hosp Psychiatry 1996; 18(1):61–5.

71. Sauve MJ, Lewis WR, Blankenbiller M, et al. Cognitive impairments in chronic heart failure: a case controlled study. J Card Fail 2009;15(1):1–10.

72. Koenig HG. Depression outcome in inpatients with congestive heart failure. Arch Intern Med 2006; 166(9):991–6.

73. Almeida OP, Garrido GJ, Beer C, et al. Cognitive and brain changes associated with ischaemic heart disease and heart failure. Eur Heart J 2012; 33(14):1769–76.

74. Gouin JP, Connors J, Kiecolt-Glaser JK, et al. Altered expression of circadian rhythm genes among individuals with a history of depression. J Affect Disord 2010;126(1–2):161–6.

75. Soria V, Martinez-Amoros E, Escaramis G, et al. Differential association of circadian genes with mood disorders: CRY1 and NPAS2 are associated with unipolar major depression and CLOCK and VIP with bipolar disorder. Neuropsychopharmacology 2010;35(6):1279–89.

76. Karatsoreos IN, Bhagat S, Bloss EB, et al. Disruption of circadian clocks has ramifications for metabolism, brain, and behavior. Proc Natl Acad Sci U S A 2011;108(4):1657–62.

77. Pell S, D'Alonzo CA. Acute myocardial infarction in a large industrial population: report of a 6-year study of 1,356 cases. JAMA 1963;185: 831–8.

78. Muller JE, Stone PH, Turi ZG, et al. Circadian variation in the frequency of onset of acute myocardial infarction. N Engl J Med 1985; 313(21):1315–22.

79. Thompson DR, Blandford RL, Sutton TW, et al. Time of onset of chest pain in acute myocardial infarction. Int J Cardiol 1985;7(2):139–48.

80. Rocco MB, Barry J, Campbell S, et al. Circadian variation of transient myocardial ischemia in patients with coronary artery disease. Circulation 1987;75(2):395–400.

81. Nademanee K, Intarachot V, Josephson MA, et al. Circadian variation in occurrence of transient overt and silent myocardial ischemia in chronic stable angina and comparison with Prinzmetal angina in men. Am J Cardiol 1987;60(7):494–8.

82. Hjalmarson A, Gilpin EA, Nicod P, et al. Differing circadian patterns of symptom onset in subgroups of patients with acute myocardial infarction. Circulation 1989;80(2):267–75.

83. Willich SN, Linderer T, Wegscheider K, et al. Increased morning incidence of myocardial infarction in the ISAM study: absence with prior beta-adrenergic blockade. ISAM Study Group. Circulation 1989;80(4):853–8.

84. Hausmann D, Nikutta P, Trappe HJ, et al. Incidence of ventricular arrhythmias during transient myocardial ischemia in patients with stable coronary artery disease. J Am Coll Cardiol 1990;16(1):49–54.

85. Goldberg RJ, Brady P, Muller JE, et al. Time of onset of symptoms of acute myocardial infarction. Am J Cardiol 1990;66(2):140–4.

86. Ridker PM, Manson JE, Buring JE, et al. Circadian variation of acute myocardial infarction and the effect of low-dose aspirin in a randomized trial of physicians. Circulation 1990;82(3):897–902.

87. Thompson DR, Pohl JE, Sutton TW. Circadian variation in the frequency of onset of chest pain in elderly patients with acute myocardial infarction. Age Ageing 1992;21(2):99–102.

88. Tofler GH, Muller JE, Stone PH, et al. Modifiers of timing and possible triggers of acute myocardial infarction in the thrombolysis in myocardial infarction phase II (TIMI II) study group. J Am Coll Cardiol 1992;20(5):1049–55.

89. Hansen O, Johansson BW, Gullberg B. Circadian distribution of onset of acute myocardial infarction in subgroups from analysis of 10,791 patients treated in a single center. Am J Cardiol 1992; 69(12):1003–8.

90. Morning peak in the incidence of myocardial infarction: experience in the ISIS-2 trial. ISIS-2 (Second International Study of Infarct Survival) Collaborative Group. Eur Heart J 1992;13(5):594–8.

91. Behar S, Halabi M, Reicher-Reiss H, et al. Circadian variation and possible external triggers of onset of myocardial infarction. SPRINT study group. Am J Med 1993;94(4):395–400.

92. Peters RW, Zoble RG, Liebson PR, et al. Identification of a secondary peak in myocardial infarction onset 11 to 12 hours after awakening: the cardiac

arrhythmia suppression trial (CAST) experience. J Am Coll Cardiol 1993;22(4):998–1003.

93. Kono T, Morita H, Nishina T, et al. Circadian variations of onset of acute myocardial infarction and efficacy of thrombolytic therapy. J Am Coll Cardiol 1996;27(4):774–8.

94. Spielberg C, Falkenhahn D, Willich SN, et al. Circadian, day-of-week, and seasonal variability in myocardial infarction: comparison between working and retired patients. Am Heart J 1996;132(3):579–85.

95. Cannon CP, McCabe CH, Stone PH, et al. Circadian variation in the onset of unstable angina and non-Q-wave acute myocardial infarction (the TIMI III Registry and TIMI IIIB). Am J Cardiol 1997;79(3):253–8.

96. Sayer JW, Wilkinson P, Ranjadayalan K, et al. Attenuation or absence of circadian and seasonal rhythms of acute myocardial infarction. Heart 1997;77(4):325–9.

97. Zhou RH, Xi B, Gao HQ, et al. Circadian and septadian variation in the occurrence of acute myocardial infarction in a Chinese population. Jpn Circ J 1998;62(3):190–2.

98. Kinjo K, Sato H, Sato H, et al. Circadian variation of the onset of acute myocardial infarction in the Osaka area, 1998-1999: characterization of morning and nighttime peaks. Jpn Circ J 2001;65(7):617–20.

99. Yamasaki F, Seo H, Furuno T, et al. Effect of age on chronological variation of acute myocardial infarction onset: study in Japan. Clin Exp Hypertens 2002;24(1–2):1–9.

100. Rana JS, Mukamal KJ, Morgan JP, et al. Circadian variation in the onset of myocardial infarction: effect of duration of diabetes. Diabetes 2003;52(6):1464–8.

101. Manfredini R, Boari B, Bressan S, et al. Influence of circadian rhythm on mortality after myocardial infarction: data from a prospective cohort of emergency calls. Am J Emerg Med 2004;22(7):555–9.

102. López Messa JB, Garmendia Leiza JR, Aguilar Garcia MD, et al. Cardiovascular risk factors in the circadian rhythm of acute myocardial infarction. Rev Esp Cardiol 2004;57(9):850–8 [in Spanish].

103. Tanaka A, Kawarabayashi T, Fukuda D, et al. Circadian variation of plaque rupture in acute myocardial infarction. Am J Cardiol 2004;93(1):1–5.

104. Lopez F, Lee KW, Marin F, et al. Are there ethnic differences in the circadian variation in onset of acute myocardial infarction? A comparison of 3 ethnic groups in Birmingham, UK and Alicante, Spain. Int J Cardiol 2005;100(1):151–4.

105. D'Negri CE, Nicola-Siri L, Vigo DE, et al. Circadian analysis of myocardial infarction incidence in an Argentine and Uruguayan population. BMC Cardiovasc Disord 2006;6:1.

106. Sari I, Davutoglu V, Erer B, et al. Analysis of circadian variation of acute myocardial infarction: afternoon predominance in Turkish population. Int J Clin Pract 2009;63(1):82–6.

107. Holmes DR Jr, Aguirre FV, Aplin R, et al. Circadian rhythms in patients with ST-elevation myocardial infarction. Circ Cardiovasc Qual Outcomes 2010;3(4):382–9.

108. Celik M, Celik T, Iyisoy A, et al. Circadian variation of acute st segment elevation myocardial infarction by anatomic location in a Turkish cohort. Med Sci Monit 2011;17(4):CR210–5.

109. Fournier S, Eeckhout E, Mangiacapra F, et al. Circadian variations of ischemic burden among patients with myocardial infarction undergoing primary percutaneous coronary intervention. Am Heart J 2012;163(2):208–13.

110. Mogabgab O, Giugliano RP, Sabatine MS, et al. Circadian variation in patient characteristics and outcomes in ST-segment elevation myocardial infarction. Chronobiol Int 2012;29(10):1390–6.

111. Chan CM, Chen WL, Kuo HY, et al. Circadian variation of acute myocardial infarction in young people. Am J Emerg Med 2012;30(8):1461–5.

112. Ammirati E, Cristell N, Cianflone D, et al. Questing for circadian dependence in ST-segment-elevation acute myocardial infarction: a multicentric and multiethnic study. Circ Res 2013;112(10):e110–4.

113. Kanth R, Ittaman S, Rezkalla S. Circadian patterns of ST elevation myocardial infarction in the new millennium. Clin Med Res 2013;11(2):66–72.

114. Wieringa WG, Lexis CP, Mahmoud KD, et al. Time of symptom onset and value of myocardial blush and infarct size on prognosis in patients with ST-elevation myocardial infarction. Chronobiol Int 2014;31(6):797–806.

115. Rallidis LS, Triantafyllis AS, Sakadakis EA, et al. Circadian pattern of symptoms onset in patients ≤35 years presenting with ST-segment elevation acute myocardial infarction. Eur J Intern Med 2015;26(8):607–10.

116. Seneviratna A, Lim GH, Devi A, et al. Circadian dependence of infarct size and acute heart failure in ST elevation myocardial infarction. PLoS One 2015;10(6):e0128526.

117. Mahmoud KD, Nijsten MW, Wieringa WG, et al. Independent association between symptom onset time and infarct size in patients with ST-elevation myocardial infarction undergoing primary percutaneous coronary intervention. Chronobiol Int 2015;32(4):468–77.

118. Hansen O, Johansson BW, Gullberg B. The clinical outcome of acute myocardial infarction is related to the circadian rhythm of myocardial infarction onset. Angiology 1993;44(7):509–16.

119. Arroyo Ucar E, Dominguez-Rodriguez A, Abreu-Gonzalez P. Influence of diurnal variation in the

size of acute myocardial infarction. Med Intensiva 2012;36(1):11–4 [in Spanish].

120. Fournier S, Taffe P, Radovanovic D, et al. Myocardial infarct size and mortality depend on the time of day-a large multicenter study. PLoS One 2015; 10(3):e0119157.

121. Ari H, Sonmez O, Koc F, et al. Circadian rhythm of infarct size and left ventricular function evaluated with tissue doppler echocardiography in st elevation myocardial infarction. Heart Lung Circ 2016; 25(3):250–6.

122. Muller JE, Ludmer PL, Willich SN, et al. Circadian variation in the frequency of sudden cardiac death. Circulation 1987;75(1):131–8.

123. Willich SN, Levy D, Rocco MB, et al. Circadian variation in the incidence of sudden cardiac death in the Framingham Heart Study population. Am J Cardiol 1987;60(10):801–6.

124. Peters RW, Muller JE, Goldstein S, et al. Propranolol and the morning increase in the frequency of sudden cardiac death (BHAT study). Am J Cardiol 1989;63(20):1518–20.

125. Willich SN, Goldberg RJ, Maclure M, et al. Increased onset of sudden cardiac death in the first three hours after awakening. Am J Cardiol 1992;70(1):65–8.

126. Levine RL, Pepe PE, Fromm RE Jr, et al. Prospective evidence of a circadian rhythm for out-of-hospital cardiac arrests. JAMA 1992;267(21):2935–7.

127. Aronow WS, Ahn C. Circadian variation of primary cardiac arrest or sudden cardiac death in patients aged 62 to 100 years (mean 82). Am J Cardiol 1993;71(16):1455–6.

128. Arntz HR, Willich SN, Oeff M, et al. Circadian variation of sudden cardiac death reflects age-related variability in ventricular fibrillation. Circulation 1993;88(5 Pt 1):2284–9.

129. Moser DK, Stevenson WG, Woo MA, et al. Timing of sudden death in patients with heart failure. J Am Coll Cardiol 1994;24(4):963–7.

130. Lucente M, Rebuzzi AG, Lanza GA, et al. Circadian variation of ventricular tachycardia in acute myocardial infarction. Am J Cardiol 1988;62(10 Pt 1):670–4.

131. Twidale N, Taylor S, Heddle WF, et al. Morning increase in the time of onset of sustained ventricular tachycardia. Am J Cardiol 1989;64(18):1204–6.

132. Lanza GA, Cortellessa MC, Rebuzzi AG, et al. Reproducibility in circadian rhythm of ventricular premature complexes. Am J Cardiol 1990;66(15): 1099–106.

133. Zehender M, Meinertz T, Hohnloser S, et al. Prevalence of circadian variations and spontaneous variability of cardiac disorders and ECG changes suggestive of myocardial ischemia in systemic arterial hypertension. Circulation 1992;85(5): 1808–15.

134. Siegel D, Black DM, Seeley DG, et al. Circadian variation in ventricular arrhythmias in hypertensive men. Am J Cardiol 1992;69(4):344–7.

135. Valkama JO, Huikuri HV, Linnaluoto MK, et al. Circadian variation of ventricular tachycardia in patients with coronary arterial disease. Int J Cardiol 1992;34(2):173–8.

136. Lampert R, Rosenfeld L, Batsford W, et al. Circadian variation of sustained ventricular tachycardia in patients with coronary artery disease and implantable cardioverter-defibrillators. Circulation 1994;90(1):241–7.

137. Wood MA, Simpson PM, London WB, et al. Circadian pattern of ventricular tachyarrhythmias in patients with implantable cardioverter-defibrillators. J Am Coll Cardiol 1995;25(4): 901–7.

138. Tofler GH, Gebara OC, Mittleman MA, et al. Morning peak in ventricular tachyarrhythmias detected by time of implantable cardioverter/defibrillator therapy. The CPI Investigators. Circulation 1995; 92(5):1203–8.

139. Englund A, Behrens S, Wegscheider K, et al. Circadian variation of malignant ventricular arrhythmias in patients with ischemic and nonischemic heart disease after cardioverter defibrillator implantation. European 7219 Jewel Investigators. J Am Coll Cardiol 1999;34(5): 1560–8.

140. Marshall J. Diurnal variation in occurrence of strokes. Stroke 1977;8(2):230–1.

141. Tsementzis SA, Gill JS, Hitchcock ER, et al. Diurnal variation of and activity during the onset of stroke. Neurosurgery 1985;17(6):901–4.

142. van der Windt C, van Gijn J. Cerebral infarction does not occur typically at night. J Neurol Neurosurg Psychiatry 1988;51(1):109–11.

143. Marler JR, Price TR, Clark GL, et al. Morning increase in onset of ischemic stroke. Stroke 1989; 20(4):473–6.

144. Pasqualetti P, Natali G, Casale R, et al. Epidemiological chronorisk of stroke. Acta Neurol Scand 1990;81(1):71–4.

145. Argentino C, Toni D, Rasura M, et al. Circadian variation in the frequency of ischemic stroke. Stroke 1990;21(3):387–9.

146. Marsh EE 3rd, Biller J, Adams HP Jr, et al. Circadian variation in onset of acute ischemic stroke. Arch Neurol 1990;47(11):1178–80.

147. Ricci S, Celani MG, Vitali R, et al. Diurnal and seasonal variations in the occurrence of stroke: a community-based study. Neuroepidemiology 1992;11(2):59–64.

148. Wroe SJ, Sandercock P, Bamford J, et al. Diurnal variation in incidence of stroke: Oxfordshire community stroke project. BMJ 1992;304(6820): 155–7.

149. Sloan MA, Price TR, Foulkes MA, et al. Circadian rhythmicity of stroke onset. Intracerebral and subarachnoid hemorrhage. Stroke 1992;23(10): 1420–6.

150. Gallerani M, Manfredini R, Ricci L, et al. Chronobiological aspects of acute cerebrovascular diseases. Acta Neurol Scand 1993;87(6):482–7.

151. Kelly-Hayes M, Wolf PA, Kase CS, et al. Temporal patterns of stroke onset. The Framingham Study. Stroke 1995;26(8):1343–7.

152. Lago A, Geffner D, Tembl J, et al. Circadian variation in acute ischemic stroke: a hospital-based study. Stroke 1998;29(9):1873–5.

153. Chaturvedi S, Adams HP Jr, Woolson RF. Circadian variation in ischemic stroke subtypes. Stroke 1999; 30(9):1792–5.

154. Raj K, Bhatia R, Prasad K, et al. Seasonal differences and circadian variation in stroke occurrence and stroke subtypes. J Stroke Cerebrovasc Dis 2015;24(1):10–6.

Circadian Periodicity of Ischemic Heart Disease

A Systematic Review of the Literature

Fabio Fabbian, MD[a],*, Subir Bhatia, MD[b],
Afredo De Giorgi, MD[a], Elisa Maietti, CStat[c],
Sravya Bhatia, BS[d], Anusha Shanbhag, MD[e],
Abhishek Deshmukh, MD[f]

KEYWORDS

- Circadian • Myocardial infarction
- Ratios between the number of events per hour during the morning and the other hours of the day

KEY POINTS

- A circadian pattern of acute myocardial infarction with a peak in the early morning waking hours has been reported since the 1980s.
- A MEDLINE literature search to identify relevant reports published during the last 20 years and focused on circadian variation of acute myocardial infarction was performed.
- Out of 1001 studies, 32 studies evaluating 34 populations were considered.
- Ratio between events per hour during the morning and events per hour during the other intervals hours of the day was 1.56 (95% confidence interval, 1.48–1.65).

INTRODUCTION

Acute cardiovascular events follow a circadian pattern,[1] and circadian rhythms occur through the integration of oscillatory expression of multiple circadian clock genes.[2] Acute myocardial infarction (AMI) continues to be a significant health concern, as patients who suffer from coronary heart disease have worse short-term and long-term morbidity and mortality compared with the general population.[3] Circadian patterns of AMI have been known since the 1980s, and it has been found that the peak in the frequency of AMI happens between 6:00 AM and noon.[4,5] Prior studies found that AMI could be triggered by several factors, both environmental

and physiologic, including circadian variations in cardiovascular and metabolic functioning.[6]

To the best of the authors' knowledge, only 1 meta-analysis was identified of published reports analyzing the circadian variation of AMI aiming to calculate the proportion of events that were attributable to the morning excess.[7] In this meta-analysis, the authors searched medical publications from January 1985 to June 1996.

The goal of the this study was to evaluate the risk of AMI during the morning versus the other hours of the day deriving data from reports published in the last 20 years in which the number of events in the different periods of the day was reported.

Disclosure Statement: Authors declare that they do not have any commercial or financial conflicts of interest and any funding sources related to this article.

[a] Department of Medical Sciences, University of Ferrara, University Hospital St. Anna, Via Aldo Moro 8, I-44124, Cona, Ferrara, Italy; [b] Department of Internal Medicine, Mayo Clinic, 200 First Street SW, Rochester, MN 55905, USA; [c] Department of Medical Sciences, University of Ferrara, Center for Clinical Epidemiology, 44121 Ferrara, Italy; [d] School of Medicine, Duke University, 8 Duke University Medical Center Greenspace, Durham, NC 27703, USA; [e] Department of Internal Medicine, University of Arkansas for Medical Sciences, 4301 W. Markham Street, Little Rock, AR 72205, USA; [f] Division of Cardiovascular Diseases, Mayo Clinic, Rochester, Minnesota, 200 First Street Southwest, Rochester, Minnesota 55905, USA
* Corresponding author.
E-mail address: f.fabbian@ospfe.it

METHODS

The authors performed a MEDLINE literature search to identify relevant reports focused on circadian variation of AMI. The following search terms were used: "circadian" and "myocardial infarction." All systematic reviews, meta-analyses, controlled trials, cohort studies, and case-control studies that were published after 1997 were considered for inclusion. Case reports, comments, discussion letters, articles in languages other than in English, and conference abstracts or proceedings were excluded. Authors, years of publication, country, and the number of patients who suffered AMI per hour during the period between 6:00 AM and noon and during the other hours of the day were calculated. One study evaluated 3 different populations; these study populations were considered separately, and calculations were performed accordingly.[8] Because of the study design in one study, the authors defined the morning to be between 06:00 and 14:00; in 6 studies the authors defined the morning period to be between 08:00 and 16:00. The ratio between the number of events per hour during the morning and the number of events per hour during the other hours of the day was calculated. Furthermore, the weight of each study was considered based on the number of patients enrolled in the study. Mean weighted ratio and its 95% confidence intervals were graphed.

RESULTS

The authors identified 1001 reports, of which, 494 were excluded because they were published before 1997. Of 507 articles, 464 were excluded because they were not clinical studies, leaving 43 articles. Finally, 11 clinical studies were excluded because the authors did not report absolute numbers or percentages in the results section (**Fig. 1**). Therefore, 32 reports evaluating 34 different populations were considered: 16 from Asia, 10 from Europe, and 8 from the United States. The authors calculated the total number of patients with AMI in whom circadian pattern was evaluated to be 131,235. Forty-one percent (n = 53,918) of patients suffered the event during the morning. During morning, a mean of 212.3 events per hour was calculated, whereas during the other hours of the day the number of events per hour was 137.1. Data derived from each study is reported in **Table 1**[8–39] The mean ratio between the number of events per hour during the morning and the number of events per hour during the other hours of the day was 1.43 (95% confidence interval [CI], 1.33–1.53). The same weighted ratio was

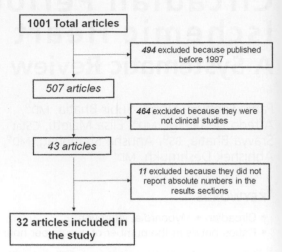

Fig. 1. Medline searching strategy using terms "circadian" and "myocardial infarction."

1.56 (95% CI, 1.48–1.65) (**Fig. 2**). Of 34 populations, only 3 showed a ratio less than 1, involving 1067 patients representing 0.81% of the number of subjects investigated.

DISCUSSION

The first report on a circadian variation for onset of AMI detecting an increased morning frequency in the period between 06:00 and 12:00 was published in 1985 by Muller and colleagues.[5] In 1997, a meta-analysis including 30 studies on AMI and 19 studies on sudden cardiac death evaluated the morning excess of AMI by investigating more than 66,000 patients. They found the incidence of AMI onset was 40% higher in the morning than throughout the rest of the day.[7] Furthermore, they estimated that more than 27% of morning AMIs and more than 22% of sudden cardiac deaths were attributable to a morning excess of risk. The current authors' results seem to confirm the previous findings with a weighted ratio between the number of events per hour during the morning and the number of events per hour during the other hours of the day to be 1.56 (95% CI, 1.48–1.65).

Although several factors have been found to modify or attenuate the circadian pattern of AMI including demographic factors,[40,41] medications,[40–44] and comorbidities,[40,41,45,46] the last 2 decades have seen major changes in lifestyle and significant improvements in medical intervention. Prior evidence shows that although the onset of AMIs is lowest during the first part of night when sleeping, the prevalence increases in the second part of night and increases further during the first hours of daytime activity.[47] The temporal relationship between AMI onset and awakening was also reported in shift workers.[48] The increased risk of AMI during the morning could be the effect of several mechanisms, all of which alter the circadian rhythm and result in decreased coronary blood flow and oxygen supply. On the other hand, factors that may be considered in the development of AMI constitute a complex interplay of internal circadian factors and physical and emotional triggers.[49] In the morning, not only does blood pressure and heart rate increase causing increased oxygen demand by the heart, but the vascular tone of coronary arteries also increases.[50]

Several factors that could trigger cardiovascular disease undergo circadian variation. Neuroendocrine mechanisms are major determinants of the normal circadian pattern, and circadian rhythms of monoaminergic systems in conjunction with those of the hypothalamic-pituitary-adrenal, hypothalamic-pituitary-thyroid, opioid, and renin-angiotensin-aldosterone systems likely contribute. Furthermore, endothelial systems and specific vasoactive peptides, such as arginine vasopressin, vasoactive intestinal peptide, melatonin, somatotropin, insulin, steroids, serotonin, corticotropin-releasing factor, adrenocorticotropic hormone, thyrotropin-releasing hormone, endogenous opioids, and prostaglandin E2 also exhibit circadian variation. As a result, physical, mental, and pathologic stimuli that activate or inhibit neuroendocrine effectors of biological rhythmicity may also interfere with, or modify, the physiologic temporal pattern.[51]

Coagulation factors have also been found to follow a circadian pattern.[52] An alteration in these factors' homeostasis may lead to an imbalance between myocardial oxygen supply and demand, potentially contributing to AMI. Therefore, circadian organization seems to impact the entire cardiovascular system, and circadian rhythms may trigger the development of acute cardiovascular events. Moreover, 24-hour recording of electrocardiograms in patients with untreated ischemic heart disease showed a circadian pattern of nonsymptomatic ischemia.[53] In these subjects, nonsymptomatic myocardial ischemia and coronary artery vasospasm was more frequent between 06:00 and 12:00.[54] Recently, Manfredini and colleagues[55] compared the time of onset of AMI and Takotsubo cardiomyopathy and found that they both seem to be more frequent during daytime. Regarding the onset of AMI, the authors analyzed 26 reports published between 1995 and 2016 involving 459,836 patients with an average of 64 years[55] and found similar results.

However, other studies found contradictory findings to ours. Reavey and colleagues[56] collected mortality data on 869,863 cardiovascular events from 1969 to 2007 and hospitalization data on 959,990 cardiovascular events from 1997 to 2008. The authors detected a circadian variation in cardiovascular mortality, with a first peak in the period 08:00 to 12:00 and a smaller second peak in the late afternoon between 14:00 and 18:00. This pattern persisted after multivariate adjustment and was more pronounced for AMI.[56] Furthermore, Seneviratna and colleagues[35] examined the circadian pattern of AMI size by assessing more than 6500 patients with ST elevation myocardial infarction from the Singapore Myocardial Infarction Registry. They found that the peak incidence of symptom onset was observed between 00:00 and 06:00. Differences in the prevalence of diabetes, infarct location, and mechanical reperfusion were found to only partially justify the circadian pattern of infarct size and acute heart failure.[35]

The contributions of external triggers that may alter the circadian rhythm have been found to be significant. Culić and colleagues[57] suggested the association between external triggering activities and AMI differ between men and women. It was postulated these gender differences might be owing to different exposures, sex-specific mechanisms, or both.[57] They reported a disproportionately higher amount of women compared with men had infarctions occurring between 06:00 and noon compared with other periods of a day. Furthermore, patients who have a larger number of cardiovascular risk factors may also have a different triggering profile, predisposing them to AMI in the early morning hours. Other research has shown, however, that trigger-related infarctions may occur more frequently in patients who have less severe coronary atherosclerosis.[58]

LIMITATIONS

Although these results confirm those of previous studies of what is already known, our study should be interpreted in light of its limitations. Several of the reports analyzed had different study designs, and few of the reports defined morning as the exact same time. Additionally, we could not evaluate circadian variation of AMI biomarkers, infarct size, type of AMI, or outcome of patients. As underlined by Cohen and colleagues,[7] we did not consider awakening and arising from bed, leading to a possible underestimation of the true risk of morning events. Fournier and colleagues[59] conducted a retrospective, registry-based study analyzing associations between peak CK, in-hospital mortality, and time of the day at symptoms onset. They evaluated more than 6000 patients with ST-elevation myocardial infarction

Table 1
Data derived from each study

Study	Country	Population	Events in the Morning	Events in the Other Periods of the Day	Events/hour in the Morning	Events/hour in the Other Periods of the Day	Ratio
Cannon et al,[9] 1997	United States	7730	2427	5303	404.5	294.6	1.37
Ku et al,[10] 1998	Taiwan	540	184	356	30.7	19.8	1.55
Kinjo et al,[11] 2001	Japan	1252	487	765	60.9	47.8	1.27
Yamasaki et al,[12] 2002	Japan	725	217	508	36.2	28.2	1.28
Rana et al,[13] 2003	United States	200	58	142	9.7	7.9	1.22
Moruzzi et al,[14] 2004	Italy	1571	467	1104	77.8	61.3	1.26
Manfredini et al,[15] 2004	Italy	442	164	278	27.3	15.4	1.76
Bhalla et al,[16] 2006	India	206	68	138	11.3	7.7	1.47
Kurisu et al,[17] 2007	Japan	544	146	398	24.3	22.1	1.10
Sari et al,[18] 2009	Turkey	476	112	364	18.7	20.2	0.92
Holmes et al,[19] 2010	United States	2143	673	1470	112.2	81.7	1.37
Li et al,[20] 2010	China	1016	340	676	56.7	37.6	1.50
Bae et al,[21] 2010	Korea	892	303	589	50.5	32.7	1.54
Matura,[22] 2010	United States	273	82	191	13.7	10.6	1.28
Park et al,[23] 2010	Korea	4573	1804	2769	225.5	173.1	1.30
Suárez-Barrientos et al,[24] 2011	Spain	811	269	542	44.8	30.1	1.48

Celik et al,[25] 2011	Turkey	465	182	283	30.3	15.7	1.92
Jia et al,[26] 2012	China	1467	469	998	78.2	55.4	1.40
Chan et al,[27] 2012	Taiwan	505	118	387	19.7	21.5	0.91
Fournier et al,[28] 2012	Switzerland	353	109	244	18.2	13.6	1.34
Mogabgab et al,[29] 2012	United States	35,492	17,391	18,101	2173.9	1131.3	1.92
Ammirati et al,[8] 2013	China	436	155	281	25.8	15.6	1.65
Ammirati et al,[8] 2013	Italy	404	157	247	26.2	13.7	1.90
Ammirati et al,[8] 2013	Scotland	254	87	167	14.5	9.3	1.56
Mogabgab et al,[30] 2013	United States	162	54	108	9.0	6.0	1.50
Isik et al,[31] 2013	Turkey	86	12	74	2.0	4.1	0.48
Mogabgab et al,[32] 2013	United States	45,218	18,721	26,497	2340.1	1656.1	1.41
Kanth et al,[33] 2013	United States	519	224	295	28.0	18.4	1.51
Wieringa et al,[34] 2014	The Netherlands	6970	2335	4635	389.2	257.5	1.51
Seneviratna et al,[35] 2015	Singapore	6710	2102	4608	350.3	256.0	1.36
Rallidis et al,[36] 2015	Greece	256	83	173	13.8	9.6	1.43
Mahmoud et al,[37] 2015	The Netherlands	6799	3198	3601	399.8	225.1	1.77
Brown et al,[38] 2015	United Kingdom	1493	623	870	77.9	54.4	1.43
Arı et al,[39] 2016	Turkey	252	97	155	16.2	8.6	1.87

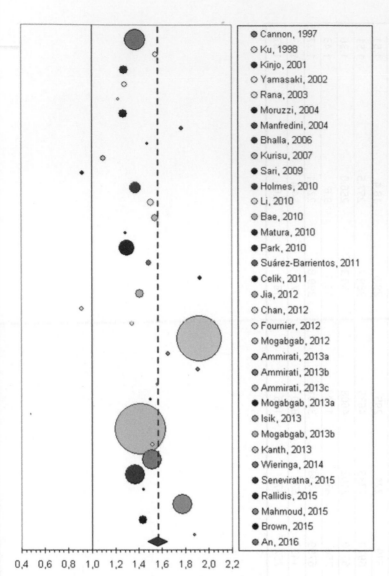

Cannon, 1997
Ku, 1998
Kinjo, 2001
Yamasaki, 2002
Rana, 2003
Moruzzi, 2004
Manfredini, 2004
Bhalla, 2006
Kurisu, 2007
Sari, 2009
Holmes, 2010
Li, 2010
Bae, 2010
Matura, 2010
Park, 2010
Suárez-Barrientos, 2011
Celik, 2011
Jia, 2012
Chan, 2012
Fournier, 2012
Mogabgab, 2012
Ammirati, 2013a
Ammirati, 2013b
Ammirati, 2013c
Mogabgab, 2013a
Isik, 2013
Mogabgab, 2013b
Kanth, 2013
Wieringa, 2014
Seneviratna, 2015
Rallidis, 2015
Mahmoud, 2015
Brown, 2015
An, 2016

0,4 0,6 0,8 1,0 1,2 1,4 1,6 1,8 2,0 2,2

Fig. 2. Weighted mean ratio between number of events per hour during the morning and number of events per hour during the other hours of the day. The diameter of every circle is proportional to the number of subjects analyzed in each population.

from 82 acute-care hospitals in Switzerland who were treated with primary angioplasty within 6 hours of symptom onset.[59] They found that the peak CK value was detected in subjects with symptoms onset at 23:00, and no correlation was found between ischemic time and circadian pattern of CK. Risk of in-hospital mortality was highest for patients with symptom onset at 00:00 and lowest for those with onset at 12:00. Our study, because of its design, could not consider CK plasma levels.

SUMMARY

Despite the optimization of interventional and medical therapy for AMI since the first reports of circadian patterns in AMI occurrence, we found that such a pattern still exists and that AMI happens most frequently in the morning hours. Further investigation into the factors contributing to early-morning risk is warranted. With better knowledge of AMI triggers, researchers, clinicians, and health care policy makers can continue to work to lessen the global burden of cardiovascular disease.

REFERENCES

1. Manfredini R, Boari B, Salmi R, et al. Twenty-four-hour patterns in occurrence and pathophysiology of acute cardiovascular events and ischemic heart disease. Chronobiol Int 2013;30:6–16.
2. Harmer SL, Panda S, Kay SA. Molecular bases of circadian rhythms. Annu Rev Cell Dev Biol 2001; 17:215–53.

3. Piironen M, Ukkola O, Huikuri H, et al. Trends in long-term prognosis after acute coronary syndrome. Eur J Prev Cardiol 2017;24(3):274–80.

4. Thompson DR, Blandford RL, Sutton TW, et al. Time of onset of chest pain in acute myocardial infarction. Int J Cardiol 1985;7:139–48.

5. Muller JE, Stone PH, Turi ZG, et al. Circadian variation in the frequency of onset of acute myocardial infarction. N Engl J Med 1985;313:1315–22.

6. Rüger M, Scheer FA. Effects of circadian disruption on the cardiometabolic system. Rev Endocr Metab Disord 2009;10:245–60.

7. Cohen MC, Rohtla KM, Lavery CE, et al. Meta-analysis of the morning excess of acute myocardial infarction and sudden cardiac death. Am J Cardiol 1997;79:1512–6.

8. Ammirati E, Cristell N, Cianflone D, et al. Questing for circadian dependence in ST-segment-elevation acute myocardial infarction: a multicentric and multi-ethnic study. Circ Res 2013;112:e110–4.

9. Cannon CP, McCabe CH, Stone PH, et al. Circadian variation in the onset of unstable angina and non-Q-wave acute myocardial infarction (the TIMI III Registry and TIMI IIIB). Am J Cardiol 1997;79:253–8.

10. Ku CS, Yang CY, Lee WJ, et al. Absence of a seasonal variation in myocardial infarction onset in a region without temperature extremes. Cardiology 1998;89:277–82.

11. Kinjo K, Sato H, Sato H, et al. Circadian variation of the onset of acute myocardial infarction in the Osaka area, 1998-1999: characterization of morning and nighttime peaks. Jpn Circ J 2001;65:617–20.

12. Yamasaki F, Seo H, Furuno T, et al. Effect of age on chronological variation of acute myocardial infarction onset: study in Japan. Clin Exp Hypertens 2002;24:1–9.

13. Rana JS, Mukamal KJ, Morgan JP, et al. Circadian variation in the onset of myocardial infarction: effect of duration of diabetes. Diabetes 2003;52:1464–8.

14. Moruzzi P, Marenzi G, Callegari S, et al. Circadian distribution of acute myocardial infarction by anatomic location and coronary artery involvement. Am J Med 2004;116:24–7.

15. Manfredini R, Boari B, Bressan S, et al. Influence of circadian rhythm on mortality after myocardial infarction: data from a prospective cohort of emergency calls. Am J Emerg Med 2004;22:555–9.

16. Bhalla A, Sachdev A, Lehl SS, et al. Ageing and circadian variation in cardiovascular events. Singapore Med J 2006;47:305–8.

17. Kurisu S, Inoue I, Kawagoe T, et al. Circadian variation in the occurrence of tako-tsubo cardiomyopathy: comparison with acute myocardial infarction. Int J Cardiol 2007;115:270–1.

18. Sari I, Davutoglu V, Erer B, et al. Analysis of circadian variation of acute myocardial infarction: afternoon predominance in Turkish population. Int J Clin Pract 2009;63:82–6.

19. Holmes DR, Aguirre FV, Aplin R, et al. Circadian rhythms in patients with ST-elevation myocardial infarction. Circ Cardiovasc Qual Outcomes 2010;3: 382–9.

20. Li J, Hua Q, Pi L, et al. Circadian variation on the onset of acute ST segment elevation myocardial infarction in diabetic subjects. J Cardiovasc Dis Res 2010;1:23–6.

21. Bae MH, Ryu HM, Lee JH, et al. The impact of circadian variation on 12-month mortality in patients with acute myocardial infarction. Korean Circ J 2010;40: 616–24.

22. Matura LA. Gender and circadian effects of myocardial infarctions. Clin Nurs Res 2010;19:55–70.

23. Park HE, Koo BK, Lee W, et al. Periodic variation and its effect on management and prognosis of Korean patients with acute myocardial infarction. Circ J 2010;74:970–6.

24. Suárez-Barrientos A, López-Romero P, Vivas D, et al. Circadian variations of infarct size in acute myocardial infarction. Heart 2011;97:970–6.

25. Celik M, Celik T, Iyisoy A, et al. Circadian variation of acute st segment elevation myocardial infarction by anatomic location in a Turkish cohort. Med Sci Monit 2011;17:CR210–5.

26. Jia EZ, Xu ZX, Cai HZ, et al. Time distribution of the onset of chest pain in subjects with acute ST-elevation myocardial infarction: an eight-year, single-center study in China. PLoS One 2012;7(3): e32478.

27. Chan CM, Chen WL, Kuo HY, et al. Circadian variation of acute myocardial infarction in young people. Am J Emerg Med 2012;30:1461–5.

28. Fournier S, Eeckhout E, Mangiacapra F, et al. Circadian variations of ischemic burden among patients with myocardial infarction undergoing primary percutaneous coronary intervention. Am Heart J 2012;163:208–13.

29. Mogabgab O, Giugliano RP, Sabatine MS, et al. Circadian variation in patient characteristics and outcomes in ST-segment elevation myocardial infarction. Chronobiol Int 2012;29:1390139–46.

30. Mogabgab O, Wiviott SD, Antman EM, et al. Relation between time of symptom onset of ST-segment elevation myocardial infarction and patient baseline characteristics: from the National Cardiovascular Data Registry. Clin Cardiol 2013; 36:222–7.

31. Isik T, Ayhan E, Uyarel H, et al. Circadian, weekly, and seasonal variation in early stent thrombosis patients who previously underwent primary percutaneous intervention with ST elevation myocardial infarction. Clin Appl Thromb Hemost 2013;19: 679–84.

32. Mogabgab O, Wiviott SD, Cannon CP, et al. Circadian variation of stent thrombosis and the effect of more robust platelet inhibition: a post hoc analysis

of the TRITON-TIMI 38 trial. J Cardiovasc Pharmacol Ther 2013;18:555–9.

33. Kanth R, Ittaman S, Rezkalla S. Circadian patterns of ST elevation myocardial infarction in the new millennium. Clin Med Res 2013;11:66–72.

34. Wieringa WG, Lexis CP, Mahmoud KD, et al. Time of symptom onset and value of myocardial blush and infarct size on prognosis in patients with ST-elevation myocardial infarction. Chronobiol Int 2014l;31:797–806.

35. Seneviratna A, Lim GH, Devi A, et al. Circadian dependence of infarct size and acute heart failure in ST elevation myocardial infarction. PLoS One 2015;10(6):e0128526.

36. Rallidis LS, Triantafyllis AS, Sakadakis EA, et al. Circadian pattern of symptoms onset in patients ≤35 years presenting with ST-segment elevation acute myocardial infarction. Eur J Intern Med 2015; 26:607–10.

37. Mahmoud KD, Nijsten MW, Wieringa WG, et al. Independent association between symptom onset time and infarct size in patients with ST-elevation myocardial infarction undergoing primary percutaneous coronary intervention. Chronobiol Int 2015;32:468–77.

38. Brown RA, Lip GY, Varma C, et al. Ethnic differences in the diurnal variation of symptom onset time for acute ST elevation myocardial infarction - An observational cohort study. Int J Cardiol 2015;187:414–6.

39. Arı H, Sonmez O, Koc F, et al. Circadian rhythm of infarct size and left ventricular function evaluated with tissue Doppler Echocardiography in ST elevation myocardial infarction. Heart Lung Circ 2016;25:250–6.

40. Gilpin EA, Hjalmarson A, Ross J Jr. Subgroups of patients with atypical circadian patterns of symptom onset in acute myocardial infarction. Am J Cardiol 1990;66:7G–11G.

41. Sayer JW, Wilkinson P, Ranjadayalan K, et al. Attenuation or absence of circadian and seasonal rhythms of acute myocardial infarction. Heart 1997; 77:325–9.

42. Willich SN, Linderer T, Wegscheider K, et al. Increased morning incidence of myocardial infarction in the ISAM Study: absence with prior beta-adrenergic blockade. ISAM Study Group. Circulation 1989;80:853–8.

43. Hansen O, Johansson BW, Gullberg B. Circadian distribution of onset of acute myocardial infarction in subgroups from analysis of 10,791 patients treated in a single center. Am J Cardiol 1992;69:1003–8.

44. Garmendia-Leiza JR, Andres-de-Llano JM, Ardura-Fernandez J, et al. Beta blocker therapy modifies circadian rhythm acute myocardial infarction. Int J Cardiol 2011;147:316–7.

45. Fava S, Azzopardi J, Muscat HA, et al. Absence of circadian variation in the onset of acute myocardial infarction in diabetic subjects. Br Heart J 1995;74: 370–2.

46. Tanaka T, Fujita M, Fudo T, et al. Modification of the circadian variation of symptom onset of acute myocardial infarction in diabetes mellitus. Coron Artery Dis 1995;6:241–4.

47. Boari B, Salmi R, Gallerani M, et al. Acute myocardial infarction: circadian, weekly, and seasonal patterns of occurrence. Biol Rhythm Res 2007;38: 155–67.

48. Knutsson A. Shift work and coronary heart disease. Scand J Soc Med 1989;44:1–36.

49. Hammoudeh AJ, Alhaddad IA. Triggers and the onset of acute myocardial infarction. Cardiol Rev 2009;17:270–4.

50. Hermida RC, Smolensky MH, Ayala DE, et al. Ambulatory blood pressure monitoring (ABPM) as the reference standard for diagnosis of hypertension and assessment of vascular risk in adults. Chronobiol Int 2015;32:1329–42.

51. Fabbian F, Smolensky MH, Tiseo R, et al. Dipper and non-dipper blood pressure 24-hour patterns: circadian rhythm-dependent physiologic and pathophysiologic mechanisms. Chronobiol Int 2013;30: 17–30.

52. Pinotti M, Bertolucci C, Portaluppi F, et al. Daily and circadian rhythms of tissue factor pathway inhibitor and factor VII activity. Arterioscler Thromb Vasc Biol 2005;25:646–9.

53. Rocco MB. Timing and triggers of transient myocardial ischemia. Am J Cardiol 1990;66:18G–21G.

54. Yasue H, Omote S, Takizawa A, et al. Circadian variation of exercise capacity in patients with Prinzmetal's variant angina: role of exercise-induced coronary arterial spasm. Circulation 1979;59: 938–48.

55. Manfredini R, Manfredini F, Fabbian F, et al. Chronobiology of Takotsubo syndrome and myocardial infarction: analogies and differences. Heart Fail Clin 2016;12:531–42.

56. Reavey M, Saner H, Paccaud F, et al. Exploring the periodicity of cardiovascular events in Switzerland: variation in deaths and hospitalizations across seasons, day of the week and hour of the day. Int J Cardiol 2013;168:2195–200.

57. Culić V, Eterović D, Mirić D, et al. Gender differences in triggering of acute myocardial infarction. Am J Cardiol 2000;85:753–6.

58. Culić V. Chronobiological rhythms of acute cardiovascular events and underlying mechanisms. Int J Cardiol 2014;174:417–9.

59. Fournier S, Taffé P, Radovanovic D, et al. Myocardial infarct size and mortality depend on the time of day-a large multicenter study. PLoS One 2015;10(3): e0119157.

Seasonal Periodicity of Ischemic Heart Disease and Heart Failure

Subir Bhatia, MD[a], Sravya Bhatia, BS[b], Jennifer Mears, BS[c],
George Dibu, MD[d], Abhishek Deshmukh, MD[c],*

KEYWORDS

- Seasonal periodicity • Ischemic heart disease • Heart failure • Myocardial infarction

KEY POINTS

- Seasonal variation for ischemic heart disease and heart failure is known.
- The interplay of environmental, biological, and physiologic changes is fascinating.
- This article highlights the seasonal periodicity of ischemic heart disease and heart failure and examines some of the potential reasons for these unique observations.

INTRODUCTION

"Look to the Seasons when Choosing Your Cures" (Hippocrates)

An increase in deaths during winter was reported as early as 1847 when William Farr described the diagnostic composition of the excess deaths occurring in that year. There has been a considerable interest in the role of climate change and its potential as a trigger for new-onset or worsening ischemic heart disease (IHD) and heart failure. The complex role of environmental factors, external biological milieu, and temporary physiologic changes is fascinating. This article highlights the seasonal periodicity of IHD and heart failure and examines some of the potential reasons for these unique observations.

ISCHEMIC HEART DISEASE
Epidemiology

An increase in mortality from acute myocardial infarction (AMI) in the winter months compared with the summer months was first reported in the 1930s.[1] Previous studies have reported seasonal

fluctuations in the onset of IHD and heart failure with a disproportionate number of admissions in the winter months compared with summer.[2–13] Far fewer studies have reported a higher incidence of AMI in the summer or no season variation.[14–20]

Furthermore, subsequent studies not only found an increase in mortality from AMI during the winter months but also from all forms of ischemic coronary disease during the winter.[21] Observational studies to determine whether cases of AMI reported to the second National Registry of Myocardial Infarction (NRMI-2) varied by season have been conducted previously as well.[22] Analysis of 259,891 cases revealed a significant peak in the winter months and a nadir in summer months. Moreover, this pattern was seen in all geographic areas, suggesting the chronobiology of season variation in AMI is independent of climate.

Analysis of 1252 patients in the Multicenter Investigation of Limitation of Infarct Size (MILIS) and Thrombolysis in Myocardial Infarction–4 (TIMI-4) trials found that mean infarct size, as measured by mean creatine-kinase in blood (CK-MB) infarct

a Department of Internal Medicine, Mayo Clinic, 200 First Street Southwest, Rochester, MN 55905, USA; b School of Medicine, Duke University, 8 Duke University Medical Center Greenspace, Durham, NC 27703, USA; c Division of Cardiovascular Diseases, Mayo Clinic, 200 First Street Southwest, Rochester, MN 55905, USA; d Division of Cardiovascular Medicine, University of Florida, 1600 SW Archer Road, Gainesville, FL 32608, USA
* Corresponding author. Division of Cardiovascular Diseases, Mayo Clinic, 200 First Street Southwest, Rochester, MN 55905.
E-mail address: Deshmukh.Abhishek@mayo.edu

Heart Failure Clin 13 (2017) 681–689
http://dx.doi.org/10.1016/j.hfc.2017.05.004
1551-7136/17/© 2017 Elsevier Inc. All rights reserved.

size index and TIMI flow grade, at 18 to 36 hours was decreased in the summer months.[23] A proposed mechanism includes an increase in vascular resistance in cold temperatures.[24–27] The subsequent increase in coronary vascular resistance would then be expected to result in reduced coronary flow. In the summer months, an increase in temperature has been hypothesized to contribute to overall reduced venous and arterial resistance, thus reducing preload as well as afterload.

Influence of Influenza

Other studies assessing potential factors contributing to seasonal fluctuations in IHD and heart failure have shown that respiratory infections are more frequent during the cold months. Given prior evidence of an association between respiratory infection and AMI,[28–30] respiratory infections may contribute to the higher rate of AMI in the winter. Vaccination against influenza has been associated with a 67% reduction in the risk of myocardial infarction during the subsequent influenza season.[31] Influenza has been shown to affect the vascular system in numerous ways. Inoculation of atherosclerotic apolipoprotein-E–deficient mice with influenza A resulted in heavy infiltration of atherosclerotic plaques by inflammatory cells as well as fibrin deposition, platelet aggregation, smooth muscle cell proliferation, and thrombosis.[32] These prothrombotic and inflammatory changes mimic those seen in coronary plaques after myocardial infarction.[33] In addition, death rates from cardiovascular disease have been noted to increase during epidemics of influenza, and it has been suggested that acute respiratory tract infections before an AMI may be a cardiovascular risk factor.[34]

Biochemical Factors

Various other factors with seasonal variation have also been identified. Studies have shown seasonal variations in coagulation factors, such as fibrinogen and activated factor VII, with a significant increase during the winter months.[35–37] Analysis of 82 subjects, 47 of whom were free of clinical signs of coronary artery disease and 35 survivors of AMI, who had measurements of various metabolic and hemostatic coronary risk factors twice in the cold months (December and March) and twice in the warm months (June and September), revealed a significantly higher body mass index, glucose, total cholesterol, low-density lipoprotein, triglycerides, lipoprotein(a) (Lp[a]), fibrinogen, and platelet counts in the colder months compared with the warm months. Other studies have shown that fibrinogen levels were significantly higher in the winter with a more pronounced difference in fibrinogen levels in

older patients (75 years of age and older) compared with subjects 55 to 75 years of age.[38]

Studies focusing on seasonal variation in cholesterol levels have also revealed total cholesterol and low-density lipoprotein cholesterol levels to be highest in wintertime.[39] A longitudinal study of seasonal variation in lipid levels in 517 healthy volunteers from a health maintenance organization serving central Massachusetts revealed a breadth of seasonal variation of 3.9 mg/dL in men, with a peak in December, and 5.4 mg/dL in women, with a peak in January.[40] Seasonal amplitude was greater in hypercholesterolemic participants compared with participants with normal cholesterol levels. Furthermore, 22% more participants had total cholesterol levels of 240 mg/dL or greater in the winter than in the summer.

Role of Air Pollution

There has been a growing amount of epidemiologic evidence underscoring a possible association between ambient air pollution and poor cardiovascular outcomes. This finding is important given the strong association between pollution levels, increased mortality, and winter months.[41–43] Specific air pollutants are implicated with an increased risk of cardiovascular disease, including carbon dioxide, oxides of nitrogen, sulfur dioxide, lead, ozone, and particulate matter less than 10 μm in diameter. These pollutants have been associated with increased hospitalizations[44,45] and mortality caused by cardiovascular disease,[46–48] with a disproportionate number of heart failures or baseline arrhythmias.[49] Exposure to fine particulate air pollutants may be associated with increased blood pressure caused by sympathetic activation.[50–52] Exposure to fine particulates has also been shown to possibly cause increase in baseline heart rate, fibrinogen levels, blood coagulation factor levels, arterial vasoconstriction, and endothelial dysfunction.[28] As a result, higher pollution levels in winter may be associated with myocardial ischemia,[29] angina pectoris, malignant ventricular arrhythmias,[30] and increased plaque vulnerability.[53]

Seasonal changes in temperature with subsequent endothelial dysfunction and changes in blood pressure may also contribute to seasonal variation in IHD. Research has shown a significant difference in seasonal variation of peak blood pressure values, with peak values in the spring and the lowest values in September.[54] Furthermore, a study of more than 17,000 European men and women found that systolic and diastolic pressures were highest in December and lowest in July, with more variation found in the elderly.[55]

Effect of Temperature

Studies have also assessed the effect of temperature alone on the risk of incident AMI. Analysis from the Worcester Heart Attack Study, a community-wide investigation of AMI in the residents of Worcester, Massachusetts, metropolitan area, found that a decrease of an interquartile range in apparent temperature was associated with an increased risk of AMI on the same day (hazard ratio, 1.15; 95% confidence interval [CI], 1.01–1.31). Extreme cold during the 2 days before an arrest was associated with a 36% increased risk of AMI (hazard ratio, 1.36; 95% CI, 1.07–1.74).[56] Further studies have suggested that the difference in temperature between summer and winter months may also play a role; previous work performed in Los Angeles by Kloner and colleagues[57] found a higher incidence of death caused by IHD in December and January compared with the summer months.

However, other studies have shown that European patients with ST-segment elevation myocardial infarction (STEMI) did not have season variations in infarct size or 1-year mortality. De Luca and colleagues[58] investigated seasonal variation in enzymatic infarct size, myocardial perfusion, and 1-year mortality in 1548 European patients who underwent primary angioplasty for STEMI. No seasonal variation was observed in patients' demographics and clinical characteristics. Furthermore, no difference was observed in the prevalence of heart failure or myocardial perfusion, enzymatic infarct size, or 1-year mortality.

Previous research has shown that seasonal variation in AMI hospitalizations may be more significant in the elderly population (65 years or older) compared with the young population (<65 years of age). Patel and colleagues[59] assessed 9,074,857 hospitalizations with a primary diagnosis of AMI in the United States from the beginning of the calendar year 2000 to the end of the calendar year 2011. The mean age was 68 years, and 60% of these patients were 65 years of age or older. There was a higher number of hospitalizations in the winter months for the elderly population compared with the summer months, with the average number of daily hospitalizations being the lowest in the month of August. However, such marked seasonal variation was not observed in the younger population.

It is thus evident that many elements may play a role in the seasonal variation seen in patients with IHD. Since the 1930s, researchers have noted the increase of illness during the winter months. Through the decades, studies have shown the influence of a multitude of factors, from temperature and air pollutants to cholesterol levels and coagulation factors, with specific factors contributing even more to older patients (>65 years of age).

HEART FAILURE
Epidemiology

Many researchers have also studied the seasonal variation in chronic heart failure (CHF). A seasonal periodicity for heart failure deaths and hospitalizations, with a peak in the winter, has been noted independent of age, major cardiovascular risk factors, gender, and outcomes.[60] Studies performed in both the southern[61–63] and northern hemispheres[64–71] have found a similar trend. Parry and colleagues[72] described the first mention of seasonality in CHF from northern Nigeria. Patients with CHF presented more frequently in cooler, dry months compared with warmer, hot months. Furthermore, early large-scale population-based studies that assessed seasonal variation in morbidity and mortality outcomes in patients with heart failure found significantly more CHF admission in winter compared with summer ($P<.00001$) with the greatest seasonal variation in patients greater than 75 years of age.[67] The largest study to date, assessing 12,077,033 hospitalizations with a primary diagnosis of heart failure in the United States from 2000 to 2011, found that the number of hospitalization was maximum in the winter months and minimum in the summer months, with an increasing trend from August to February.[73] In addition, mortalities associated with heart failure hospitalization rates were maximum in the winter months and minimum in the summer months.[73] It has been proposed that lower summer admissions compared with winter may be caused by bed closures during the summer as well as a reduction of local populations for summer vacations (**Table 1**).[69]

However, some studies of non-American patients have found contrasting results. A study consisting of 661 Japanese patients with acute heart failure admitted to the intensive care unit found that hospitalization in the summer (between July and September) was associated with more severe rates of heart failure, decreased left ventricular ejection fraction, and the use of dobutamine.[74] In addition, the cardiovascular death rate was significantly higher in the summer than in other months in this study.

Infectious Disease and Tachyarrhythmia

Numerous studies have also analyzed the influence of infectious diseases and tachyarrhythmia in seasonal variation in heart failure. A seasonal pattern of

Table 1
Seasonal trends in ischemic heart disease

	Author, Year	Country	Cases (n)	Age (y)	Peak
Ischemic heart disease	Rosahn,[1] 1937	United States	612	62	Winter–spring
	Heyer et al,[14] 1953	United States	1386	NA	Summer
	Ku et al,[15] 1998	Taiwan	540	NA	No peak
	Spencer et al,[22] 1998	United States	259,891	66	Winter
	Kloner et al,[23] 1999	United States	222,265	NA	Winter
	Sheth et al,[2] 1999	Canada	159,884	—	Winter
	Grech et al,[3] 2001	Malta	2157	62 (M), 72 (F)	Winter
	Yamasaki et al,[16] 2002	Japan	725	67 ± 12	No peak
	González Hernández et al,[4] 2004	Spain	8400	65 ± 12	Winter
	Azegami et al,[17] 2005	Japan	195	20–83	Summer
	Gerber et al,[18] 2006	United States	2676	68 ± 14	No peak
	Rumana et al,[5] 2008	Japan	335	68 ± 13 (M), 75 ± 10 (F)	Winter
	Abrignani et al,[6] 2009	Italy	3918	67 ± 8	Winter
	Kriszbacher et al,[7] 2009	Hungary	81,956	NA	Spring
	Manfredini et al,[8] 2009	Italy	64,191	68 ± 13 (M), 71 ± 11 (F)	Winter
	Mahmoud et al,[19] 2011	Netherlands	124	63 ± 13	Summer
	Ishikawa et al,[20] 2012	Japan	343	67 ± 13	No peak
	Verberkmoes et al,[9] 2012	Netherlands	11,389	64 (M), 71 (F)	Winter
	Reavey et al,[10] 2013	Switzerland	361322	NA	November–December
	Hong & Kang,[11] 2014	Korea	265935	—	Winter
	Lashari et al,[12] 2015	Pakistan	428	49 ± 10	Winter
	Sen et al,[13] 2015	Turkey	402	62 ± 12	Winter

Abbreviations: F, female; M, male; NA, not available.

infectious disease, specifically respiratory infections, was considered a possible trigger of heart failure.[75] Prior research has also shown that influenza is more prominent in the late fall and winter months and may contribute to heart failure exacerbations.[76] In addition, acute arrhythmias, another known trigger for heart failure exacerbations, were also found to follow seasonal variations.[77,78] Specifically, tachyarrhythmic episodes in patients with an implantable cardioverter-defibrillator were not distributed equally over the year.[79,80] These events tended to occur more frequently in the winter months, regardless of climate[57] or hemisphere.[81] Given the possibility that stressors such as the holiday season could explain the variation in tachyarrhythmia, and that these results were also observed in animal models,[82] it has been

hypothesized that periods of increased vulnerability caused by changes in circadian rhythm may play a role in initiation of tachyarrhythmia.[83]

Hemodynamics

Patients with CHF have reduced physiologic reserve to compensate for an increase in cardiac workload. Reduction in temperature may result in physiologic changes causing decompensation via volume overload secondary to tachycardia, increased peripheral vascular resistance, increased blood pressure, and higher rates of arrhythmias.[64,84] Additional studies have found seasonal variation in hemodynamics, which may also contribute to the seasonal variation in heart failure exacerbations. An early study showed increases in heart rate and total peripheral resistance but decreased cardiac output in the winter, suggesting that increased afterload may cause acute pulmonary edema by overloading the left ventricle.[85] Other studies have found that factors other than temperature may contribute, including changes in adrenal and thyroid function.[86,87] Furthermore, an increase in caloric intake during the winter,[86] alcohol consumption, and vitamin D deficiency may also precipitate heart failure. Increased sodium intake could lead to volume overload status, and, because patients with heart failure are typically more sedentary than patients without heart failure, they may have a decreased exposure to sunlight in winter, thus leading to greater risk for vitamin D deficiency.[88] An increase in alcohol consumption during the winter has also been noted and may contribute to heart failure hospitalization caused by decreased myocardial contractility and induction of atrial fibrillation.[77]

Effect of Weather

Weather changes associated with heart failure hospitalizations have also been proposed. Poisson regression models constructed to evaluate associations between temperature, precipitation, and days of extreme heat with hospitalizations for congestive heart failure as well as acute coronary syndrome and stroke found that temperature changes (defined as a 3°C decrease in maximum temperature or a 3°C increase in minimum temperature) increased hospitalizations for congestive heart failure by 6% to 11%.[89] Other studies have assessed the relationship between the average daily temperature as well as diurnal temperature range with emergency room visits for IHD in Taichung City, Taiwan.[90] Admissions for IHD increased 30% to 70% when the average daily temperature was lower than 26.2°C. In contrast, investigation of the effect of diurnal temperature on hospital admissions for cardiovascular and respiratory-related diseases in 4 metropolitan areas in Korea from 2003 to 2006 revealed that the effects on heart failure and asthma significantly increased by 3% per 1°C increment in the diurnal temperature range. The diurnal temperature range effect on admissions was greater in patients aged 75 years or older compared with those less than 75 years of age.[91] It has been proposed that the resulting neurohormonal activation and hemodynamic stress from cold activation may predispose individuals to myocardial ischemia as well as lethal arrhythmias, leading to a risk of heart failure exacerbation.[92–94]

Other explanations for increased heart failure in winter months include an increase in resting heart rate, plasma norepinephrine level, and blood pressure secondary to the colder temperature in winter.[92,95] It has been shown that patients with CHF have altered hemodynamic factors, including stroke volume, as well as hormonal factors that affect the regulation of heart rate and peripheral vascular resistance. Thus, these dysfunctional responses may blunt the thermoregulatory responses in patients with heart failure by limiting their ability to perfuse their peripheral tissues during excessive heat, predisposing them to heat stroke.[96,97] Furthermore, in heat stress, individuals with CHF may not generate a sufficient cardiac output to adequately perfuse the peripheral circulation.[98] Typically, the cutaneous circulation receives 5% to 10% of resting cardiac output, but in heat stress the cutaneous circulation requires 50% to 70% of resting cardiac output.[99] A study assessing cutaneous vasodilatation and sweat rate comparing patients with stable class II to III CHF with matched healthy subjects during whole-body sweating[100] found that patients with CHF had attenuated cutaneous vasodilator responses to both whole-body and local heating but preserved sweat response, providing further evidence that attenuated vasodilatation is a potential mechanism for heat intolerance in patients with CHF.

Effect of Air Pollution

Other studies have found that seasonal changes throughout the year affect air pollution, which may contribute to a higher incidence of heart failure. Increasing amounts of pollution and worse morbidity and mortality outcomes of patients with dilated cardiomyopathy has been well documented.[101,102] Some studies have suggested that higher pollutant levels in winter specifically may contribute to congestive heart disease.[103,104] Studies from the APHEA2 (A Study of Air Pollution and Health: European Approach 2), conducted in 29 European cities, found that temperature and humidity were effect modifiers for the impact of ambient particles on mortality.[105,106] The effects of air pollution on emergency ischemic hospital admission across different seasons and varying humidity levels from 1998 to 2007 have also been considered.[107] Season and relative humidity both modified the associations between ambient pollution and IHD admissions, resulting in more IHD admissions in the cool and dry season compared with the warm and humid season.

Overall, studies of the seasonality of heart failure exacerbations and hospitalizations have indicated that the dry winter months may contribute to the increased incidence of heart failure secondary to multiple factors. Environmental factors, such as temperature changes, air pollution, vitamin D deficiency, and weather, as well as changes in the cardiac function, such as tachyarrhythmia and hemodynamic instability, have been found to influence the seasonality of heart failure.

The complex dynamics of cardiovascular function with a reduced physiologic reserve and other environmental factors seem to play an integral role in this winter effect. Although these findings are interesting and provoking, whether specific counseling is necessary for patients for the winter effect is not clear. Further studies designed for risk factor modification specifically in winter months and assessing clinical outcomes need to be performed.

REFERENCES

1. Rosahn PD. Incidence of coronary thrombosis in relation to climate. JAMA 1937;109:1294‑9.
2. Sheth T, Nair C, Muller J, et al. Increased winter mortality from acute myocardial infarction and stroke: the effect of age. J Am Coll Cardiol 1999; 33:1916‑9.
3. Grech V, Aquilina O, Pace J. Gender differences in seasonality of acute myocardial infarction admissions and mortality in a population-based study. J Epidemiol Community Health 2001;55: 147‑8.
4. González Hernández E, Cabadeés O'Callaghan A, Cebriaán Doménech J, et al. Seasonal variations in admissions for acute myocardial infarction. The PRIMVAC study. Rev Esp Cardiol 2004;57:12‑9.
5. Rumana N, Kita Y, Turin TC, et al. Seasonal pattern of incidence and case fatality of acute myocardial infarction in a Japanese population (from the Takashima AMI Registry, 1988 to 2003). Am J Cardiol 2008;102:1307‑11.
6. Abrignani MG, Corrao S, Biondo GB, et al. Influence of climatic variables on acute myocardial infarction hospital admissions. Int J Cardiol 2009; 137:123‑9.
7. Kriszbacher I, Bódis J, Csoboth I, et al. The occurrence of acute myocardial infarction in relation to weather conditions. Int J Cardiol 2009;135:136‑8.
8. Manfredini R, Manfredini F, Boari B, et al. Seasonal and weekly patterns of hospital admissions for nonfatal and fatal myocardial infarction. Am J Emerg Med 2009;27:1097‑103.
9. Verberkmoes NJ, Soliman Hamad MA, Ter Woorst JF, et al. Impact of temperature and atmospheric pressure on the incidence of major acute cardiovascular events. Neth Heart J 2012;20:193‑6.
10. Reavey M, Saner H, Paccaud F, et al. Exploring the periodicity of cardiovascular events in Switzerland: variation in deaths and hospitalizations across seasons, day of the week and hour of the day. Int J Cardiol 2013;168:2195‑200.
11. Hong JS, Kang HC. Seasonal variation in case fatality rate in Korean patients with acute myocardial infarction using the 1997-2006 Korean National Health Insurance Claims Database. Acta Cardiol 2014;69:513‑21.
12. Lashari MN, Alam MT, Khan MS, et al. Variation in admission rates of acute coronary syndrome patients in coronary care unit according to different seasons. J Coll Physicians Surg Pak 2015;25:91‑4.
13. Sen T, Astarcioglu MA, Asarcikli LD, et al. The effects of air pollution and weather conditions on the incidence of acute myocardial infarction. Am J Emerg Med 2016;34(3):449‑54.
14. Heyer HE, Teng HC, Barris W. The increased frequency of acute myocardial infarction during summer months in a warm climate; a study of 1,386 cases from Dallas, Texas. Am Heart J 1953;45: 741‑8.
15. Ku CS, Yang CY, Lee WJ, et al. Absence of a seasonal variation in myocardial infarction onset in a region without temperature extremes. Cardiology 1998;89:277‑82.
16. Yamasaki F, Seo H, Furuno T, et al. Effect of age on chronological variation of acute myocardial infarction onset: study in Japan. Clin Exp Hypertens 2002;24:1‑9.
17. Azegami M, Hongo M, Yazaki Y, et al. Seasonal difference in onset of coronary heart disease in young Japanese patients: a comparison with older patients. Circ J 2005;69:1176‑9.
18. Gerber Y, Jacobsen SJ, Killian JM, et al. Seasonality and daily weather conditions in relation to myocardial infarction and sudden cardiac death in Olmsted County, Minnesota, 1979 to 2002. J Am Coll Cardiol 2006;48:287‑92.
19. Mahmoud KD, Lennon RJ, Ting HH, et al. Circadian variation in coronary stent thrombosis. JACC Cardiovasc Interv 2011;4:183‑90.
20. Ishikawa K, Niwa M, Tanaka T. Difference of intensity and disparity in impact of climate on several vascular diseases. Heart Vessels 2012;27:1‑9.
21. Rogers WJ, Bowlby LJ, Chandra NC, et al. Treatment of myocardial infarction in the United States (1990 to 1993): observations from the National Registry of Myocardial Infarction. Circulation 1994;90:2103‑14.
22. Spencer FA, Goldberg RJ, Becker RC, et al. Seasonal distribution of acute myocardial infarction in the second National Registry of Myocardial Infarction. J Am Coll Cardiol 1998;31(6):1226‑33.
23. Kloner RA, Das S, Poole K, et al. Seasonal variation of myocardial infarction size. Am J Cardiol 2001;88: 1021‑4.
24. Argiles A, Mourad G, Mion C. Seasonal changes in blood pressure in patients with end-stage renal

disease treated with hemodialysis. N Engl J Med 1998;339:1364–70.

25. Spodick DH, Flessas AP, Johnson MM. Association of acute respiratory symptoms with onset of acute myocardial infarction: prospective investigation of 150 consecutive patients and matched control patients. Am J Cardiol 1984;53:481–2.

26. Meier CR, Jick SS, Derby LE, et al. Acute respiratory-tract infections and risk of first-time acute myocardial infarction. Lancet 1998;351:1467–71.

27. Mattila KJ, Valtonen VV, Nieminen MS, et al. Role of infection as a risk for atherosclerosis, myocardial infarction, and stroke. Clin Infect Dis 1998;26:719–34.

28. Donaldson K, Stone V, Seaton A, et al. Ambient particle inhalation and the cardiovascular system: potential mechanisms. Environ Health Perspect 2001;109(Suppl 4):523–7.

29. Pekkanen J, Peters A, Hoek G, et al. Particulate air pollution and risk of ST-segment depression during repeated submaximal exercise tests among subjects with coronary heart disease: the Exposure and Risk Assessment for Fine and Ultrafine Particles in Ambient Air (ULTRA) study. Circulation 2002;106:933–8.

30. Peters A, Liu E, Verrier RL, et al. Air pollution and incidence of cardiac arrhythmia. Epidemiology 2000;11:11–7.

31. Naghavi M, Barlas Z, Siadaty S, et al. Association of influenza vaccination and reduced risk of recurrent myocardial infarction. Circulation 2000;102:3039–45.

32. Naghavi M, Wyde P, Litovsky S, et al. Influenza infection exerts prominent inflammatory and thrombotic effects on the atherosclerotic plaques of apolipoprotein E-deficient mice. Circulation 2003;107:762–8.

33. Virmani R, Kolodgie FD, Burke AP, et al. Lessons from sudden coronary death: a comprehensive morphological classification scheme for atherosclerotic lesions. Arterioscler Thromb Vasc Biol 2000;20:1262–75.

34. Tillett HE, Smith JWG, Gooch CD. Excess deaths attributable to influenza in England and Wales: age at death and certified cause. Int J Epidemiol 1983;12:344–52.

35. Thakur CP, Anand MP, Shahi MP. Cold weather and myocardial infarction. Int J Cardiol 1987;16:19–25.

36. Mavri A, Guzic-Salobir B, Salobir-Pajnic B, et al. Seasonal variation of some metabolic and haemostatic risk factors in subjects with and without coronary artery disease. Blood Coagul Fibrinolysis 2001;12:359–65.

37. Crawford VL, McNerlan SE, Stout RW. Seasonal changes in platelets, fibrinogen and factor VII in elderly people. Age Ageing 2003;32:661–5.

38. van der Bom JG, de Maat MP, Bots ML, et al. Seasonal variation in fibrinogen in the Rotterdam Study. Thromb Haemost 1997;78:1059–62.

39. Manfredini R, Manfredini F, Malagoni AM, et al. Chronobiology of vascular disorders: a "seasonal" link between arterial and venous thrombotic diseases? J Coagul Disord 2010;2:61–7.

40. Ockene IS, Chiriboga DE, Stanek EJ 3rd, et al. Seasonal variation in serum cholesterol levels: treatment implications and possible mechanisms. Arch Intern Med 2004;164(8):863–70.

41. Peng RD, Dominici F, Pastor-Barriuso R, et al. Seasonal analyses of air pollution and mortality in 100 US cities. Am J Epidemiol 2005;161(6):585–94.

42. Dominici F, Peng RD, Bell ML, et al. Fine particulate air pollution and hospital admission for cardiovascular and respiratory diseases. JAMA 2006;295(10):1127–34.

43. Grundström M, Linderholm HW, Klingberg J, et al. Urban NO_2 and NO pollution in relation to the North Atlantic Oscillation NAO. Atmos Environ 2011;45(4):883.

44. Schwartz J. Air pollution and hospital admissions for heart disease in eight US counties. Epidemiology 1999;10(1):17–22.

45. Poloniecki JD, Atkinson RW, de Leon AP, et al. Daily time series for cardiovascular hospital admissions and previous day's air pollution in London, UK. Occup Environ Med 1997;54:535–40.

46. Samet JM, Dominici F, Curriero FC, et al. Fine particulate air pollution and mortality in 20 U.S. cities, 1987–1994. N Engl J Med 2000;343:1742–9.

47. Pope CA, Burnett RT, Thun MJ, et al. Lung cancer, cardiopulmonary mortality, and long-term exposure to fine particulate air pollution. JAMA 2002;287:1132–41.

48. Pope CA, Burnett RT, Thurston GD, et al. Cardiovascular mortality and long-term exposure to particulate air pollution: epidemiological evidence of general pathophysiological pathways of disease. Circulation 2004;109:71–7.

49. Mann JK, Tager IB, Lurmann F, et al. Air pollution and hospital admissions for ischemic heart disease in persons with congestive heart failure or arrhythmia. Environ Health Perspect 2002;110:1247–52.

50. Magari SR, Hauser R, Schwartz J, et al. Association of heart rate variability with occupational and environmental exposure to particulate air pollution. Circulation 2001;104:986–91.

51. Devlin RB, Ghio AJ, Kehrl H, et al. Elderly humans exposed to concentrated air pollution particles have decreased heart rate variability. Eur Respir J Suppl 2003;40:76s–80s.

52. Urch B, Silverman F, Corey P, et al. Acute blood pressure responses in healthy adults during controlled air pollution exposures. Environ Health Perspect 2005;113:1052–5.

53. Spengler JD. Long-term measurements of respirable sulfates and particles inside and outside homes. Atmos Environ 1981;15:23–30.

54. Rose G. Seasonal variation in blood pressure in man. Nature 1961;189:235.

55. Brennan PJ, Greenberg G, Miall WE, et al. Seasonal variation in arterial blood pressure. BMJ 1982;285:919–23.

56. Madrigano J, Mittleman MA, Baccarelli A, et al. Temperature, myocardial infarction, and mortality: effect modification by individual- and area-level characteristics. Epidemiology 2013;24(3):439–46.

57. Kloner RA, Poole WK, Perritt RL. When throughout the year is coronary death most likely to occur? A 12-year population-based analysis of more than 220,000 cases. Circulation 1999;100:1630–4.

58. De Luca G, Suryapranata H, Ottervanger JP, et al. Absence of seasonal variation in myocardial infarction, enzymatic infarct size, and mortality in patients with ST-segment elevation treated with primary angioplasty. Am J Cardiol 2005;95:1459–61.

59. Patel NJ, Pant S, Deshmukh AJ, et al. Seasonal variation of acute myocardial infarction related hospitalizations in the United States: perspective over the last decade. Int J Cardiol 2014;172(3):e441–2.

60. Gallerani M, Boari B, Manfredini F, et al. Seasonal variation in heart failure hospitalization. Clin Cardiol 2011;34(6):389–94.

61. Isezuo SA. Seasonal variation in hospitalization for hypertension-related morbidities in Soko, northwestern Nigeria. Int J Circumpolar Health 2003;62:397–409.

62. Diaz A, Ferrante D, Badra R, et al. Seasonal variation and trends in heart failure morbidity and mortality on a South American community hospital. Congest Heart Fail 2007;13:263–6.

63. Ansa VO, Ekott JU, Essien IO, et al. Seasonal variation in admission for heart failure, hypertension and stroke in Uyo, South Eastern Nigeria. Ann Afr Med 2008;7:62–6.

64. Boulay F, Berthier F, Sisteron O, et al. Seasonal variation in chronic heart failure hospitalizations and mortality in France. Circulation 1999;100:280–6.

65. Allegra JR, Cochrane DG, Biglow R. Monthly, weekly, and daily patterns in the incidence of congestive heart failure. Acad Emerg Med 2001;8:682–5.

66. Montes Santiago J, Rey Garcia G, Mediero Dominguez A, et al. Seasonal changes in hospitalization and mortality resulting from chronic heart failure in Vigo. An Med Interna 2001;18:578–81.

67. Steward S, McIntyre K, Capewell S, et al. Heart failure in a cold climate. Seasonal variation in heart failure-related morbidity and mortality. J Am Coll Cardiol 2002;39:760–6.

68. Tepper D. Frontiers in congestive heart failure: heart failure in a cold climate. Seasonal variation in heart failure-related morbidity and mortality. Congest Heart Fail 2002;8:90.

69. Feldman DE, Platt R, Dery V, et al. Seasonal congestive heart failure mortality and hospitalization trends, Quebec 1990-1998. J Epidemiol Community Health 2004;58:129–30.

70. Ogawa M, Tanaka F, Onoda T, et al, The Northern Iwate Heart Disease Registry Consortium. A community based epidemiological and clinical study of hospitalization of patients with congestive heart failure in Northern Iwate, Japan. Circ J 2008;71:455–9.

71. Oktay C, Luk JH, Allegra JR, et al. The effect of temperature on illness severity in emergency department congestive heart failure patients. Ann Acad Med Singapore 2009;38:1081–4.

72. Parry EH, Ladipo GO, Davidson NM, et al. Seasonal variation of cardiac failure in northern Nigeria. Lancet 1977;1:1023–5.

73. Patel NJ, Nalluri N, Deshmukh A, et al. Seasonal trends of heart failure hospitalizations in the United States: a national perspective from 2000 to 2011. Int J Cardiol 2014;173(3):562–3.

74. Yamamoto Y, Shirakabe A, Hata N, et al. Seasonal variation in patients with acute heart failure: prognostic impact of admission in the summer. Heart Vessels 2015;30(2):193–203.

75. Rosenwaike I. Seasonal variation of deaths in the United States, 1951–1960. J Am Stat Assoc 1966;61:706–19.

76. Fleming DM. The contribution of influenza to combined acute respiratory infections, hospital admissions, and deaths in winter. Commun Dis Public Health 2000;3:32–8.

77. Kupari M, Koskinen P. Seasonal variation in occurrence of acute atrial fibrillation and relation to air temperature and sale of alcohol. Am J Cardiol 1990;15:1519–20.

78. Fries RP, Heisel AG, Jung JK, et al. Circannual variation of malignant ventricular tachyarrhythmias in patients with implantable cardioverter-defibrillators and either coronary artery disease or idiopathic dilated cardiomyopathy. Am J Cardiol 1997;79:1194–7.

79. Mittelman RS, Zhang X, Stanek EJ, et al. Ventricular tachyarrhythmias occur more frequently in winter and less frequently in spring than in other seasons: report from a multicenter implantable cardioverter defibrillator (ICD) database (abstr). J Am Coll Cardiol 1996;27(Suppl 2):97A.

80. Sideris A, Anderson M, Prasad K, et al. Seasonal variation in shock frequency in patients with implantable cardioverter defibrillators (abstr). J Am Coll Cardiol 1996;27(Suppl 2):348A.

81. Van der Palen J, Doggen CJ, Beaglehole R. Variation in time and day of onset of myocardial infarction and sudden death. N Z Med J 1995;108: 332–4.

82. Spear JF, Moore EN. Gender and seasonally related difference in myocardial recovery and susceptibility to sotalol-induced arrhythmias in isolated rabbit hearts. J Cardiovasc Electrophysiol 2000;11: 880–7.

83. Zipes DP. Warning: The short days of winter may be hazardous to your health. Circulation 1999; 100:1590–2.

84. Martinez-Selles M, Garcia Robles JA, Prieto L, et al. Annual rates of admission and seasonal variations in hospitalizations for heart failure. Eur J Heart Fail 2002;4:779–86.

85. Izzo JL, Larrabee PS, Sander E, et al. Hemodynamics of seasonal adaptation. Am J Hypertens 1990;3:405–7.

86. Hata T, Ogihara T, Maruyama A, et al. The seasonal variation of blood pressure in patients with essential hypertension. Clin Exp Hypertens 1982;A4: 341–54.

87. Nicolau GY, Haus E. Chronobiology of the endocrine system. Endocrinology 1989;27:153–83.

88. Barnett AG, de Looper M, Fraser JF. The seasonality in heart failure deaths and total cardiovascular deaths. Aust N Z J Public Health 2008;32:408–13.

89. Ebi KL, Exuzides KA, Lau E, et al. Weather changes associated with hospitalizations for cardiovascular diseases and stroke in California, 1983-1998. Int J Biometeorol 2004;49:48–58.

90. Liang WM, Liu WP, Chou SY, et al. Ambient temperature and emergency room admissions for acute coronary syndrome in Taiwan. Int J Biometeorol 2008;52:223–9.

91. Lim YH, Hong YC, Kim H. Effects of diurnal temperature range on cardiovascular and respiratory hospital admissions in Korea. Sci Total Environ 2012; 417-418:55–60.

92. Westheim A, Os I, Thaulow E, et al. Haemodynamic and neurohumoral effects of cold pressor test in severe heart failure. Clin Physiol 1992;12:95–106.

93. Raven PB, Wilkerson JE, Horvath SM, et al. Thermal, metabolic and cardiovascular responses to various degrees of cold stress. Can J Physiol Pharmacol 1975;53:292–8.

94. Lassvik CT, Areskog N. Angina in cold environment. Reactions to exercise. Br Heart J 1979;42: 396–401.

95. Hayward JM, Holmes WF, Gooden BA. Cardiovascular responses in man to a stream of cold air. Cardiovasc Res 1976;10:691–6.

96. Grassi G, Seravalle G, Cattaneo BM, et al. Sympathetic activation and loss of reflex sympathetic control in mild congestive heart failure. Circulation 1995;92:3206–11.

97. Leimbach WN Jr, Wallin BG, Victor RG, et al. Direct evidence from intraneural recordings for increased central sympathetic outflow in patients with heart failure. Circulation 1986;73:913–9.

98. Tei C, Horikiri Y, Park JC, et al. Acute hemodynamic improvement by thermal vasodilation in congestive heart failure. Circulation 1995;91:2582–90.

99. Rowell LB. Circulatory adjustments to dynamic exercise and heat stress: competing controls. In: Rowell LB, editor. Human circulation regulation during physical stress. New York: Oxford University Press; 1986. p. 363–406.

100. Cui J, Arbab-Zadeh A, Prasad A, et al. Effects of heat stress on thermoregulatory responses in congestive heart failure patients. Circulation 2005; 112:2286–92.

101. Maitre A, Bonneterre V, Huillard L, et al. Impact of urban atmospheric pollution on coronary disease. Eur Heart J 2006;27:2275–84.

102. Bhaskaran K, Hajat S, Haines A, et al. Effects of air pollution on the incidence of myocardial infarction. Heart 2009;95:1746–59.

103. Bell ML, Ebisu K, Peng RD, et al. Seasonal and regional short-term effects of fine particles on hospital admissions in 202 US counties, 1999–2005. Am J Epidemiol 2008;168:1301–10.

104. Morris RD, Naumova EN. Carbon monoxide and hospital admissions for congestive heart failure: evidence of an increased effect at low temperatures. Environ Health Perspect 1998;106:649–53.

105. Aga E, Samoli E, Touloumi G, et al. Short-term effects of ambient particles on mortality in the elderly: results from 28 cities in the APHEA2 project. Eur Respir J 2003;21:28S–33S.

106. Katsouyanni K, Touloumi G, Samoli E, et al. Confounding and effect modification in the short-term effects of ambient particles on total mortality: results from 29 European cities within the APHEA2 project. Epidemiology 2001;12:521–31.

107. Qiu H, Yu ITS, Wang XR, et al. Cool and dry weather enhances the effects of air pollution on emergency IHD hospital admissions. Int J Cardiol 2013;168:500–5.

Chronobiologic Aspects of Venous Thromboembolism

Chiara Fantoni, MD, Francesco Dentali, MD,
Walter Ageno, MD*

KEYWORDS

- Deep vein thrombosis • Pulmonary embolism • Chronobiology • Circadian • Circannual

KEY POINTS

- Venous thromboembolism is a common vascular disease affecting apparently healthy individuals and patients with traditional risk factors, such as surgery, immobilization, and trauma.
- Several studies suggest a seasonal variation in the incidence of venous thromboembolism, with a peak incidence in the winter, but available evidence is not entirely consistent.
- More convincing evidence shows a circadian variability in the onset of venous thromboembolism, with a peak incidence in the morning.
- Changes in hemostatic parameters observed in the winter, possibly also favored by air pollution and peaks of respiratory infections, and in the morning may explain the observed patterns.

INTRODUCTION

Venous thromboembolism (VTE), comprising pulmonary embolism (PE) and deep vein thrombosis (DVT), is the third most frequent cardiovascular disease after myocardial infraction and stroke.[1] The incidence of first VTE varies from 71 to 117 cases per 100,000 persons each year in the United States, with an increasing rate after 60 years of age.[2]

The pathophysiologic mechanism leading to thromboembolic events is traditionally explained in the Virchow triad: vascular endothelial damage, stasis of blood flow, and blood hypercoagulability. The most important risk factors for VTE include increasing age, prolonged immobility, major surgery or trauma, malignancy, prior VTE, presence of central venous lines, hormone therapy, chronic heart failure, and disturbance of hemostasis

leading to a thrombophilic status.[3] Recent studies have suggested that some traditional cardiovascular risk factors, such as arterial hypertension or dyslipidemia, could also be considered independent risk factors for thromboembolic events.[4]

In the past years, several studies have demonstrated the circadian (from the Latin circa-diem, approximately 24 hours) and seasonal pattern of onset of many cardiovascular diseases, such as myocardial infraction,[5,6] sudden cardiac death,[7,8] aortic dissection,[9,10] and stroke.[11,12] Several studies have also addressed the seasonal variation in the onset and mortality for PE and DVT, but the results obtained are not univocal. As regards daily variation, several investigations have demonstrated an increased rate of VTE during morning hours.

Several factors have been proposed to explain the chronobiologic variation in DVT and PE

Disclosures: The authors have no conflicts of interest related to this article to disclose.
Department of Medicine and Surgery, Research Center on Thromboembolic Diseases and Antithrombotic Therapies, University of Insubria, Ospedale di Circolo, Via Guicciardini 9, Varese 21100, Italy
* Corresponding author. Department of Medicine and Surgery, University of Insubria - Ospedale di Circolo, Via Guicciardini 9, Varese 21100, Italy.
E-mail address: walter.ageno@uninsubria.it

Heart Failure Clin 13 (2017) 691–696
http://dx.doi.org/10.1016/j.hfc.2017.05.005
1551-7136/17/© 2017 Elsevier Inc. All rights reserved.

heartfailure.theclinics.com

including seasonal and daily fluctuation of coagulation factors,[13,14] the influence of physical activity,[15] and the variation of meteorologic parameters.[16] Some studies have also hypothesized a potential role of air pollution exposure in causing thromboembolic events.[17]

This article summarizes the available evidence regarding chronobiologic aspects of VTE and discusses the potential causes of this phenomenon.

CHRONOBIOLOGY OF INCIDENCE AND MORTALITY FOR VENOUS THROMBOEMBOLIC EVENTS
Seasonal Variability

Seasonal variation in VTE has been investigated by several epidemiologic studies, but the results seemed to be conflicting and difficult to compare because of the different statistical methods used and the different sample size. Most investigations are retrospective and the data are derived from hospital discharge databases and registries.

The largest study published so far was conducted by Stein and colleagues[18] and collected data on hospital discharges over 21 years in the United States. This study showed no seasonal pattern in the incidence of VTE; however, the authors considered quarter of years rather than seasons and the statistical method used was not suitable for detecting periodic oscillations. No seasonal pattern in the incidence of DVT of the legs has also been documented in two small studies conducted by Bounameaux and coworkers[19] in Switzerland and Galle and coworkers[20] in Belgium. In a small study conducted in the north of Italy, no seasonal variation in the incidence of DVT and nonfatal PE was observed, with just a tendency toward an increased incidence of events during winter and summer, whereas a weekly rhythm was found with a peak on Saturdays and during the morning.[21]

In a prospective multicenter Italian study including 2119 patients with thromboembolic events, VTE was more frequent in autumn, in particular in September and October, and less frequent during spring with nadir in June. The same annual distribution was observed in all subgroups divided by gender, age, type of event (PE, DVT of the upper and lower limb, secondary or idiopathic), and different risk factors (previous VTE, no prophylaxis, immobilization, surgery).[22]

In a systematic review and meta-analysis conducted by our group including 35,000 patients and 12 studies, we showed a significantly increased incidence of VTE in the winter, with a relative risk of 1.143 (99% confidence interval [CI], 1.141–1.144), and a monthly variation of VTE with an increased incidence in January with a relative risk of 1.194 (99% CI, 1.186–1.203). These results were also confirmed in the subgroup analysis considering hospitalized patients only.[23]

More recent studies supported the presence of seasonal variation in the incidence of VTE. In a time-series analysis including 162,032 patients hospitalized for PE in Spain, Guijarro and colleagues[24] showed a significant seasonal pattern of admission for PE with a peak in winter months, in particular in January and February, and a lower incidence in June and July, with a difference between February and June of 29%. In a large nationwide study conducted by Zöller and colleagues,[25] 194,708 patients with a first episode of TVE were identified in the Swedish Hospital Discharge registry from 1964 to 2010. In this analysis a seasonal variation in VTE was observed in both sexes, with a peak during winter. The peak-to-low ratio was 1.15, with a higher risk in December. In this study the seasonal variation was stronger in patients aged 50 years or older, whereas among young individuals with a family history of VTE (0–25 years), the peak of incidence was in July (peak-to-low ratio, 1.20). This difference was explained by considering that genetic disorders are more likely to manifest in young patients, whereas in older patients the effect of familiarity is less prominent.

With regard to family history and genetic predisposition, a small study conducted by Bilora and colleagues,[26] including 44 patients with protein C or protein S deficiency, showed a seasonal variation in the incidence of thrombotic events with a peak during winter.

Finally, the influence of age on the seasonal pattern of PE was investigated in a nationwide retrospective analysis conducted in France by Olié and Bonaldi.[27] In this study information on hospitalization and mortality for PE was collected, including greater than 599,000 patients hospitalized for PE and 150,000 deaths caused by PE. The analysis showed a winter peak in the incidence of PE with an average 28.6% (95% CI, 26.5–30.8) increase in hospitalization rates and 30.4% (95% CI, 27.4–33.4) increase in mortality rates compared with summer. The risk of being hospitalized for PE in the colder season showed a similar pattern for males and females, and increased with age until 75 years old (+36%; 95% CI, 34–39).

Regarding seasonal variation in the mortality for PE, several studies have shown nonunivocal results. In two small studies conducted by Colantonio and coworkers[28] and Gallerani and coworkers,[29] circannual rhythm was found for fatal PE with a peak during winter. Similar results were obtained analyzing the seasonal variation of fatal PE after total hip arthroplasty, including more than 18,000 patients.[30] Conversely, in a large study conducted by Stein and colleagues[31] reporting data of the US National Center for Health Statistics, no seasonal variation was observed in PE mortality rates. Similarly, no seasonality for fatal PE was observed by Kosacka and colleagues[32] in Poland; of interest, this study found a peak of incidence of PE during spring. In these two investigations the authors categorized data using quarter of years rather than seasons and this categorization, as previously described, could influence the results obtained. Finally, in a large Chinese study on seasonal variations of mortality from cardiovascular diseases, the risk of death for pulmonary heart disease was higher in winter compared with summer months in patients older than 65 years (relative risk, 1.42; 95% CI, 1.10–1.83).[33]

Circadian Variability

The circadian rhythmicity of VTE has been investigated in several studies, showing an increased incidence during morning hours. As previously described, Bilora and colleagues[21] demonstrated a daily variation in DVT and nonfatal PE, with a significant peak in the morning (12.26 hours for DVT and 10.26 hours for PE).

In a retrospective investigation including 248 hospitalized patients, Sharma and colleagues[34] described a circadian pattern of onset of nonfatal PE with a peak in the morning, with a three-time higher prevalence compared with evening hours. Similar results have been obtained regarding fatal PE. In a small study including 152 patients, Colantonio and colleagues[35] demonstrated a circadian and circannual pattern of onset of fatal PE, with an increased risk in wintertime and in the morning. Gallerani and colleagues[36] showed a significant morning pattern for fatal PE in inpatients and outpatients, with an acrophase between 11.0 hours and 13.30 hours.

The same author described a circadian rhythmicity of sudden cardiac death from PE in 48 outpatients, with a significant acrophase in the morning (11.46 hours).[29] Similar temporal variation has been demonstrated in fatal postsurgical PE in orthopedic and general surgery patients.[37,38]

PATHOPHYSIOLOGY OF SEASONAL VARIATION OF VENOUS THROMBOEMBOLISM

The pathophysiologic mechanism leading to the seasonal variation of VTE is not completely understood, but several factors might contribute to this phenomenon.

Seasonal changes in ambient temperature are considered the main cause of the circannual variation of many cardiovascular diseases, probably caused by the variation in the main pathogenetic factors. The association between low temperature, morbidity, and mortality for cardiovascular and pulmonary diseases has been well recognized,[39,40] with an increase in mortality rate in winter of 30% compared with summer.[41]

Several studies have also demonstrated the influence of low temperatures, low atmospheric pressure, and humidity in the incidence of VTE.[42,43] In particular in a retrospective large study conducted in Scotland a positive correlation was described between high wind speed, low atmospheric pressure, and low temperature and increased risk of DVT.[16] In Italy, Masotti and colleagues[44] showed an inverse correlation between ambient temperature, barometric pressure, and onset and mortality for PE. They also described higher blood levels of polymerase chain reaction, D dimer, platelets, and fibrinogen in patients hospitalized for PE during cold months compared with the warm season.

In the past, several studies have demonstrated an increase of some hemostatic parameters associated with low temperatures. Keatinge and colleagues[45] showed a rise in blood viscosity, red cells, and platelets count with mild surface cooling. Bull and colleagues[46] described a positive correlation between low temperature, blood viscosity, and coagulation factors. Other studies described seasonal variation with a winter peak of fibrinogen levels, factor VII, protein C, and other coagulation factors.[13,47,48] Changes in coagulation factors during the winter might also occur as a consequence of inflammatory conditions related to peak incidences of some infectious diseases. For example, infections of the respiratory tract, which are more frequent during the cold months, are associated with increased fibrinogen levels.[49] The elevation of coagulation protein levels during the cold months can lead to a hypercoagulable states and influence the onset of thromboembolic and cardiovascular events during the cold season.

Traditional cardiovascular risk factors, such as hypertension and dyslipidemia, have been reported to be independently associated with venous thromboembolic disease.[4] Several studies have demonstrated a seasonal pattern with a winter peak for serum cholesterol levels and arterial blood pressure, caused by variation in hormones and vasoactive substance concentration.[50] The variation of these cardiovascular risk factors plays an important role on the seasonal changes of cardiovascular diseases and could also influence the onset of venous thromboembolic events. In addition, during the cold months physical activity is extremely limited, especially in elderly patients, and this could favor prothrombotic changes and lead to an increase in the incidence of DVT and PE.[15]

Recently, there has been a growing interest in the role of air pollution as a risk factor for thromboembolic events. Air pollution is composed by gaseous pollutants (ozone, carbon monoxide, sulfur dioxide, nitrogen oxides) and particulate matter (PM), presenting in different size and compositions. In several studies, the short- and long-term exposure to inhalable particulates has been associated with an increase in all-cause mortality and morbidity, in particular for respiratory, cardiovascular, and cerebrovascular diseases.[51-53]

In the last years, several studies investigated the influence of air pollution on the incidence of DVT and PE. Recently Franchini and colleagues[17] conducted a systematic literature review to elucidate the possible association between exposure to air pollution and development of VTE. Eleven studies have been analyzed, involving more than 500,000 patients. In 8 of 11 studies a positive correlation was found between short- or long-term exposure to air pollution and the incidence of VTE, with different risks ranging from 1.05 to 5.24. Because of the heterogeneity in sample size, design, follow-up, and statistical methods of the included studies, no additional analysis could be done.[17] In a case-crossover analysis conducted in the United Kingdom, Milojevic and colleagues[54] also found a positive correlation between increased levels of $PM_{2.5}$ and PE-related mortality.

The mechanism connecting air pollution and arterial and venous thrombosis remains not completely understood. Air pollutants seem to have a pulmonary and systemic proinflammatory and pro-oxidant effect; they can also influence the coagulation cascade and platelet function, increasing levels of coagulation proteins.[55,56] During winter months, air pollution levels are more elevated, in particular near the big cities, and this might influence the incidence of cardiovascular and thromboembolic events.

The daily variation of VTE can be explained considering the circadian morning peak of several parameters, such as blood viscosity,[57] hematocrit,[58] platelet aggregation, and adhesiveness.[14] An increased activity of some coagulation factors, such as fibrinogen, factor VII, factor VIII, and factor IX, has been documented in the morning.[59-61] Some studies demonstrated lower values of prothrombin time and activated partial thromboplastin time in the morning, with a difference between 8 AM

and 4 PM of 10%.[62] Furthermore, fibrinolysis presents wide oscillations during the day, with a minimum in activity during the morning and a relative hypercoagulable state.[14] Other conditions, considered triggers of thrombus detachment, occur in the first hours of the morning. These include the increase of sympathetic activity,[63] arterial hypertension, and heart rate.[64]

DISCUSSION

The seasonal variation of venous thromboembolic disease has been well investigated in the literature, but available results are not univocal. Despite differences among investigations, most studies showed a seasonal variability in the incidence and mortality of VTE, with a peak during wintertime. The mechanism leading to this phenomenon is not completely understood, but it is connected to the increase in coagulation proteins, caused by air pollution and meteorologic parameters.

Regarding circadian variation of thromboembolic events, several studies have shown an increased rate during morning hours in the occurrence of VTE and VTE-related mortality. The investigations showed the same diurnal pattern in hospitalized patients, outpatients, and surgical patients.

In light of this evidence, the "time factor" can be considered an additional factor to consider in the risk assessment of patients to better identify individuals at increased risk and to adopt the best prophylactic strategies. More studies are warranted to consolidate these findings and clarify their clinical implication.

REFERENCES

1. Goldhaber SZ. Venous thromboembolism: epidemiology and magnitude of the problem. Best Pract Res Clin Haematol 2012;25(3):235–42.
2. White RH. The epidemiology of venous thromboembolism. Circulation 2003;107:I4–8.
3. Anderson FA Jr, Spencer FA. Risk factors for venous thromboembolism. Circulation 2003;107(23 Suppl 1):I9–16.
4. Ageno W, Becattini C, Brighton T, et al. Cardiovascular risk factors and venous thromboembolism: a meta-analysis. Circulation 2008;117(1):93–102.
5. Muller JE, Stone PH, Turi ZG, et al. Circadian variation in the frequency of onset of acute myocardial infarction. N Engl J Med 1985;313:1315–22.
6. Ornato JP, Peberdy MA, Chandra NC, et al. Seasonal pattern of acute myocardial infarction in the National Registry of Myocardial Infarctions. J Am Coll Cardiol 1996;28:1684–8.

7. Cohen MC, Rohtla KM, Lavery CE, et al. Meta-analysis of the morning excess of acute myocardial infarction and sudden cardiac death. Am J Cardiol 1997;79(11):1512–6.

8. Gallerani M, Manfredini R, Ricci L, et al. Sudden death may show a circadian time of risk depending on its anatomo-clinical causes and age. Jpn Heart J 1993;34(6):729–39.

9. Mehta RH, Manfredini R, Hassan F, et al. Chronobiological patterns of acute aortic dissection. Circulation 2002;106:1110–5.

10. Mehta RH, Manfredini R, Bossone E, et al. The winter peak in the occurrence of acute aortic dissection is independent by climate. Chronobiol Int 2005;22: 723–9.

11. Gallerani M, Manfredini R, Ricci L, et al. Chronobiological aspects of acute cerebrovascular diseases. Acta Neurol Scand 1993;87:482–7.

12. Gallerani M, Portaluppi F, Maida G, et al. Circadian and circannual rhythmicity in the occurrence of subarachnoid hemorrhage. Stroke 1996;27:1793–7.

13. Stout RW, Crawford V. Seasonal variations in fibrinogen concentrations among elderly people. Lancet 1991;338:9–13.

14. Haus E. Chronobiology of hemostasis and inferences for the chronotherapy of coagulation disorders and thrombosis prevention. Adv Drug Deliv Rev 2007;59(9–10):966–84.

15. Rosenfeld BA, Faraday N, Campbell D, et al. The effects of bed rest on circadian changes in hemostasis. Thromb Haemost 1994;72:281–4.

16. Brown HK, Simpson AJ, Murchison JT. The influence of meteorological variables on the development of deep venous thrombosis. Thromb Haemost 2009; 102(4):676–82.

17. Franchini M, Mengoli C, Cruciani M, et al. Association between particulate air pollution and venous thromboembolism: a systematic literature review. Eur J Intern Med 2016;27:10–3.

18. Stein PD, Kayali F, Olson RE. Analysis of occurrence of venous thromboembolic disease in the four seasons. Am J Cardiol 2004;93:511–3.

19. Bounameaux H, Hicklin L, Desmarais S. Seasonal variation in deep vein thrombosis. BMJ 1996;312:284–5.

20. Galle C, Wautrecht JC, Motte S, et al. The role of season in the incidence of deep venous thrombosis. J Mal Vasc 1998;23(2):99–101.

21. Bilora F, Manfredini R, Petrobelli F, et al. Chronobiology of non fatal pulmonary thromboembolism. Panminerva Med 2001;43(1):7–10.

22. Manfredini R, Imberti D, Gallerani M, et al. Seasonal variation in the occurrence of venous thromboembolism: data from the MASTER registry. Clin Appl Thromb Hemost 2009;15(3):309–15.

23. Dentali F, Ageno W, Rancan E, et al. Seasonal and monthly variability in the incidence of venous thromboembolism. A systematic review and a meta-analysis of the literature. Thromb Haemost 2011; 106(3):439–47.

24. Guijarro R, Trujillo-Santos J, Bernal-Lopez MR, et al. Trend and seasonality in hospitalizations for pulmonary embolism: a time-series analysis. J Thromb Haemost 2015;13(1):23–30.

25. Zöller B, Li X, Ohlsson H, et al. Age-and sex-specific seasonal variation of venous thromboembolism in patients with and without family history: a nationwide family study in Sweden. Thromb Haemost 2013; 110(6):1164–71.

26. Bilora F, Boccioletti V, Manfredini E, et al. Seasonal variation in the incidence of deep vein thrombosis in patients with deficiency of protein C or protein S. Clin Appl Thromb Hemost 2002;8(3):231–7.

27. Olié V, Bonaldi C. Pulmonary embolism: does the seasonal effect depend on age? A 12-year nationwide analysis of hospitalization and mortality. Thromb Res 2017;150:96–100.

28. Colantonio D, Casale R, Natali G, et al. Seasonal periodicity in fatal pulmonary thromboembolism. Lancet 1990;335(8680):56–7.

29. Gallerani M, Manfredini R, Ricci L, et al. Sudden death from pulmonary thromboembolism: chronobiological aspects. Eur Heart J 1992;13(5):661–5.

30. Wroblewski BM, Siney PD, White R. Fatal pulmonary embolism after total hip arthroplasty. Seasonal variation. Clin Orthop Relat Res 1992;276:222–4.

31. Stein PD, Kayali F, Beemath A, et al. Mortality from acute pulmonary embolism according to season. Chest 2005;128(5):3156–8.

32. Kosacka U, Kiluk IE, Milewski R, et al. Variation in the incidence of pulmonary embolism and related mortality depending on the season and day of the week. Pol Arch Med Wewn 2015;125(1–2):92–4.

33. Xu B, Liu H, Su N, et al. Association between winter season and risk of death from cardiovascular diseases: a study in more than half a million inpatients in Beijing, China. BMC Cardiovasc Disord 2013;13:93.

34. Sharma GV, Frisbie JH, Tow DE, et al. Circadian and circannual rhythm of nonfatal pulmonary embolism. Am J Cardiol 2001;87(7):922–4.

35. Colantonio D, Casale R, Lorenzetti G, et al. Chrono-risks in the episodes of fatal pulmonary thromboembolism. G Clin Med 1990;71:563e7 [in Italian].

36. Gallerani M, Manfredini R, Portaluppi F, et al. Circadian variation in the occurrence of fatal pulmonary embolism. Differences depending on sex and age. Jpn Heart J 1994;35(6):765–70.

37. Wroblewski BM, Siney PD, Fleming PA. Fatal pulmonary embolism after total hip arthroplasty: diurnal variations. Orthopedics 1998;21(12):1269–71.

38. Belcaro G, Nicolaides AN, Geroulakos G, et al. Circadian pattern of post-surgical fatal pulmonary embolism. Vasa 1997;26:287e90.

39. Lin S, Soim A, Gleason KA, et al. Association between low temperature during winter season and

40. Wilmshurst P. Temperature and cardiovascular mortality. BMJ 1994;309(6961):1029–30.

41. Gemmell I, McLoone P, Boddy FA, et al. Seasonal variation in mortality in Scotland. Int J Epidemiol 2000;29(2):274–9.

42. Meral M, Mirici A, Aslan S, et al. Barometric pressure and the incidence of pulmonary embolism. Chest 2005;128(4):2190–4.

43. Staskiewicz G, Torres K, Czekajska-Chehab E, et al. Low atmospheric pressure and humidity are related with more frequent pulmonary embolism episodes in male patients. Ann Agric Environ Med 2010;17(1):163–7.

44. Masotti L, Ceccarelli E, Forconi S, et al. Seasonal variations of pulmonary embolism in hospitalized patients. Respir Med 2005;99(11):1469–73.

45. Keatinge WR, Coleshaw SR, Cotter F, et al. Increases in platelet and red cell counts, blood viscosity, and arterial pressure during mild surface cooling: factors in mortality from coronary and cerebral thrombosis in winter. Br Med J (Clin Res Ed) 1984; 289(6456):1405–8.

46. Bull GM, Brozovic M, Chakrabarti R, et al. Relationship of air temperature to various chemical, haematological, and haemostatic variables. J Clin Pathol 1979;32(1):16–20.

47. van der Bom JG, de Maat MP, Bots ML, et al. Seasonal variation in fibrinogen in the Rotterdam Study. Thromb Haemost 1997;78(3):1059–62.

48. Rudnicka AR, Rumley A, Lowe GD, et al. Diurnal, seasonal, and blood-processing patterns in levels of circulating fibrinogen, fibrin D-dimer, C-reactive protein, tissue plasminogen activator, and von Willebrand factor in a 45-year-old population. Circulation 2007;115(8):996–1003.

49. Woodhouse PR, Khaw KT, Plummer M, et al. Seasonal variations of plasma fibrinogen and factor VII activity in the elderly: winter infections and death from cardiovascular disease. Lancet 1994; 343(8895):435–9.

50. Fares A. Winter cardiovascular diseases phenomenon. N Am J Med Sci 2013;5(4):266–79.

51. Dockery DW, Pope CA 3rd, Xu X, et al. An association between air pollution and mortality in six U.S. cities. N Engl J Med 1993;329(24):1753–9.

52. Hoek G, Krishnan RM, Beelen R, et al. Long-term air pollution exposure and cardio- respiratory mortality: a review. Environ Health 2013;12(1):43.

53. Newby DE, Mannucci PM, Tell GS, et al. Expert position paper on air pollution and cardiovascular disease. Eur Heart J 2015;36(2):83–93b.

54. Milojevic A, Wilkinson P, Armstrong B, et al. Short-term effects of air pollution on a range of cardiovascular events in England and Wales: case-crossover analysis of the MINAP database, hospital admissions and mortality. Heart 2014;100(14):1093–8.

55. Mills NL, Donaldson K, Hadoke PW, et al. Adverse cardiovascular effects of air pollution. Nat Clin Pract Cardiovasc Med 2009;6(1):36–44.

56. Baccarelli A, Zanobetti A, Martinelli I, et al. Effects of exposure to air pollution on blood coagulation. J Thromb Haemost 2007;5(2):252–60.

57. Ehrly AM, Jung G. Circadian rhythm of human blood viscosity. Biorheology 1973;10(4):577–83.

58. Seaman GVF, Engel R, Swank RL, et al. Circadian periodicity in some physicochemical parameters of circulating blood. Nature 1965;4999:833–5.

59. Kapiotis S, Jilma B, Quehenberger P, et al. Morning hypercoagulability and hypofibrinolysis. Diurnal variations in circulating activated factor VII, prothrombin fragment F1+2, and plasmin-plasmin inhibitor complex. Circulation 1997;96(1):19–21.

60. Petralito A, Mangiafico RA, Gibiino S, et al. Daily modifications of plasma fibrinogen platelets aggregation, Howell's time, PTT, TT, and antithrombin II in normal subjects and in patients with vascular disease. Chronobiologia 1982;9(2):195–201.

61. Akiyama Y, Kazama M, Tahara C, et al. Reference values of hemostasis related factors of healthy Japanese adults. I: circadian fluctuation. Thromb Res 1990;60(4):281–9.

62. Haus E, Cusulos M, Sackett-Lundeen L, et al. Circadian variations in blood coagulation parameters, alpha-antitrypsin antigen and platelet aggregation and retention in clinically healthy subjects. Chronobiol Int 1990;7(3):203–16.

63. Muller JE. Circadian variation and triggering of acute coronary events. Am Heart J 1999;137(4 Pt 2):S1–8.

64. Millar-Craig MW, Bishop CN, Raftery EB. Circadian variation of blood-pressure. Lancet 1978;1(8068): 795–7.

Chronobiology of Acute Aortic Syndromes

Hasan K. Siddiqi, MD, MSCR[a],*, Eduardo Bossone, MD, PhD, FESC[b], Reed E. Pyeritz, MD, PhD[c], Kim A. Eagle, MD, MACC[d]

KEYWORDS

- Chronobiology • Acute aortic syndrome • Aortic dissection • Aortic disease

KEY POINTS

- Acute aortic syndromes have a high morbidity and mortality, with the need for quick recognition and treatment.
- The chronobiology of acute aortic syndromes seems to mirror that of several other cardiovascular conditions, with a peak in the winter months and in the morning hours of the day.
- There are several proposed mechanisms for the pathobiology behind the unique chronobiology of acute aortic dissection, with differential circadian and seasonal effects playing a role in the vascular and endothelial milieu leading to the cascade that ultimately results in the acute aortic syndrome.

INTRODUCTION

Acute aortic syndromes, and particularly acute aortic dissection (AAD), are highly morbid conditions that require prompt diagnosis and management. Dissection of the thoracic aorta, especially the ascending portion, has an extremely high mortality, with a death rate of 1% to 2% per hour for the first 24 hours in patients who do not receive treatment.[1] In recent years, for those patients who survive to reach a hospital, the mean hospital mortality for AAD is still about 25%.[2]

Chronobiology is a field of medicine and biology that studies the presence of rhythms and their effects on physiology. Many cardiovascular conditions show rhythmic patterns, with notable peaks at certain points in the 24-hour day as well as weekly and seasonal variations. Previous studies have described these cycles in myocardial infarction,[3] stroke,[4] pulmonary embolism,[5] ventricular arrhythmias[6] and, more recently, takotsubo cardiomyopathy.[7] This issue outlines expert reviews on many of these conditions. Although several studies examined the chronobiology of AAD in the general population, further investigations are needed to discover its pathophysiology and how the risk for dissection in the population can be minimized.[8]

REVIEW OF THE LITERATURE

Several studies have examined AAD in relation to circadian and seasonal variation. The seminal article on this topic was from the International Registry for Acute Aortic Dissection (IRAD) consortium in 2002.[9] IRAD is the world's largest registry of AADs, and encompasses more than 45 international sites. In their 2002 article on the chronobiology of AADs, the IRAD group analyzed data from 689 patients for circadian rhythms and 932 patients for seasonal analysis. There was a higher frequency of AAD in the morning (6:00 AM to 12:00

[a] Cardiovascular Medicine, Brigham and Women's Hospital, 75 Francis Street, Boston, MA 02115, USA; [b] "Cava de' Tirreni" Cardiology Unit, Heart Department, Scuola Medica Salernitana, University Hospital, Via Pr. Amedeo, 36, Lauro (AV), Salerno 83023, Italy; [c] Department of Medicine, Leonard Davis Institute of Health Economics, Smilow Center for Translational Research, Perelman School of Medicine, University of Pennsylvania, 11-133, 3400 Civic Center Boulevard, Philadelphia, PA 19104, USA; [d] Division of Cardiology, University of Michigan School of Public Health, Domino's Farms, University of Michigan, 24 Frank Lloyd Wright Drive, Ann Arbor, MI 48105, USA

* Corresponding author. 33 Pond Avenue, Apartment B 1013, Brookline, MA 02445.
E-mail address: hsiddiqi@partners.org

Heart Failure Clin 13 (2017) 697–701
http://dx.doi.org/10.1016/j.hfc.2017.05.006
1551-7136/17/© 2017 Elsevier Inc. All rights reserved.

PM) as well as during the winter months (December 21 to March 20) in the general population, as seen in **Figs. 1** and **2**, respectively.[9] Moreover, data from the IRAD Registry also showed the lack of significantly different rates of clinical outcomes (including mortality) during the 24-hour and seasonal periods.[9]

In a separate analysis of the IRAD database, the presence of a winter peak in AAD occurred in both cold and warm climate settings, giving credence to the hypothesis that there was a specific seasonal influence on the incidence of AAD.[10] DeAnda and colleagues[11] analyzed data from hospitals in the Unites States and United Kingdom, compared with those in Argentina, Australia, and New Zealand, and found a winter peak of AAD in both the northern and southern hemispheres, further strengthening the hypothesis that there is a seasonal effect on incidence of AAD.

A recent meta-analysis found 42 studies and a total of more than 80,000 patients that reported on the chronobiology of AAD.[8] Ten studies including 58,954 patients were used in the analysis of seasonal distribution, 14 studies with 46,231 patients were used in the analysis of monthly distribution, 5 studies including 22,731 patients were used in the day-of-week analysis, and 7 studies with 1,695 patients were used for hourly

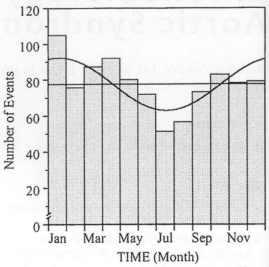

Fig. 2. IRAD data for seasonal variation in onset of AAD. Histograms represent number of total events occurring in each month of the year. Superimposed is overall best-fitting curve calculated by rhythm analysis resulting from single component with period of 8766 hours. (*From* Mehta RH, Manfredini R, Hassan F, et al, International Registry of Acute Aortic Dissection (IRAD) Investigators. Chronobiological patterns of acute aortic dissection. Circulation 2002;106(9):1113; with permission.)

distribution analysis.[8] Similar to the findings in most individual studies, the meta-analysis showed an increased incidence of AAD in winter, with a relative risk of 1.17 compared with all other seasons, and 1.33 compared with summer. Monthly meta-analysis showed that December had a peak in AAD, with a relative risk of 1.14 compared with other months. Weekly analysis of AAD showed an increased incidence on Mondays compared with all other days of the week, with a relative risk of 1.21. Circadian analysis of hourly variation in AAD, grouped by 6-hour intervals, showed a peak from 6 AM to noon, with a relative risk of 1.58 compared with the remaining intervals of the day.[8] **Fig. 3** shows a summary of these data from the meta-analysis.

A study combining patients with Marfan syndrome (MFS) from IRAD and the National Registry of Genetically Triggered Thoracic Aortic Aneurysms and Cardiovascular Conditions (GenTAC) examined the chronobiology of AAD in patients with genetic conditions.[12] The aim of this study was to evaluate whether AAD in this higher risk population followed the chronobiological patterns seen in the general population, as described earlier. The results of this study included 257 unique subjects with MFS, and replicated findings similar to that of the general population. Specifically, this study

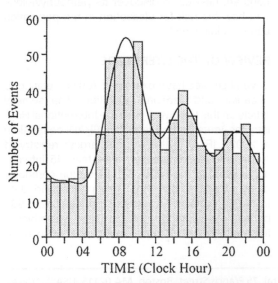

Fig. 1. IRAD data for circadian variation in onset of AAD. Histograms represent number of total events occurring in each hour of the day. Superimposed is overall best-fitting curve calculated by rhythm analysis, resulting from 4 significant harmonics with 24-hour, 12-hour, 8-hour, and 6-hour periods. (*From* Mehta RH, Manfredini R, Hassan F, et al, International Registry of Acute Aortic Dissection (IRAD) Investigators. Chronobiological patterns of acute aortic dissection. Circulation 2002;106(9):1112; with permission.)

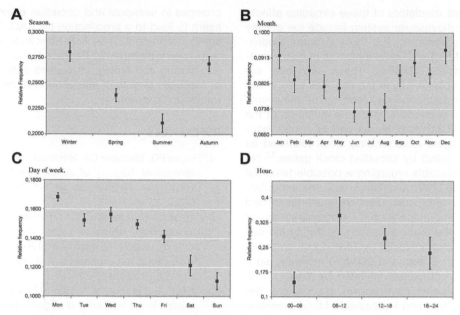

Fig. 3. Meta-analysis of available studies regarding AAD showing relative frequency of AAD with average variation (99% CI) by (*A*) season, (*B*) month, (*C*) day of week, (*D*) hour. (*From* Vitale J, Manfredini R, Gallerani M, et al. Chronobiology of acute aortic rupture or dissection: a systematic review and a meta-analysis of the literature. Chronobiol Int 2015;32(3):385–94; with permission.)

showed that AAD was more likely in the winter/spring season (November–April) than in the other half of the year (57% vs 43%; $P = .05$), and during the daytime hours, with 65% of dissections occurring from 6 AM to 6 PM ($P = .001$). Therefore, despite having a genetic predisposition to aortic aneurysms and dissection, the MFS population reflects a chronobiology of AAD that is similar to that of the general population.[12]

PROPOSED PATHOPHYSIOLOGY

The cardiovascular system shows multiple levels of chronobiologic variation, including arterial blood pressure, heart rate, vascular tone, coagulation, and fibrinolysis.[13] **Fig. 4** shows the various possible modulators of this chronobiological pattern.[14] Chronobiological patterns in other diseases and organ systems may shed light on how daily and seasonal variations alter disorders and physiology. The most frequently studied and understood chronobiological rhythm is the circadian rhythm, a 24-hour cycle that is regulated by multiple internal and external cues (zeitgebers).[15] Light is the most significant zeitgeber, and regulates various physiologic effects through its action on the suprachiasmatic nucleus of the hypothalamus. Important in this system are various neurohormonal regulators of the cardiovascular system, including melatonin,[16] aldosterone, glucocorticoids,[17] catecholamines,[18] and growth

hormone.[19] Through these mediators and others, the activity of multiple genes throughout the body and cardiovascular system is regulated.[20] The genes implicated in this regulatory mechanism include *clock*, casein kinase 1ε (*CK1ε*), period (*per1, per2*), arntl (*bmal1*), rev/erb-a, and cryptochromes.[21] None are known to interact specifically with fibrillin-1 or the transforming growth factor beta signaling pathway, which are particularly involved in the pathophysiology of MFS.

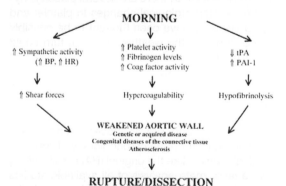

Fig. 4. Concurrent pathophysiologic mechanisms underlying circadian variation of aortic rupture or dissection. BP, blood pressure; coag, coagulation; HR, heart rate; PAI-1, plasminogen activator inhibitor-1; tPA, tissue plasminogen activator. (*From* Manfredini R, Boari B, Gallerani M, et al. Chronobiology of rupture and dissection of aortic aneurysms. J Vasc Surg 2004;40:385; with permission.)

Important mediators of these circadian effects on the cardiovascular system include the activity of multiple enzymes, like the matrix metalloproteases (MMPs) and tissue inhibitors of matrix metalloproteinases (TIMPs). These enzymes are thought to play a role in the changes seen in the aortic wall during the development of aneurysms and before dissection.[22] Various members of the MMP and TIMP families, as well as genes regulating collagen, have recently been identified as being controlled by circadian clock genes.[23] No data are available regarding a possible temporal variation of MMP and TIMP, with the exception of patients with ocular diseases, such as corneal erosions and ulceration.[24] Concentrations of MMP-9 in the tears are negligible during the day and completely inhibited by TIMP-1 but, on awakening, MMP-9 shows a 200-fold increase, so it cannot be completely inhibited by TIMP-1.[24] In addition, studies have shown associations between variation and increases in blood pressure, heart rate, vascular tone, platelet aggregability, and hematocrit, leading to altered plasma viscosity and the incidence of cardiovascular events.[9,13] **Fig. 4** shows some proposed mechanisms that could be involved in this circadian pattern of AAD.

Seasonal rhythms are also important in the incidence of various physiologic and pathophysiologic conditions. In the cardiovascular system, multiple studies have established that there is a clear seasonal pattern to the incidence of coronary events[25] and acute myocardial infarction.[26] Similarly, recent work has described seasonal changes in protein expression patterns associated with the immune system.[27] Although the pathophysiology of the increase in cardiac disorders in the winter months is not clear, there are several plausible hypotheses. Hematological changes in platelet and blood viscosity have been thought to be possibly associated with the weather, which in turn could affect the forces acting on a vulnerable aorta that could lead to an AAD.[28]

SUMMARY

Retrospective and registry-based studies have shed some light on the chronobiology of AAD. Individual studies, like the original IRAD study, along with a large meta-analysis of all available studies have shown that AAD seems to share a similar chronobiology to many other cardiovascular maladies. Specifically, there is an increased incidence of reported AAD during the morning hours (6 AM–12 PM), as well as in the winter months. Although the pathobiology behind these chronobiological patterns is not well elucidated, the interaction of various internal cues and clocks along with

changes in seasonal and circadian environments seem to lead to a predilection for AAD. These insights are important clinically because they may help inform therapeutic decisions about medication dosing and timing, as well as shedding light on possible targets of intervention to prevent this catastrophic event.

REFERENCES

1. Hagan PG, Nienaber CA, Isselbacher EM, et al. The International Registry of Acute Aortic Dissection (IRAD): new insights into an old disease. JAMA 2000;283(7):897–903.
2. Trimarchi S, Nienaber CA, Rampoldi V, et al. Contemporary results of surgery in acute type A aortic dissection: the International Registry of Acute Aortic Dissection experience. J Thorac Cardiovasc Surg 2005;129(1):112–22.
3. Muller JE, Ludmer PL, Willich SN, et al. Circadian variation in the frequency of sudden cardiac death. Circulation 1987;75(3):131–8.
4. Elliott WJ. Circadian variation in the timing of stroke onset: a meta-analysis. Stroke 1998;29(5):992–6.
5. Dentali F, Ageno W, Rancan E, et al. Seasonal and monthly variability in the incidence of venous thromboembolism. A systematic review and a meta-analysis of the literature. Thromb Haemost 2011; 106(3):439–47.
6. Raeder EA, Hohnloser SH, Grayboys TB, et al. Spontaneous variability and circadian distribution of ectopic activity in patients with malignant ventricular arrhythmia. J Am Coll Cardiol 1988;12(3): 656–61.
7. Manfredini R, Salmi R, Fabbian F, et al. Breaking heart: chronobiologic insights into Takotsubo cardiomyopathy. Heart Fail Clin 2013;9(2):147–56.
8. Vitale J, Manfredini R, Gallerani M, et al. Chronobiology of acute aortic rupture or dissection: a systematic review and a meta-analysis of the literature. Chronobiol Int 2015;32(3):385–94.
9. Mehta RH, Manfredini R, Hassan F, et al, International Registry of Acute Aortic Dissection (IRAD) Investigators. Chronobiological patterns of acute aortic dissection. Circulation 2002;106(9):1110–5.
10. Mehta RH, Manfredini R, Bossone E, et al. Does circadian and seasonal variation in occurrence of aortic dissection influence in-hospital outcomes? Chronobiol Int 2005;22(2):343–51.
11. DeAnda A, Grossi EA, Balsam LB, et al. The chronobiology of Stanford type A aortic dissections: a comparison of northern versus southern hemispheres. Aorta (Stamford) 2015;3(6):182–6.
12. Siddiqi HK, Luminais SN, Montgomery D, et al. Chronobiology of acute aortic dissection in the Marfan syndrome (from the National Registry of Genetically Triggered Thoracic Aortic Aneurysm and

Cardiovascular Conditions and the International Registry of Acute Aortic Dissection). Am J Cardiol 2017;119(5):785–9.

13. Portaluppi F, Manfredini R, Fersini C. From a static to a dynamic concept of risk: the circadian epidemiology of cardiovascular events. Chronobiol Int 1999;16(1):33–49.

14. Manfredini R, Boari B, Gallerani M, et al. Chronobiology of rupture and dissection of aortic aneurysms. J Vasc Surg 2004;40:382–8.

15. Martino TA, Sole MJ. Molecular time: an often overlooked dimension to cardiovascular disease. Circ Res 2009;105(11):1047–61.

16. Brzezinski A. Melatonin in humans. N Engl J Med 1997;336(3):186–95.

17. Charloux A, Gronfier C, Lonsdorfer-Wolf E, et al. Aldosterone release during the sleep-wake cycle in humans. Am J Physiol 1999;276(1 pt 1):E43–9.

18. Lightman SL, James VH, Linsell C, et al. Studies of diurnal changes in plasma renin activity, and plasma noradrenaline, aldosterone and cortisol concentrations in man. Clin Endocrinol (Oxf) 1981;14(3): 213–23.

19. Obal F Jr, Krueger JM. GHRH and sleep. Sleep Med Rev 2004;8(5):367–77.

20. Young ME. The circadian clock within the heart: potential influence on myocardial gene expression, metabolism, and function. Am J Physiol Heart Circ Physiol 2006;290(1):H1–16.

21. Bjarnason GA, Jordan RC, Wood PA, et al. Circadian expression of clock genes in human oral mucosa

and skin: association with specific cell-cycle phases. Am J Pathol 2001;158(5):1793–801.

22. Duellman T, Warren CL, Peissig P, et al. Matrix metalloproteinase for abdominal aortic aneurysm. Circ Cardiovasc Genet 2012;5(5):529–37.

23. Bray MS, Shaw CA, Moore MW, et al. Disruption of the circadian clock within the cardiomyocyte influences myocardial contractile function; metabolism; and gene expression. Am J Physiol Heart Circ Physiol 2008;294(2):H1036–47.

24. Markoulli M, Papas E, Cole N, et al. The diurnal variation of matrix metalloproteinase-9 and its associated factors in human tears. Invest Ophthalmol Vis Sci 2012;53(3):1479–84.

25. Pell JP, Cobbe SM. Seasonal variations in coronary heart disease. QJM 1999;92(12):689–96.

26. Ornato JP, Peberdy MA, Chandra NC, et al. Seasonal pattern of acute myocardial infarction in the National Registry of Myocardial Infarction. J Am Coll Cardiol 1996;28(7):1684–8.

27. Dopico XC, Evangelou M, Ferreira RC, et al. Widespread seasonal gene expression reveals annual differences in human immunity and physiology. Nat Commun 2015;6:7000.

28. Keatinge WR, Coleshaw SR, Cotter F, et al. Increases in platelet and red cell counts, blood viscosity, and arterial pressure during mild surface cooling: factors in mortality from coronary and cerebral thrombosis in winter. Br Med J 1984;289(6456): 1405–8.

Circaseptan Periodicity of Cardiovascular Diseases

Massimo Gallerani, MD[a], Marco Pala, MD[a], Ugo Fedeli, MD[b],*

KEYWORDS

- Periodicity • Circaseptan chronobiology • Weekend • Day of week • Cardiovascular diseases

KEY POINTS

- A Monday peak has been observed in studies investigating incidence and hospitalization for cardiovascular disorders.
- Among patients hospitalized on weekends, a higher short-term mortality has been reported, at least partly associated with organization of health care.
- Further research is warranted to investigate variations by day of week not only for in-hospital mortality, but for several process of care and outcome measures.

INTRODUCTION

The analysis of chronobiology of cardiovascular events initially focused on the circadian and seasonal variability. The research on triggering mechanisms highlighted the need to assess also issues related to the activity and/or organization of the working week. Early studies on acute myocardial infarction and sudden cardiac death showed a different distribution in the occurrence of events during the week. Because the week is socially constructed, the likely mechanisms driving circaseptan rhythms in illness are psychosocial and therefore associated with health behaviors.

In a second instance, evidence emerged in the scientific literature addressing variations in the quality of delivered care and related short-term outcomes according to day of week of admission, with unfavorable outcomes among patients admitted on weekends.

In the first section of the article, circaseptan variability in the occurrence of cardiovascular events is reviewed, and the second section is devoted to the so-called "weekend effect."

CIRCASEPTAN PERIODICITY

Monday represents a critical day for several cardiovascular events and other diseases.[1] The first studies carried out by Gnecchi-Ruscone and colleagues[2] in Italy, and Willich and colleagues[3] in Germany, reported an increased risk of acute myocardial infarction on Monday. In particular, Willich and colleagues[3] found that a weekly variation with a Monday peak was present only in the working but not in the nonworking population. However, another study from Germany[4] confirmed a higher frequency of events on Monday, but with no differences between working or retired patients. Some years later, a Japanese study found a main Monday peak in the onset of myocardial infarction in working men and a peak on Saturday for women, hypothesizing the existence of a higher stressful burden for women related to family roles during weekends.[5]

A meta-analysis[6] estimated the excess risk associated with the Monday peak in cardiac mortality and reported an increased pooled odds ratio of 1.19, without significant differences between

Disclosures: The authors have no conflicts of interest related to this article to disclose.
[a] Department of Internal Medicine, Hospital of Ferrara, Azienda Ospedaliero-Universitaria, Via Aldo Moro 8, Ferrara 44124, Italy; [b] Epidemiological Department, Veneto Region, Passaggio Gaudenzio 1, Padova 35131, Italy
* Corresponding author.
E-mail address: ugo.fedeli@regione.veneto.it

subgroups by age and gender. Another meta-analysis of 28 community-based studies[7] confirmed a statistically significant excess in coronary events on Mondays in more than 70% of studies (20 of 28). The Monday excess in events was observed in both fatal and nonfatal events, men and women, and was greater in younger than in older subjects. However, the magnitude of the Monday peak was limited.

More recently, the Monday preference was confirmed in other studies,[8–10] although such excess did not always reach statistical significance. The weekly peak of acute myocardial infarction was detected on the first workday of the week, with a gradually decreasing tendency until the end of the week. Moreover, there was a significant difference between the number of events on workdays and weekends, but with no difference between workers younger than 65 and retired subjects older than 65 or between the 2 genders.[11] Finally, Collart and colleagues[12] observed that the Monday peak of events was more pronounced in patients aged 35 to 44 and then decreased up to ages of 65 to 69.

Monday represents a critical day for onset of stroke as well,[13–18] independent of the presence or not of common risk factors.[19,20] A study on more than 56,000 cases[21] confirmed that ischemic stroke had a peak on Monday and a trough on Sunday (16.6% vs 12.9%, respectively), with no significant differences between fatal or nonfatal cases. Interestingly, transient ischemic attacks showed the same pattern (16.1% vs 11.6%).[22] The incidence of cerebral hemorrhage and subarachnoid hemorrhage was not significantly different among days of the week.[20] More recently a Spanish study[23] found that number of hospital admissions due to stroke remains stable from Monday to Friday, whereas it abruptly decreases during the weekends, reaching its minimum values on Sunday.

In analyses of causes of death records, overall cardiovascular mortality, and specifically mortality from ischemic cardiac and cerebrovascular diseases, was highest on Mondays.[24]

Among studies analyzing the weekly pattern of out-of-hospital cardiac arrest (OHCAs), most found a greater incidence on Saturdays[25] and Mondays.[6,26–31] Lopez-Messa and colleagues[32] reported instead a peak on Wednesdays. Also ventricular arrhythmias displayed a main peak of onset on Monday.[33]

Few data are available on the weekly distribution of worsening heart failure, although Allegra and colleagues[34] found a higher number of hospitalizations on Monday.

A limited number of studies is available on the circaseptan variability of takotsubo cardiomyopathy.

Two studies confirmed a Monday peak,[35,36] one found a non–statistically significant peak on Tuesday,[37] and another did not demonstrate any weekly periodicity.[38]

Last, a Monday peak was found in subjects with acute aortic diseases,[39] aortic rupture or dissection were reported to have a higher incidence on Monday.[40,41] Other studies did not find a weekly variation in the distribution of events,[42,43] but a review confirmed the Monday preference for aortic rupture/dissection.[44]

It must be remarked that acute myocardial infarction and cerebrovascular events occur on the basis of atherosclerosis as a result of yearly accumulation of risk factors. Therefore, if different cardiovascular events occur more frequently on a specific day of the week, it is assumed that in addition to traditional long-acting risk factors, other "triggering factors" may explain such circaseptan periodicity. Similarly, a lower incidence on a specific day of the week may be the consequence of "delaying factors." Several potential triggering factors might explain such Monday preference for cardiovascular events; for example, stress from commencing the weekly working activities,[3] higher blood pressure levels,[45,46] and unfavorable biochemical status.[47] Morning blood pressure surge, evaluated by means of 24-hour ambulatory monitoring, was the greatest on Monday,[45] and significant differences have been reported in blood parameters, characterized by unfavorable profile on Monday compared with non-Monday values.[47]

The role of stress associated with commencing weekly activities is supported by the fact that another well-known stress-related cardiac disease that clinically mimics acute myocardial infarction, takotsubo cardiomyopathy, has been found to exhibit a Monday peak.[35] A further interesting confirmation of the association between stress and Monday comes from a Korean study demonstrating differences in adrenocortical activities between workdays and nonworkdays.[48] In full-time Monday through Saturday working subjects, in fact, the molar cortisol-to-dehydroepiandrosterone ratio, measured after awakening from salivary samples, was significantly higher on Monday and Tuesday and significantly lower on Sunday than on the other days.[48] On the other hand, a lower incidence on Sunday could be explained by "delaying factors," such as less stress, lower anxiety, and sufficient time to sleep and rest.[49,50]

Although the reasons remain speculative, several changes in behavior around weekends, including alcohol intake, sleep/wake cycle, and physical activity may further partly explain the observed weekly variability.[31,51]

WEEKEND EFFECT

Weekend admission may be associated with worse outcomes because of shortage of staff, lower experience of personnel, and limited availability of therapeutic and diagnostic procedures, a phenomenon known as "weekend effect" or "off-hour effect" (extending to weekends, holidays, and nights). The first reports that hospital mortality was higher during weekends appeared in the 1970s. Such a weekend effect was confirmed by Bell and Redelmeier[52] in a study of adult admissions to Canadian hospitals. The investigators reported that mortality was higher for one-fourth of the 100 conditions that comprised the most frequent causes of death, although for most conditions, no such effect was apparent. Many studies have subsequently demonstrated the existence of the weekend effect,[53–55] although not all agree it exists.[56,57]

A systematic review published in 2010[58] and several more recent studies confirmed unfavorable outcomes for admissions on weekends; the overall increase in the risk of mortality for unselected emergency admissions could be estimated at approximately 10% to 15%, translating in many thousands of additional deaths each year (**Table 1**). Two major explanations have been forwarded,[54] which are not mutually exclusive: patients admitted over the weekend are sicker than their weekday counterparts, and/or that patients admitted over the weekend experience poorer quality of care.

A recent systematic review confirmed an increased mortality risk among patients admitted off-hours for many neoplastic, respiratory, gastrointestinal, and circulatory diseases.[79] Short-term mortality (risk estimates expressed as odds ratio [OR] with 95% confidence interval [CI]) was higher in patients admitted off-hours for aortic aneurysm (6 studies, OR 1.52, CI 1.30–1.77), pulmonary embolism (8 studies, OR 1.20, 1.13–1.28), major arrhythmia and cardiac arrest (10 studies, OR 1.19, 1.09–1.29), subarachnoid hemorrhage (4 studies, OR 1.10, 1.01–1.19), intracerebral hemorrhage (8 studies, OR 1.10, 1.04–1.17), heart failure (7 studies, OR 1.10, 1.01–1.21), stroke (32 studies, OR 1.10, 1.06–1.14), and myocardial infarction (56 studies, OR 1.06, 1.04–1.09).[79]

Weekend Effect: Acute Myocardial Infarction

Sorita and colleagues[80] examined 36 studies on short-term mortality among patients with acute myocardial infarction: overall, off-hour presentation was associated with a significantly increased mortality, especially for ST elevation myocardial infarction (STEMI), and for reports outside Northern America; the effect was even larger in more recent publications. For admissions on weekends with respect to weekdays, the OR was equal to 1.06 (CI 1.03–1.09). Such increased mortality risk paralleled with longer door to balloon times among patients with STEMI admitted off-hours across 30 reviewed studies,[80] suggesting a strong association between increased mortality and worse quality of care. Magid and colleagues[81] already reported that in the United States the increased risk of mortality for patients admitted off-hours disappeared after adjustment for reperfusion treatment time. Also analyses on inpatient databases from New Jersey[82] and Korea[83] demonstrated that the weekend effect became nonsignificant after adjustment for therapeutic procedures. Although residual confounding due to differences in case-mix cannot be completely ruled out, myocardial infarction represents a clinical setting in which increased mortality is more clearly associated with the factors acting after hospital admission, including availability of cardiologists and skilled staff for the cardiac catheterization laboratory. Even if the relative increase in risk is limited, the impact at the population level for a such common disease is substantial.[80] Analyses of recent US hospitalization records show a decrease over time in the disparity in the risk of death for patients admitted on the weekend versus on weekdays both for STEMI and for other acute coronary syndromes.[84] Also other reports demonstrated that when the weekend effect is examined over time within a single country, the magnitude of the weekend effect tends to decrease, possibly due to improvements in the adherence to current guidelines.[85]

Weekend Effect: Stroke

Sorita and colleagues[86] reviewed 21 studies investigating outcomes in patients admitted off-hours for ischemic stroke. Off-hour presentation was associated with all investigated outcomes: in-hospital mortality, 7-day mortality, 30-day mortality, and worse Ranking Scale at discharge. Specifically, from 19 studies reporting short-term mortality among patients admitted on weekends versus weekdays, the overall OR was equal to 1.11 (CI 1.06–1.18). The effect was significant both in studies based on clinical registries and on administrative data, and was somewhat larger in reports from Europe and Asia with respect to North America. Studies reporting short-term mortality for hemorrhagic stroke are summarized in **Table 2**: most found an increased mortality risk among patients admitted on weekends; according to analyses of US discharges for intracerebral

Table 1
Weekend (WE) admission and risk of mortality (in-hospital, 7-day, or 30-day mortality): synopsis of the available studies

Author, Publication Year	Country	Study Period	Number of Admissions	WE (Relative Risk with 95% Confidence Interval)	Notes
Bell & Redelmeier et al,[52] 2001	Inpatient database, Ontario, Canada	1988–1997	3,789,917	—	Increased mortality for patients admitted on WE with selected serious medical conditions
Cram et al,[53] 2004	Inpatient database, California, USA	1998	1,100,984	All admissions 1.20 (1.17–1.23) Unscheduled 1.21 (1.11–1.16) Emergency room admissions 1.03 (1.01–1.06)	
Ensminger et al,[59] 2004	Mayo Clinic, USA	1994–2002	29,084	1.70 (1.55–1.85)	Patients admitted to medical, surgical, and multispecialty intensive care units (ICUs)
Arias et al,[60] 2004	15 Pediatric ICUs, USA	1995–2001	20,547	1.00 (0.78–1.28)	Mortality within 48 h
Schmulewitz et al,[57] 2005	Royal Infirmary of Edinburgh, UK	2001	3244	Ranging from 0.61 to 3.13, depending on diagnosis	Patients with 6 medical conditions
Barba et al,[61] 2006	Emergency adult admissions, single hospital Spain	1999–2003	35,993	1.40 (1.13–1.62)	Deaths within 48 h
Arabi et al,[62] 2006	ICU admissions, single hospital, Saudi Arabia	1999–2003	2093	No difference between weekdays, weeknights, and WE	
Laupland et al,[63] 2008	ICU admissions, Calgary Health Region, Canada	2000–2006	20,466	1.05 (0.95–1.17)	
Schilling et al,[64] 2010	Admissions to 39 Michigan hospitals, USA	2003–2006	166,920	1.08 (1.03–1.13)	
Aylin et al,[55] 2010	Inpatient database, public acute hospitals, England	2005/2006	4,317,866	1.10 (1.08–1.11)	Emergency admissions
Marco et al,[65] 2010	Emergency admissions to internal medicine, Spain	2005	429,880	In hospital 1.07 (1.05–1.10) Within 2 d 1.28 (1.22–1.33)	
Cavallazzi et al,[58] 2010	Pooled analysis of 6 studies on ICU admission	—	180,600	1.08 (1.04–1.13)	Studies including Ensminger et al,[59]; Laupland et al[63]
Kuijsten et al,[66] 2010	National ICU registry, the Netherlands	2002–2008	149,894	1.10 (1.07–1.14)	

Study	Data source	Years	N	Result	Notes
Ricciardi et al,[67] 2011	Nationwide inpatient sample, nonelective admission, US	2003–2007	29,991,621	1.10 (1.10–1.11)	
Mikulich et al,[68] 2011	Emergency medical admissions, single hospital, Ireland	2002–2009	49,337	1.05 (0.88–1.24)	
Freemantle et al,[69] 2012	Inpatient database, England	2009–2010	14,217,640	Sunday vs Wednesday 1.16 (1.14–1.18) Saturday vs Wednesday 1.11 (1.09–1.13)	
Mohammed et al,[70] 2012	Inpatient database, England	2008–2009	4,640,516	Elective admission 1.32 (1.23–1.41) Emergency admission 1.09 (1.05–1.13)	
Ricciardi et al,[71] 2014	Nationwide Inpatient Sample (NIS) United States	2003–2008	26,051,775	1.1 (1.0–1.1)	Agency for Healthcare Research and Quality
De Giorgi et al,[72] 2015	Ferrara Hospital inpatient database, Italy	2000–2013	411,588	1.41 (1.36–1.47)	
Freemantle et al,[73] 2015	Inpatient database, England	2013–2014	14,818,374	Sunday vs Wednesday 1.15 (1.14–1.17) Saturday vs Wednesday 1.10 (1.08–1.11)	
Meacock et al,[74] 2016	Accident and emergency attendances and emergency admissions, England	2013–2014	12,670,788 attendances, 4,656,586 admissions	Accident and emergency attendances 1.01 (0.99–1.02) Admission through accident and emergency 1.05 (1.04–1.07) Direct admission 1.21 (1.16, 1.26)	
Anselmi et al,[75] 2016	Linked hospitalization and Accident and emergency attendances, England	2013–2014	3,027,946	Sunday vs Wednesday 1.06 (1.03–1.09), Sunday night, Saturday day/night not significant	Adjusted for mode of arrival
Aldridge et al,[76] 2016	Survey on 115 trusts, England	June 2014	—	1.10 (1.08–1.11)	
Huang et al,[77] 2016	Database on 17 medical centers, Taiwan	2007–2009	82,340	1.19 (1.09–1.30)	
Mohammed et al,[78] 2016	Emergency admissions, 3 acute hospitals, England	2014	58,481	1.00 (0.92–1.08)	

hemorrhage, the magnitude of the effect is declining over time, and is larger in nonteaching hospitals.[95]

The weekend effect found in analyses of administrative data was not confirmed based on the local stroke registry in Oxfordshire, UK, with multiple reasons explaining such discrepancy.[100] Patients with less severe symptoms are less likely to present for medical attention on weekends, with a larger proportion of major strokes at the weekend with respect to weekdays; also in a previous report the weekend effect disappeared after adjustment for admission latency.[101] Furthermore, a number of elective admissions during weekdays for procedures or further investigations were miscoded in hospital records as acute stroke.[100] In a report from the Canadian Stroke Network, patients with minor stroke were less likely than those with major stroke to present on weekends and more likely to present on Monday, suggesting delays in hospital presentation in those with minor stroke symptoms; nonetheless, case fatality was higher in patients admitted on weekends also after adjustment for stroke severity.[102] Overall, the weekend effect in stroke admissions has been confirmed in many studies, and could represent a simplification of the several patterns of time variation occurring in stroke care: according to an audit program form England and Wales, different indicators of quality of care displayed a diurnal pattern, a day of week pattern, or an off-hour pattern.[103]

Weekend Effect: Other Cardiovascular Diseases

In the original report from Bell and Redelmeier,[52] weekend admissions for several other cardiovascular disorders were associated with increased mortality, including pulmonary embolism, ruptured abdominal aortic aneurysms, cardiac dysrhythmia, and cardiac conduction disorders.

A concerning association has been found between hospital admission on weekends for pulmonary embolism and in-hospital mortality. In fact, a significantly increased risk of in-hospital mortality has been found in studies carried out in Canada,[52] the United States,[104,105] the Emilia Romagna region in Italy,[106] England and Wales,[107] and Australia.[108] For 2 other recent studies, such increase was not statistically significant due to a limited sample size.[109,110]

An overview of studies on aortic aneurysm/dissection is provided in **Table 3**. Bell and Redelmeier[52] found that ruptured abdominal aneurysm was associated with a significantly higher mortality in patients admitted during weekends (42% vs 36% in weekdays). Similar results were reported

by subsequent studies based on analyses of inpatient databases carried out in the United States and England; in Italy, admission for aortic aneurysm rupture or dissection was associated with an increased risk of death both at the regional and national levels.

Earlier reports on hospitalization for heart failure based both on administrative and registry-based data failed to demonstrate an association between weekend admission and short-term mortality (**Table 4**). By contrast, in Get With the Guidelines–heart failure registry, weekend admission was associated with increased in-hospital mortality and slightly longer in-hospital length of stay compared with weekday admission.[115] This latter finding was confirmed by more recent analyses of inpatient archives from Italy, England, and Australia. Differences in disease severity and prevalence of comorbidities based on clinical data between patients admitted on weekends or on weekdays were evidenced in some reports,[117] but negligible in others.[115] It was supposed that the differences between reports might be due to the differences in the health care system, specifically the reduction of the territorial level of assistance during weekends and holidays.

The first reports based on administrative databases showed an association between admission for cardiac arrest/arrhythmia on weekends and short-term mortality.[52,53,55] Koike and colleagues[118] analyzed 173,137 patients with out of hospital cardiac arrest in Japan; after adjusting for potential confounding factors the day of admission (weekday vs weekend/holiday), had no significant effect on rates of 1-month survival or neurologically favorable 1-month survival. Similar results were reported from studies carried out in the United States and Canada.[31,119,120] With regard to hospital cardiac arrests, studies reported conflicting results on the weekend effect,[108,121,122] which was instead confirmed among admissions for atrial fibrillation.[123,124]

An increased risk was found for sudden infant death syndrome,[125–128] pediatric out-of-hospital cardiac arrests (OHCAs),[129,130] and pediatric in-hospital cardiac arrests,[131] but not in all studies.[132,133] It was hypothesized that infants may receive less attention on weekends[127] and that parents may be less willing to seek medical help on the weekend for apparently minor illnesses.[134]

WEEKEND EFFECT: SUMMARY

Although hospitals are open all time, their activities (including staffing levels and service offerings) vary over the course of the week with fluctuations in

Table 2
Weekend (WE) admission for *hemorrhagic stroke* and risk of mortality (in-hospital, 7-day or 30-day mortality): synopsis of the available studies

Author, Publication Year	Country	Study Period	Number of Cases	WE (Relative Risk with 95% Confidence Interval)	Notes
Intracerebral hemorrhage					
Bell and Redelmeier,[52] 2001	Inpatient database Ontario, Canada	1988–1997	10,987	1.01 (0.93–1.11)	
Cram et al,[53] 2004	Inpatient database, California, USA	1998	6210	0.98 (0.87–1.10)	Emergency admissions
Crowley et al,[87] 2009	Nationwide inpatient sample, USA	2004	13,821	1.12 (1.05–1.20)	
Reeves et al,[88] 2009	GWGT-Stroke Program, USA	2003–2007	34,945	1.19[a] (1.12–1.27)	Intracerebral hemorrhage + sub-arachnoid hemorrhage
Clarke et al,[89] 2010	Inpatient database, Queensland, Australia	2002–2007	1781	1.01 (0.86–1.16)	
O'Brien et al,[90] 2011	Stroke events in ARIC cohort study, USA	1987–2004	108	0.37 (0.11–1.26)	
Jiang et al,[91] 2011	Single teaching hospital, China	2007–2009	313	not reported	Weekday 22%, WE 18%, $P = .315$
McDowell et al,[92] 2014	Single neurologic intensive care unit, USA	2006–2009	200	1.02 (0.91–1.14)	Hypertensive intracerebral hemorrhage
Béjot et al,[93] 2013	Dijon stroke registry, France	1985–2010	557	1.00 (0.72–1.39)	
Roberts et al,[94] 2015	Linked archives, Wales, UK	2004–2012	4041	1.08 (0.99–1.18)	
Patel et al,[95] 2016	Nationwide inpatient sample, USA	2002–2011	485,329	Whole period: 1.11 (1.09–1.13) 2008–2011: 1.05 (1.02–1.08)	2008–2011: teaching 1.02 (0.98–1.06) Nonteaching 1.10 (1.05–1.15)

(continued on next page)

Table 2
(continued)

Author, Publication Year	Country	Study Period	Number of Cases	WE (Relative Risk with 95% Confidence Interval)	Notes
Subarachnoid hemorrhage					
Bell and Redelmeier,[52] 2001	Inpatient database Ontario, Canada	1988–1997	6247	1.10 (0.97–1.25)	
Cram et al,[53] 2004	Inpatient database, California, USA	1998	1819	0.98 (0.79–1.21)	Emergency admissions
Crowley et al,[96] 2009	Nationwide inpatient sample, USA	2004	5667	1.03 (0.92–1.16)	
Zhang et al,[97] 2011	Single teaching hospital, China	2006–2009	183	1.77 (0.83–1.77)	
Deshmuk et al,[98] 2016	Multicenter audit, England	2009–2011	385	2.01 (1.13–4.0)	
Other hemorrhage					
Bell and Redelmeier,[52] 2001	Inpatient database Ontario, Canada	1988–1997	3535	1.23 (0.98–1.48)	Other nontraumatic intracranial hemorrhage
Cram et al,[53] 2004	Inpatient database, California, USA	1998	1459	1.15 (0.89–1.50)	Other nontraumatic intracranial hemorrhage, Emergency admissions
Busl and Prabhakaran,[99] 2013	Nationwide Inpatient Sample, USA	2007–2009	14,093	1.19 (1.02–1.38)	Nontraumatic subdural hematoma
Roberts et al,[94] 2015	Linked archives, Wales, UK	2004–2012	1548	1.27 (0.96–1.67)	Other nontraumatic intracranial hemorrhage

Abbreviation: ARIC, Atherosclerosis Risk in Communities.
[a] Off-Hours: weekends + weekday night shifts.

Table 3

Weekend (WE) admission for *aortic aneurysm/dissection* and risk of mortality (in-hospital, 7-day, or 30-day mortality): synopsis of the available studies

Author, Publication Year	Country	Study Period	Number of Cases	WE (Relative Risk with 95% Confidence Interval)	Notes
Bell and Redelmeier,[52] 2001	Inpatient database Ontario, Canada	1988–1997	5454	1.28 (1.13–1.46)	Ruptured abdominal aortic aneurysm
Cram et al,[53] 2004	Inpatient database, California, USA	1998	1682	1.13 (0.90–1.41)	Aortic aneurysm – emergency admissions
Aylin et al,[55] 2010	Inpatient database, England	2005/2006	5573	1.45 (1.26–1.66)	Aortic, peripheral and visceral artery aneurysms
Gallerani et al,[111] 2012	Inpatient database, Emilia Romagna Region, Italy	1999–2009	4461	1.32 (1.14–1.51)	Aortic aneurysm rupture or dissection
Gallerani et al,[41] 2013	National inpatient database, Italy	2008–2010	15,137	1.34 (1.24–1.44)	Aortic aneurysm rupture or dissection
Groves et al,[112] 2014	Nationwide inpatient sample, USA	2009	7200	Thoracic 2.55 (1.77–3.68) Abdominal 1.32 (1.13–1.55)	Ruptured aortic aneurysm
Kumar et al,[113] 2016	Nationwide inpatient sample, USA	2004–2012	21,156	1.17 (1.06–1.28)	Acute aortic dissection

Table 4
Weekend (WE) admission for *heart failure* and risk of mortality (in-hospital, 7-day, or 30-day mortality): synopsis of the available studies

Author, Publication Year	Country	Study Period	Number of Cases	WE (Relative Risk with 95% Confidence Interval)	Notes
Bell and Redelmeier,[52] 2001	Inpatient database Ontario, Canada	1988–1997	141,687	1.00 (0.96–1.04)	
Cram et al,[53] 2004	Inpatient database, California, USA	1998	55,835	1.05 (0.96–1.16)	Emergency admissions
Fonarow et al,[114] 2008	Optimize-Heart Failure registry USA	2003–2004	48,612	0.99 (0.84–1.17)	
Horwich et al,[115] 2009	Get With the Guidelines (GWTG)-HF, USA	2005–2008	81,810	1.13 (1.02–1.27)	
Aylin et al,[55] 2010	Inpatient database, England	2005/2006	56,394	1.11 (1.05–1.17)	
Gallerani et al,[116] 2011	Ferrara Hospital, Italy	2002–2009	9657	1.33 (1.15–1.53)	
Freemantle et al,[69] 2012	Inpatient database, England	2009–2010	7247 deaths	Sunday vs Wednesday 1.10 (1.01–1.21) Saturday vs Wednesday 1.16 (1.06–1.27)	
Hamaguchi et al,[117] 2014	Japanese Cardiac Registry of Heart Failure	2004–2005	1620	1.12 (0.63–2.00)	
Concha et al,[108] 2014	Emergency department admissions, New South Wales, Australia	2000–2007	14,598	1.16 (1.07–1.26)	Heart failure and shock, in-hospital mortality

demand. Elective hospital-based services are typically scheduled during the day-time hours of the working week. By contrast, hospitals face a more uniform burden of acutely ill patients who require urgent medical attention.[54] Hospital wards suffer a dramatic decrease in number and seniority of staff members during weekends, and this increased staff workload can lead to a decrease in quality.[52,127] When studies carried out in 2010 compared mortality for the entire patient population admitted during weekends versus weekdays, a 10% to 15% higher risk for weekend admissions was found.[135] However, these analyses were based on administrative databases that have little information about the clinical state of patients at the time of admission. Recent reports from the United Kingdom failed to demonstrate a higher mortality for weekend hospitalizations, attributing previous findings to coding errors and inadequate adjustment for disease severity and comorbidities.[78,135,136] To determine if the widely held concerns about a weekend effect are justified, investigations should focus on multiple dimensions of the quality of care, such as health outcomes (not only mortality, but also morbidity, quality of life), safety (falls, hospital-acquired infections), patients' experience (delays in diagnosis, not receiving sufficient information), and poorer operational efficiency (delayed discharges).[71,74,100,101,135]

REFERENCES

1. Brillman JC, Burr T, Forslund D, et al. Modeling emergency department visit patterns for infectious disease complaints: results and application to disease surveillance. BMC Med Inform Decis Mak 2005;5:4.

2. Gnecchi-Ruscone T, Piccaluga E, Guzzetti S, et al. Morning and Monday: critical periods for the onset of acute myocardial infarction. Eur Heart J 1994;15: 882–7.

3. Willich SN, Lowel H, Lewis M, et al. Weekly variation of acute myocardial infarction. Increased Monday risk in the working population. Circulation 1994;90:87–93.

4. Spielberg C, Falkenhahn D, Willich SN, et al. Circadian, day-of-week, and seasonal variability in myocardial infarction: comparison between working and retired patients. Am Heart J 1996;132:579–85.

5. Kinjo K, Sato H, Sato H, et al. Variation during the week in the incidence of acute myocardial infarction: increased risk for Japanese women on Saturdays. Heart 2003;89:398–403.

6. Witte DR, Grobbee DR, Bots ML, et al. A meta-analysis of excess cardiac mortality on Monday. Eur J Epidemiol 2005;20:401–6.

7. Barnett AG, Dobson AJ. Excess in cardiovascular events on Mondays: a meta-analysis and perspective study. J Epidemiol Community Health 2005;59: 109–14.

8. Kriszbacher I, Boncz I, Koppan M, et al. Seasonal variations in the occurrence of acute myocardial infarction in Hungary between 2000 and 2004. Int J Cardiol 2008;129:251–4.

9. Manfredini R, Manfredini F, Boari B, et al. Seasonal and weekly patterns of hospital admissions for nonfatal and fatal myocardial infarction. Am J Emerg Med 2009;27:1097–103.

10. Reavey M, Saner H, Paccaud F, et al. Exploring the periodicity of cardiovascular events in Switzerland: variation in deaths and hospitalizations across seasons, day of the week and hour of the day. Int J Cardiol 2013;168:2195–200.

11. Bodis J, Boncz I, Kriszbacher I. Permanent stress may be trigger of an acute myocardial infarction on the first work-day of the week. Int J Cardiol 2010;144:423–5.

12. Collart P, Coppieters Y, Godin I, et al. Day-of-the-week variations in myocardial infarction onset over a 27-year period: the importance of age and other risk factors. Am J Emerg Med 2014;32:558–62.

13. Pasqualetti P, Natali G, Casale R, et al. Epidemiological chronorisk of stroke. Acta Neurol Scand 1990;81:71–4.

14. Kelly-Hayes M, Wolf PA, Kase CS, et al. Temporal patterns of stroke onset. The Framingham Study. Stroke 1995;26:1343–7.

15. Manfredini R, Casetta I, Paolino E, et al. Monday preference in onset of ischemic stroke. Am J Med 2001;111:401–3.

16. Wang H, Sekine M, Chen X, et al. A study of weekly and seasonal variation of stroke onset. Int J Biometeorol 2002;47:13–20.

17. Jakovljevic D. Day of the week and ischemic stroke: is it Monday high or Sunday low? Stroke 2004;35:2089–93.

18. Turin TC, Kita Y, Murakami Y, et al. Increase of stroke incidence after weekend regardless of traditional risk factors: Takashima Stroke Registry, Japan; 1988–2003. Cerebrovasc Dis 2007;24:328–37.

19. Manfredini R, Manfredini F, Boari B, et al. The Monday peak in the onset of ischemic stroke is independent of major risk factors. Am J Emerg Med 2009;27:244–6.

20. Shigematsu K, Watanabe Y, Nakano H, Kyoto Stroke Registry Committee. Weekly variations of stroke occurrence: an observational cohort study based on the Kyoto Stroke Registry, Japan. BMJ Open 2015;5:e006294.

21. Manfredini R, Manfredini F, Malagoni AM, et al. Day-of-week distribution of fatal and nonfatal stroke in elderly subjects. J Am Geriatr Soc 2009;57: 1511–3.

22. Manfredini R, Manfredini F, Boari B, et al. Temporal patterns of hospital admissions for transient ischemic attack: a retrospective population-based study in the Emilia-Romagna region of Italy. Clin Appl Thromb Hemost 2010;16:153–60.

23. Santurtún A, Ruiz PB, López-Delgado L, et al. Stroke: temporal trends and association with atmospheric variables and air pollutants in Northern Spain. Cardiovasc Toxicol 2016. http://dx.doi.org/10.1007/s12012-016-9395-6.

24. Capodaglio G, Gallerani M, Fedeli U, et al. Contemporary burden of excess cardiovascular mortality on Monday. A retrospective study in the Veneto region of Italy. Int J Cardiol 2016;214:307–9.

25. Savopoulos C, Ziakas A, Hatzitolios A, et al. Circadian rhythm in sudden cardiac death: a retrospective study of 2,665 cases. Angiology 2006;57: 197–204.

26. Peckova M, Fahrenbruch CE, Cobb LA, et al. Weekly and seasonal variation in the incidence of cardiac arrests. Am Heart J 1999;137:512–5.

27. Arntz HR, Willich SN, Schreiber C, et al. Diurnal, weekly and seasonal variation of sudden death. Population-based analysis of 24,061 consecutive cases. Eur Heart J 2000;21:315–20.

28. Allegra JR, Cochrane DG, Allegra EM, et al. Calendar patterns in the occurrence of cardiac arrest. Am J Emerg Med 2002;20:513–7.

29. Herlitz J, Eek M, Holmberg M, et al. Diurnal, weekly and seasonal rhythm of out of hospital cardiac arrest in Sweden. Resuscitation 2002;54:133–8.

30. Gruska M, Gaul GB, Winkler M, et al. Increased occurrence of out-of-hospital cardiac arrest on Mondays in a community-based study. Chronobiol Int 2005;22:107–20.

31. Bagai A, McNally BF, Al-Khatib SM, et al. Temporal differences in out-of-hospital cardiac arrest incidence and survival. Circulation 2013;128: 2595–602.

32. López-Messa JB, Alonso-Fernández JI, Andrés-de Llano JM, et al. Circadian rhythm and time variations in out-hospital sudden cardiac arrest. Med Intensiva 2012;36:402–9.

33. Peters RW, McQuillan S, Resnick SK, et al. Increased Monday incidence of life-threatening ventricular arrhythmias. Experience with a third-generation implantable defibrillator. Circulation 1996;94:1346–9.

34. Allegra JR, Cochrane DG, Biglow R. Monthly, weekly, and daily patterns in the incidence of congestive heart failure. Acad Emerg Med 2001; 8:682–5.

35. Manfredini R, Citro R, Previtali M, et al. Monday preference in onset of takotsubo cardiomyopathy. Am J Emerg Med 2010;28:715–9.

36. Song BG, Oh JH, Kim HJ, et al. Chronobiological variation in the occurrence of Tako-tsubo cardiomyopathy: experiences of two tertiary cardiovascular centers. Heart Lung 2013;42:40–7.

37. Sharkey SW, Lesser JR, Garberich RF, et al. Comparison of circadian rhythm patterns in Takotsubo cardiomyopathy versus ST-segment elevation myocardial infarction. Am J Cardiol 2012;110: 795–9.

38. Parodi G, Bellandi B, Del Pace S, et al. Natural history of tako-tsubo cardiomyopathy. Chest 2011; 139:887–92.

39. Manfredini R, Boari B, Salmi R, et al. Day-of-week variability in the occurrence and outcome of aortic diseases: does it exist? Am J Emerg Med 2008;26: 363–6.

40. Lasica RM, Perunicic J, Mrdovic I, et al. Temporal variations at the onset of spontaneous acute aortic dissection. Int Heart J 2006;47:585–95.

41. Gallerani M, Volpato S, Boari B, et al. Outcomes of weekend versus weekday admission for acute aortic dissection or rupture: a retrospective study on the Italian National Hospital Database. Int J Cardiol 2013;168:3117–9.

42. Benouaich V, Soler P, Gourraud PA, et al. Impact of meteorological conditions on the occurrence of acute type A aortic dissections. Interact Cardiovasc Thorac Surg 2010;10:403–7.

43. Ryu HM, Lee JH, Kwon YS, et al. Examining the relationship between triggering activities and the 10; circadian distribution of acute aortic dissection. Korean Circ J 2010;40:565–72.

44. Vitale J, Manfredini R, Gallerani M, et al. Chronobiology of acute aortic rupture or dissection: a systematic review and a meta-analysis of the literature. Chronobiol Int 2015;32:385–94.

45. Murakami S, Otsuka K, Kubo Y, et al. Repeated ambulatory monitoring reveals a Monday morning surge in blood pressure in a community-dwelling population. Am J Hypertens 2004;17:1179–83.

46. Pieper C, Warren K, Pickering TC. A comparison of ambulatory blood pressure and heart rate at home on work and nonwork days. J Hypertens 1993;11: 177–83.

47. Urdal P, Anderssen SA, Holme I, et al. Monday and non-Monday concentrations of lifestyle-related blood components in the Oslo diet and exercise study. J Intern Med 1998;244:507–13.

48. Kim MS, Lee YJ, Ahn RS. Day-to-day differences in cortisol levels and molar cortisol-to-DHEA ratios among working individuals. Yonsei Med J 2010; 51:212–8.

49. Jood K, Redfors P, Rosengren A, et al. Self-perceived psychological stress and ischemic stroke: a case-control study. BMC Med 2009;7:53.

50. Ernst E, Weihmayr T, Schmid M, et al. Cardiovascular risk factors and hemorheology. Physical fitness, stress and obesity. Atherosclerosis 1986;59:263–9.

51. Nishiyama C, Iwami T, Nichol G, et al. Association of out-of-hospital cardiac arrest with prior activity and ambient temperature. Resuscitation 2011;82: 1008–12.

52. Bell CM, Redelmeier DA. Mortality among patients admitted to hospitals on weekends as compared with weekdays. N Engl J Med 2001;345:663–8.

53. Cram P, Hillis SL, Barnett M, et al. Effects of weekend admission and hospital teaching status on in-hospital mortality. Am J Med 2004;117:151–7.

54. Becker D. Weekend hospitalization and mortality: a critical review. Expert Rev Pharmacoecon Outcomes Res 2008;8:23–6.

55. Aylin P, Yunus A, Bottle A, et al. Weekend mortality for emergency admissions. A large, multicentre study. Qual Saf Health Care 2010;19:213–7.

56. Wunsch H, Mapstone J, Brady T, et al. Hospital mortality associated with day and time of admission to intensive care units. Intensive Care Med 2004;30:895–901.

57. Schmulewitz L, Proudfoot A, Bell D. The impact of weekends on outcome for emergency patients. Clin Med (Lond) 2005;5:621–5.

58. Cavallazzi R, Marik PE, Hirani A, et al. Association between time of admission to the ICU and mortality: a systematic review and metaanalysis. Chest 2010;138:68–75.

59. Ensminger SA, Morales IJ, Peters SG, et al. The hospital mortality of patients admitted to the ICU on weekends. Chest 2004;126:1292–8.

60. Arias Y, Taylor DS, Marcin JP. Association between evening admissions and higher mortality rates in the pediatric intensive care unit. Pediatrics 2004; 113:e530–4.

61. Barba R, Losa JE, Velasco M, et al. Mortality among adult patients admitted to the hospital on weekends. Eur J Intern Med 2006;17:322–4.

62. Arabi Y, Alshimemeri A, Taher S. Weekend and weeknight admissions have the same outcome of weekday admissions to an intensive care unit with onsite intensivist coverage. Crit Care Med 2006; 34:605–11.

63. Laupland KB, Shahpori R, Kirkpatrick AW, et al. Hospital mortality among adults admitted to and discharged from intensive care on weekends and evenings. J Crit Care 2008;23:317–24.

64. Schilling PL, Campbell DA Jr, Englesbe MJ, et al. A comparison of in-hospital mortality risk conferred by high hospital occupancy, differences in nurse staffing levels, weekend admission, and seasonal influenza. Med Care 2010;48:224–32.

65. Marco J, Barba R, Plaza S, et al. Analysis of the mortality of patients admitted to internal medicine wards over the weekend. Am J Med Qual 2010; 25:312–8.

66. Kuijsten HA, Brinkman S, Meynaar IA, et al. Hospital mortality is associated with ICU admission time. Intensive Care Med 2010;36:1765–71.

67. Ricciardi R, Roberts PL, Read TE, et al. Mortality rate after non-elective hospital admission. Arch Surg 2011;146:545–51.

68. Mikulich O, Callaly E, Bennett K, et al. The increased mortality associated with a weekend emergency admission is due to increased illness severity and altered case-mix. Acute Med 2011; 10:182–7.

69. Freemantle N, Richardson M, Wood J, et al. Weekend hospitalization and additional risk of death: an analysis of inpatient data. J R Soc Med 2012;105: 74–84.

70. Mohammed MA, Sidhu KS, Rudge G, et al. Weekend admission to hospital has a higher risk of death in the elective setting than in the emergency setting: a retrospective database study of national health service hospitals in England. BMC Health Serv Res 2012;12:87.

71. Ricciardi R, Nelson J, Roberts PL, et al. Is the presence of medical trainees associated with increased mortality with weekend admission? BMC Med Educ 2014;14:4.

72. De Giorgi A, Fabbian F, Tiseo R, et al. Weekend hospitalization and inhospital mortality: a gender effect? Am J Emerg Med 2015;33:1701–3.

73. Freemantle N, Ray D, McNulty D, et al. Increased mortality associated with weekend hospital admission: a case for expanded seven day services? BMJ 2015;351:h4596.

74. Meacock R, Anselmi L, Kristensen SR, et al. Higher mortality rates amongst emergency patients admitted to hospital at weekends reflect a lower probability of admission. J Health Serv Res Policy 2017;22(1):12–9.

75. Anselmi L, Meacock R, Kristensen SR, et al. Arrival by ambulance explains variation in mortality by time of admission: retrospective study of admissions to hospital following emergency department attendance in England. BMJ Qual Saf 2016. http://dx.doi.org/10.1136/bmjqs-2016-005680.

76. Aldridge C, Bion J, Boyal A, et al. Weekend specialist intensity and admission mortality in acute hospital trusts in England: a cross-sectional study. Lancet 2016;388:178–86.

77. Huang CC, Huang YT, Hsu NC, et al. Effect of weekend admissions on the treatment process and outcomes of internal medicine patients: a nationwide cross-sectional study. Medicine (Baltimore) 2016;95:e2643.

78. Mohammed MA, Faisal M, Richardson D, et al. Adjusting for illness severity shows there is no difference in patient mortality at weekends or weekdays for emergency medical admissions. QJM 2016 [pii:hcw104]. [Epub ahead of print].

79. Zhou Y, Li W, Herath C, et al. Off-hour admission and mortality risk for 28 specific diseases: a systematic review and meta-analysis of 251 cohorts. J Am Heart Assoc 2016;5:e003102.

80. Sorita A, Ahmed A, Starr SR, et al. Off-hour presentation and outcomes in patients with acute myocardial infarction: systematic review and meta-analysis. BMJ 2014;348:f7393.

81. Magid DJ, Wang Y, Herrin J, et al. Relationship between time of day, day of week, timeliness of reperfusion, and in-hospital mortality for patients with acute ST-segment elevation myocardial infarction. JAMA 2005;294:803–12.

82. Kostis WJ, Demissie K, Marcella SW, et al. Weekend versus weekday admission and mortality from myocardial infarction. N Engl J Med 2007; 356:1099–109.

83. Hong JS, Kang HC, Lee SH. Comparison of case fatality rates for acute myocardial infarction in weekday vs weekend admissions in South Korea. Circ J 2010;74:496–502.

84. Khoshchehreh M, Groves EM, Tehrani D, et al. Changes in mortality on weekend versus weekday admissions for Acute Coronary Syndrome in the United States over the past decade. Int J Cardiol 2016;210:164–72.

85. Hansen KW, Hvelplund A, Abildstrøm SZ, et al. Prognosis and treatment in patients admitted with acute myocardial infarction on weekends and weekdays from 1997 to 2009. Int J Cardiol 2013;168:1167–73.

86. Sorita A, Ahmed A, Starr SR, et al. Off-hour presentation and outcomes in patients with acute

ischemic stroke: a systematic review and meta-analysis. Eur J Intern Med 2014;25:394–400.

87. Crowley RW, Yeoh HK, Stukenborg GJ, et al. Influence of weekend hospital admission on short-term mortality after intracerebral hemorrhage. Stroke 2009;40:2387–92.

88. Reeves MJ, Smith E, Fonarow G, et al. Off-hour admission and in-hospital stroke case fatality in the get with the guidelines-stroke program. Stroke 2009;40:569–76.

89. Clarke MS, Wills RA, Bowman RV, et al. Exploratory study of the 'weekend effect' for acute medical admissions to public hospitals in Queensland, Australia. Intern Med J 2010;40:777–83.

90. O'Brien EC, Rose KM, Shahar E, et al. Stroke mortality, clinical presentation and day of arrival: the Atherosclerosis Risk in Communities (ARIC) study. Stroke Res Treat 2011;2011:383012.

91. Jiang F, Zhang JH, Qin X. "Weekend effects" in patients with intracerebral hemorrhage. Acta Neurochir Suppl 2011;111:333–6.

92. McDowell MM, Kellner CP, Sussman ES, et al. The role of admission timing in the outcome of intracerebral hemorrhage patients at a specialized stroke center. Neurol Res 2014;36:95–101.

93. Béjot Y, Aboa-Eboulé C, Jacquin A, et al. Stroke care organization overcomes the deleterious 'weekend effect' on 1-month stroke mortality: a population-based study. Eur J Neurol 2013;20: 1177–83.

94. Roberts SE, Thorne K, Akbari A, et al. Mortality following stroke, the weekend effect and related factors: record linkage study. PLoS One 2015;10: e0131836.

95. Patel AA, Mahajan A, Benjo A, et al. A nationwide analysis of outcomes of weekend admissions for intracerebral hemorrhage shows disparities based on hospital teaching status. Neurohospitalist 2016; 6:51–8.

96. Crowley RW, Yeoh HK, Stukenborg GJ, et al. Influence of weekend versus weekday hospital admission on mortality following subarachnoid hemorrhage. Clinical article. J Neurosurg 2009;111:60–6.

97. Zhang G, Zhang JH, Qin X. Effect of weekend admission on in-hospital mortality after subarachnoid hemorrhage in Chongqing China. Acta Neurochir Suppl 2011;110:229–32.

98. Deshmukh H, Hinkley M, Dulhanty L, et al. Effect of weekend admission on in-hospital mortality and functional outcomes for patients with acute subarachnoid haemorrhage (SAH). Acta Neurochir (Wien) 2016;158:829–35.

99. Busl KM, Prabhakaran S. Predictors of mortality in nontraumatic subdural hematoma. J Neurosurg 2013;119:1296–301.

100. Li L, Rothwell PM. Oxford Vascular Study. Biases in detection of apparent "weekend effect" on outcome with administrative coding data: population based study of stroke. BMJ 2016;353:i2648.

101. Jauss M, Oertel W, Allendoerfer J, et al. Bias in request for medical care and impact on outcome during office and non-office hours in stroke patients. Eur J Neurol 2009;16:1165–7.

102. Fang J, Saposnik G, Silver FL, et al, Investigators of the Registry of the Canadian Stroke Network. Association between weekend hospital presentation and stroke fatality. Neurology 2010;75: 1589–96.

103. Bray BD, Cloud GC, James MA, et al. Weekly variation in health-care quality by day and time of admission: a nationwide, registry-based, prospective cohort study of acute stroke care. Lancet 2016;388:170–7.

104. Aujesky D, Jiménez D, Mor MK, et al. Weekend versus weekday admission and mortality after acute pulmonary embolism. Circulation 2009;119: 962–8.

105. Nanchal R, Kumar G, Taneja A, et al. Pulmonary embolism: the weekend effect. Chest 2012;142: 690–6.

106. Gallerani M, Imberti D, Ageno W, et al. Higher mortality rate in patients hospitalised for acute pulmonary embolism during weekends. Thromb Haemost 2011;106:83–9.

107. Roberts SE, Thorne K, Akbari A, et al. Weekend emergency admissions and mortality in England and Wales. Lancet 2015;385:1829.

108. Concha OP, Gallego B, Hillman K, et al. Do variations in hospital mortality patterns after weekend admission reflect reduced quality of care or different patient cohorts? A population-based study. BMJ Qual Saf 2014;23:215–22.

109. Giri S, Pathak R, Aryal MR, et al. Lack of "weekend effect" on mortality for pulmonary embolism admissions in 2011: data from nationwide inpatient sample. Int J Cardiol 2015;180:151–3.

110. Coleman CI, Brunault RD, Saulsberry WJ. Association between weekend admission and in-hospital mortality for pulmonary embolism: an observational study and meta-analysis. Int J Cardiol 2015;194: 72–4.

111. Gallerani M, Imberti D, Bossone E, et al. Higher mortality in patients hospitalized for acute aortic rupture or dissection during weekends. J Vasc Surg 2012;55:1247–54.

112. Groves EM, Khoshchehreh M, Le C, et al. Effects of weekend admission on the outcomes and management of ruptured aortic aneurysms. J Vasc Surg 2014;60:318–24.

113. Kumar N, Venkatraman A, Pandey A, et al. Weekend hospitalizations for acute aortic dissection have a higher risk of in-hospital mortality compared to weekday hospitalizations. Int J Cardiol 2016;214: 448–50.

114. Fonarow GC, Abraham WT, Albert NM, et al. Day of admission and clinical outcomes for patients hospitalized for heart failure: findings from the organized program to initiate lifesaving treatment in hospitalized patients with heart failure (OPTIMIZE-HF). Circ Heart Fail 2008;1:50–7.

115. Horwich TB, Hernandez AF, Liang L, et al. Weekend hospital admission and discharge for heart failure: association with quality of care and clinical outcomes. Am Heart J 2009;158:451–8.

116. Gallerani M, Boari B, Manfredini F, et al. Weekend versus weekday hospital admissions for acute heart failure. Int J Cardiol 2011;146:444–7.

117. Hamaguchi S, Kinugawa S, Tsuchihashi-Makaya M, et al. Weekend versus weekday hospital admission and outcomes during hospitalization for patients due to worsening heart failure: a report from Japanese Cardiac Registry of Heart Failure in Cardiology (JCARE-CARD). Heart Vessels 2014; 29:328–35.

118. Koike S, Tanabe S, Ogawa T, et al. Effect of time and day of admission on 1-month survival and neurologically favourable 1-month survival in out-of-hospital cardiopulmonary arrest patients. Resuscitation 2011;82:863–8.

119. Brooks SC, Schmicker RH, Rea TD, et al. Out-of-hospital cardiac arrest frequency and survival: evidence for temporal variability. Resuscitation 2010; 81:175–81.

120. Qureshi SA, Ahern T, O'Shea R, et al. A standardized code blue team eliminates variable survival from in-hospital cardiac arrest. J Emerg Med 2012;42:74–8.

121. Peberdy MA, Ornato JP, Larkin GL, et al. Survival from in-hospital cardiac arrest during nights and weekends. JAMA 2008;299:785–92.

122. Robinson EJ, Smith GB, Power GS, et al. Risk-adjusted survival for adults following in-hospital cardiac arrest by day of week and time of day: observational cohort study. BMJ Qual Saf 2016; 25(11):832–41.

123. Deshmukh A, Pant S, Kumar G, et al. Comparison of outcomes of weekend versus weekday admissions for atrial fibrillation. Am J Cardiol 2012;110: 208–11.

124. Weeda ER, Hodgdon N, Do T, et al. Association between weekend admission for atrial fibrillation or flutter and in-hospital mortality, procedure utilization, length-of-stay and treatment costs. Int J Cardiol 2016;202:427–9.

125. Brooke H, Gibson A, Tappin D, et al. Case-control study of sudden infant death syndrome in Scotland, 1992–95. BMJ 1997;314:1516.

126. Williams SM, Mitchell EA, Scragg R, et al. Why is sudden infant death syndrome more common at weekends? Arch Dis Child 1997;77:415–9.

127. Alm B, Norvenius SG, Wennergren G, et al. Changes in the epidemiology of sudden infant death syndrome in Sweden 1973–1996. Arch Dis Child 2001;84:24–30.

128. Mooney JA, Helms PJ, Jolliffe IT. Higher incidence of SIDS at weekends, especially in younger infants. Arch Dis Child 2004;89:670–2.

129. Moler FW, Donaldson AE, Meert K, et al. Multicenter cohort study of out-of-hospital pediatric cardiac arrest. Crit Care Med 2011;39:141–9.

130. Kitamura T, Kiyohara K, Nitta M, et al. Survival following witnessed pediatric out-of-hospital cardiac arrests during nights and weekends. Resuscitation 2014;85:1692–8.

131. Meert KL, Donaldson A, Nadkarni V, et al. Pediatric emergency care applied research network multicenter cohort study of in-hospital pediatric cardiac arrest. Pediatr Crit Care Med 2009;10:544–53.

132. Leach CEA, Blair PS, Fleming PJ, et al. Epidemiology of SIDS and explained sudden infant deaths. Pediatrics 1999;104:e43.

133. Spiers PS, Guntheroth WG. The effect of weekend on the risk of sudden infant death syndrome. Pediatrics 1999;104:e58.

134. Dattani N, Cooper N. Trends in cot deaths. Health Stat Q 2000;5:10–6.

135. Black N. Higher mortality in weekend admissions to the hospital: true, false, or uncertain? JAMA 2016; 316:2593–4.

136. Hogan H, Zipfel R, Neuburger J, et al. Avoidability of hospital deaths and association with hospital-wide mortality ratios: retrospective case record review and regression analysis. BMJ 2015;351: h3239.

Sex and Circadian Periodicity of Cardiovascular Diseases
Are Women Sufficiently Represented in Chronobiological Studies?

Roberto Manfredini, MD[a],*, Raffaella Salmi, MD[b],
Rosaria Cappadona, MW[c], Fulvia Signani, PsyD[d],
Stefania Basili, MD[e], Niki Katsiki, MD, MSc, PhD, FRSPH[f]

KEYWORDS

- Biological rhythms • Circadian rhythm • Sex • Clinical studies • Myocardial infarction
- Aortic aneurysm, rupture and dissection • Cerebrovascular disease • Stroke
- Sudden cardiac death

KEY POINTS

- Women are often excluded or underrepresented in clinical trials. Moreover, many studies do not report the number of men/women participants or provide analysis by sex.
- The onset of many life-threatening cardiovascular acute events respects a circadian (~24 hour) periodicity.
- Although 44% of the chronobiologic studies provided separate analysis by sex, these studies included 85% of total cases.
- Morning hours represent a critical time for the onset of acute cardiovascular diseases in men and women.

CLINICAL TRIALS AND SEX DISPARITIES

The problem of exclusion or underrepresentation of women in clinical trials has remained an open question over time. In his special report published in the *New England Journal of Medicine* more than 2 decades ago, Jean-Claude Bennet wrote that, "although the inclusion of women and minorities in medical research is necessary for valid inferences about health and disease in these groups, both women and members of minority groups have been excluded from or underrepresented in many clinical trials."[1] Over that time, the US Food and Drug Administration adopted specific

Disclosure Statement: N. Katsiki has given talks, attended conferences, and participated in trials sponsored by Amgen, Angelini, AstraZeneca, Boehringer Ingelheim, Galenica, MSD, Novartis, Novo Nordisk, Sanofi, and WinMedica, The other authors have nothing to disclose.
[a] Department of Medical Sciences, School of Medicine, Pharmacy and Prevention, University of Ferrara, via L. Ariosto 35, I-41121 Ferrara, Italy; [b] Second Internal Medicine Unit, Azienda Ospedaliera-Universitaria 'S. Anna', Ferrara, Italy; [c] Department of Morphology, Surgery and Experimental Medicine, School of Medicine, Pharmacy and Prevention, University of Ferrara, Ferrara, Italy; [d] Azienda Sanitaria Locale, Ferrara, Italy; [e] Department of Internal Medicine and Medical Specialties, Sapienza University of Rome, Rome, Italy; [f] Second Department of Propaedeutic Internal Medicine, Medical School, Aristotle University of Thessaloniki, Thessaloniki, Greece
* Corresponding author. Department of Medical Sciences, School of Medicine, Pharmacy and Prevention, University of Ferrara, via L. Ariosto 35, I-41121 Ferrara, Italy.
E-mail address: roberto.manfredini@unife.it

Heart Failure Clin 13 (2017) 719–738
http://dx.doi.org/10.1016/j.hfc.2017.05.008
1551-7136/17/© 2017 Elsevier Inc. All rights reserved.

measures aimed at improving and ensuring the representativeness of women participating in clinical trials. In detail, the National Institutes of Health Revitalization (1993) required that National Institutes of Health–funded clinical trials should include women and minorities. Later, in 1998, the US Food and Drug Administration issued the "demographic rule," requiring drug manufacturers to report the age, sex, and race of clinical trial participants in their annual reports to the agency.[2] A study by Geller and colleagues[3] aimed to determine the level of compliance with these guidelines for the inclusion, analysis, and reporting of sex and race/ethnicity in federally funded randomized controlled trials and to compare the current level of compliance with that from 2004. After a PubMed search, 86 articles were included in the analysis (30 were sex specific, and 56 included both men and women). The median enrollment of women in these latter studies was slightly more than one-third (37%), and 75% of the studies did not report any outcomes by sex. Compared with 2004, no significant changes in inclusion or reporting of sex or race/ethnicity were found. A cross-sectional study of 86 novel therapeutics approved by the US Food and Drug Administration (2011–2013) on the basis of 206 pivotal trials was recently done.[4] A similar proportion of pivotal trial participants was found for males and females (mean 50.3% and 49.7%, respectively). Thus, progress has been made since the early 2000s, when the participation of women in clinical research was limited.[4] Even if much has changed since the U.S. federal law mandating the inclusion of women as well as men in clinical trials and analyzing the results by sex, such progress is not considered sufficient by some authors.[5]

CIRCADIAN PERIODICITY OF CARDIOVASCULAR DISEASES

Chronobiology is the biomedical science aimed to study biological rhythms. According to the cycle length, such rhythms may be divided into 3 main types: (a) ultradian (<24 hours, eg, hours, minutes or even seconds), (b) circadian (approximately 24 hours), and (c) infradian (>24 hours, eg, days, weeks, months, or seasons).[6] Circadian rhythms, driven by specific clocks, are the most commonly and widely studied biological rhythms; this topic is the subject of other articles in this special issue.[7,8] In conditions of both health and disease, the cardiovascular system is organized in nature according to a oscillatory circadian order, and several pathophysiological factors, not so harmful if considered alone, are capable to trigger unfavorable, events if they present all together within the same temporal window. This phenomenon opened up the new concept of 'chronorisk.'[9] As a consequence, since the early 1980s a series of studies demonstrated that the occurrence of cardiovascular events is not evenly distributed in time, but shows specific temporal patterns varying with the time of the day.[10,11] In this special issue, specific articles are devoted to circadian and other temporal rhythmic oscillations (eg, weekly, seasonal) for several diseases of the cardiovascular system, such as ischemic heart disease, acute aortic syndromes, and venous thromboembolism.[12–15]

Quoting Berlin and Ellenberg,[16] we aimed to try to answer their questions. Do the results of chronobiological studies apply consistently and equally across all clinically meaningful subclasses of patients enrolled in the studies? In other words, are women sufficiently represented in the studies exploring the circadian periodicity of acute cardiovascular diseases? Can the results of these studies be extrapolated to sex subgroups of patients who did not participate sufficiently in the original research? Thus, a PubMed search was performed, investigating the papers published between 1996 and 2015, focusing on the circadian periodicity of acute myocardial infarction (AMI), sudden cardiac death (SCD) and cardiac arrest, rupture or dissection of aortic aneurysms, and cerebrovascular events (eg, stroke, ischemic and hemorrhagic, intracerebral and subarachnoid hemorrhage). For each of these diseases, data on published studies were collected, including authors, country and year of publication, as well as clinical trial characteristics, including number of patients, age, number of men and women, circadian peak time of occurrence, and analysis by sex (when performed) with respective peak times. Moreover, for each of these diseases a figure showed the weighted mean ratio between number of events per hour during the 24 hours of the day, roughly splitting the day in 2 parts (such as midnight to noon, and noon to midnight) both for men and women. In these figures, the diameter of each circle is proportional to the number of subjects analyzed in each study.

ACUTE MYOCARDIAL INFARCTION

Awareness of a clinical condition represents a crucial point. Although coronary heart disease (CHD) awareness among women has increased over the last decades, it is still suboptimal. In this context, the 2012 American Heart Association National Women's Survey showed that only 56% of women respondents cited CHD as the leading cause of death in women, and only 48% of women considered themselves very well or well informed about CHD.[17] This is confirmed by the results of a study conducted in 3501 young (aged 18–55 years) AMI patients in both sexes, aimed to compare cardiac risk factor prevalence, risk perceptions, and health care provider feedback on CHD and risk modification.[18] Overall, only 53% of patients considered themselves at risk for CHD, 46% reported being told they were at risk, whereas 49% reported that their health care provider had discussed CHD and risk modification. In particular, despite a similar or even greater burden of risk compared with men, women were 11% less likely to report that their health care providers had told them they were at risk for CHD before the index AMI event and 16% less likely to report having had a health care provider discussing with them about CHD and risk reduction strategies.[18] Furthermore, risk factors, symptoms, and treatments of AMI are not always the same for women. Recent statements from the American Heart Association were dedicated to sex-specific differences in the presentation, mechanisms, prevention, and outcomes of AMI in women.[19,20] Of note, sex differences have been reported in atherosclerotic and nonatherosclerotic CHD prevalence,[21] as well as in cardiovascular risk factors and their treatment.[22]

In their milestone study published in the *New England Journal of Medicine* more than 30 years ago, Muller and colleagues[23] first reported an evident 24-hour distribution of AMI, characterized by a morning peak between 6 AM and noon. Such a morning excess of AMI incidence was also found in a later metaanalysis from the same research group from the Harvard University, reporting than 1 in every 11 AMIs is attributed to the morning peak of cardiovascular events.[24] Muller and colleagues[25] reported a series of possible triggers of AMI and its circadian variation, such as physical or mental stress, and hypercoagulation status and coronary vasoconstriction, induced by daily activities. Culic and colleagues[26] analyzed a cohort of AMI patients with or without triggers. A greater proportion of AMIs occurred in the morning (6 AM to noon), and this was more prominent in women than in men, and in patients with triggers. The independent predictors of morning-related AMI included female sex (odds ratio [OR], 1.3; 95% CI, 1.0–1.7), previous angina (OR, 1.24; 95% CI, 1.0–1.9), presence of diabetes mellitus (OR, 1.4; 95% CI, 1.1–2.1), and no use of antiischemic drugs in the previous 24 hours (OR, 1.52; 95%, CI 1.1–2.5). Thus, the association between triggering activities and AMI seems to differ between men and women. These sex differences could be due to different exposure to AMI triggers, as well as

sex-specific mechanisms in triggering AMI, or both.[26]

The results of our search are reported in **Table 1**.[27–53] Twenty-seven studies were included, of which 12 were performed in Europe, 6 in Japan, 5 in the United States, 3 in China, and 1 in India, accounting for nearly 550,000 cases. All studies reported the number of men and women included, and 12 (44%) provided a separate analysis by sex (**Fig. 1**). A marked difference was observed between the earlier (before 2000) studies (7/7 with no analysis by sex) and the more recent ones (12/17, 71%). However, the studies with analysis by sex accounted for 95% of the overall sample.

The presence of a morning peak of AMI was reported in 25 of 27 studies (93%). In 2 and 3 studies (in men and women, respectively) demonstrating a morning peak in the overall sample, the subanalysis by sex did not identify significant rhythmicity. However, a sample of more than 200,000 cases of AMI in women provided strong evidence that, during the morning hours, individuals of both sexes are at the greatest risk of AMI occurrence. A more in-depth knowledge of the precise time frame in which the risk of AMI occurrence is highest (6 AM to noon) could be a precious tool for both patients and health care providers.

SUDDEN CARDIAC DEATH AND CARDIAC ARREST

SCD is an unexpected witnessed death, occurring within 1 hour of the onset of acute symptoms.[54] The underlying etiopathologic factors are not fully known, because different entities may have SCD as the final clinical outcome. A study on a consecutive series of 732 SCD cases, referring to the emergency department and undergoing necropsy, was performed in Italy a couple of decades ago.[55] In 403 of 732 cases (55%), the pathologist identified the final cause of death. The 4 main causes were AMI (55.1%), pulmonary emboli (7.5%), rupture of an aortic aneurysm (3.8%), and stroke (2.3%).[55]

We identified 10 studies, 5 performed in Europe, 2 in Japan, 2 in the United States, and 1 in China (**Table 2**), accounting for 71,000 SCD cases.[40,56–64] All studies reported the number of men and women included, but only 4 (40%) provided a separate analysis by sex (**Fig. 2**). Studies with analysis by sex accounted for only 10% of the overall sample. The presence of a morning peak of SCD onset was reported in 9 of 10 studies (90%). For the 4 studies with analysis by sex, 2 of the 4 showed different patterns (morning

Table 1
Studies on circadian periodicity of acute myocardial infarction (PubMed search 1996–2015)

Author, Year, Country	Cases (n)	M/W	Peak (Overall)	Analysis by Sex	Peak (M)	Peak (W)
Kono et al,[27] 1996, Japan	608	465/143	7 AM and 8–10 AM	No	No analysis	No analysis
Krantz et al,[28] 1996, USA	63	54/9	6–11 AM and 2–6 PM	No	No analysis	No analysis
Spielberg et al,[29] 1996, Germany	1901	1242/659	10 AM	No	No analysis	No analysis
Cannon et al,[30] 1997, USA	7730	4510/3220	6 AM–12 PM	No	No analysis	No analysis
Sayer et al,[31] 1997, UK	1225	900/325	9 AM	No	No analysis	No analysis
Zhou et al,[32] 1998, China	428	267/161	1–7 AM	No	No analysis	No analysis
Kinjo et al,[33] 2001, Japan	1252	956/296	8 AM–12 PM	Yes	<65 y: night	≥65 y: morning
Yamasaki et al,[34] 2002, Japan	725	495/230	6–12 AM	No	No analysis	No analysis
López-Messa et al,[35] 2004, Spain	54,249	40,988/13,261	10 AM	Yes	10 AM	10 AM
Manfredini et al,[36] 2004, Italy	442	320/122	8–9 AM	Yes	8–9 AM	No peak
Tanaka et al,[37] 2004, Japan	174	134/40	6 AM–12 PM	No	No analysis	No analysis
Bhalla et al,[38] 2006, India	459	295/164	6 AM–12 PM and 6 AM–12 PM	No	No analysis	No analysis
Tamura et al,[39] 2006, Japan	21	16/5	6 AM–12 PM	No	No analysis	No analysis

			8 PM–12 AM	Yes	8 PM and 12 AM / 8 AM–12 PM	Not Significant
Savopoulos et al,[40] 2006, Greece	2665	2113/552				
Leiza et al,[41] 2007, Spain	41,244	31,295/9942	10 AM	Yes	10 AM	10 AM
Mahmoud et al,[42] 2011, USA	124	88/36	7 AM	No	No analysis	No analysis
Itaya et al,[43] 2012, Japan	522	272/250	7–10 AM and 7–9 PM	Yes	5–6 AM	7–8 PM
Jia et al,[44] 2012, China	1467	1159/308	7–9 AM	Yes	7–9 AM	7–9 AM
Kanth et al,[45] 2013, USA	519	358/161	11 AM–12 PM	Yes	10–11 AM	10–11 AM
Reavey et al,[46] 2013, Switzerland	361322	201,618/159,704	8–9 AM and 5–6 PM	Yes	<65 y: 10 AM and 4 PM / ≥65 y: 9 AM and 5 PM	<65 y: 8 AM and 6 PM / ≥65 y: 8 AM and 6 PM
Mogabgab et al,[47] 2013, USA	45,218	31,908/13,310	6 AM and 2 PM	Yes	6 AM–2 PM	10 PM–6 AM
Wieringa et al,[48] 2014, Netherlands	6970	5053/1917	9 AM	Yes	12 AM–6 AM	No peak
Rallidis et al,[49] 2015, Greece	256	224/32	6 AM–12 PM	No	No analysis	No analysis
Seneviratna et al,[50] 2015, Singapore	6710	5333/1337	12 AM–6 AM	No	No analysis	No analysis
Fournier et al,[51] 2015, Switzerland	6223	4953/1270	12 AM	No	No analysis	No analysis
Mahmoud et al,[52] 2015, Netherlands	6799	4943/1280	3 AM	Yes	No peak	No peak
Ari et al,[53] 2016, Turkey	252	209/43	6 AM–12 PM	No	No analysis	No analysis

Per chronobiologic definition, 12 AM is intended as midnight, 12 PM as noon.
Abbreviations: M, men; W, women.

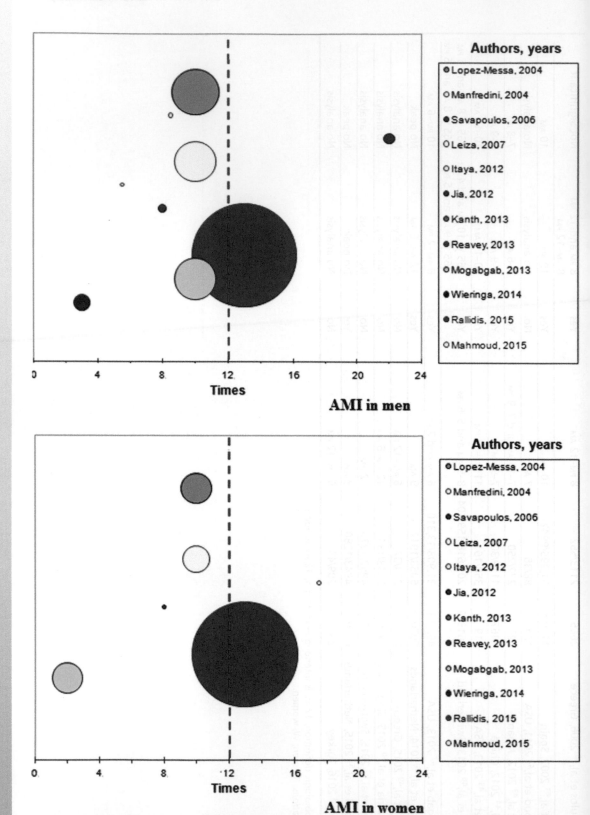

Fig. 1. Acute myocardial infarction (AMI): studies with analysis by sex. Weighted mean ratio between number of events per hour during the 24 hours of the day (midnight to noon, and noon to midnight) both for men and women. The diameter of each circle is proportional to the number of subjects analyzed in study population.

Table 2
Studies on circadian periodicity of sudden cardiac death and cardiac arrest (PubMed search 1996–2015)

Author, Year, Country	Cases (n)	M/W	Peak (Overall)	Analysis by Sex	Peak (M)	Peak (W)
Thakur et al,[56] 1996, USA	2250	1487/763	6 AM–12 PM	Yes	6 AM–12 PM	5–6 PM
Peckova et al,[57] 1998, USA	3690	2425/1264	8–10 AM and 5–7 PM	No	No analysis	No analysis
Arntz et al,[58] 2000, Germany	24,061	12,950/1111	10–11 AM	No	No analysis	No analysis
Soo et al,[59] 2000, UK	748	502/246	No peak	Yes	No peak	No peak
Savopoulos et al,[40] 2006, Greece	2665	2113/552	8–12 PM	Yes	8–12 PM	No peak
Lateef et al,[60] 2008, Singapore	2167	1472/695	8 AM and 7 PM	No	No analysis	No analysis
Pleskot et al,[61] 2008, Czech Republic	495	373/122	6–10 AM	No	No analysis	No analysis
Kriszbacher et al,[62] 2010, Hungary	32,329	17,558/14,771	6 AM and 12 PM	No	No analysis	No analysis
Tsukada et al,[63] 2010, Japan	1293	819/474	6–10 AM and 7–9 PM	Yes	8 AM and 5 PM	5–7 PM
Nakanishi et al,[64] 2011, Japan	1396	803/593	8 AM and 7 PM	No	No analysis	No analysis

Per chronobiologic definition, 12 AM is intended as midnight, 12 PM as noon.
Abbreviations: M, men; W, women.

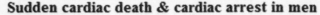

Sudden cardiac death & cardiac arrest in men

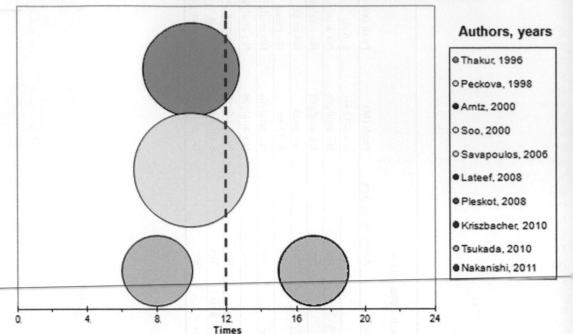

Sudden cardiac death & cardiac arrest in women

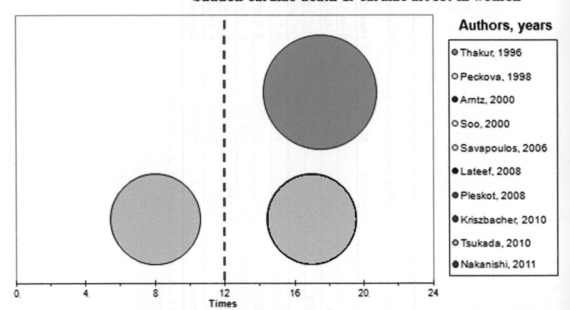

Fig. 2. Sudden cardiac death and cardiac arrest: studies with analysis by sex. Weighted mean ratio between number of events per hour during the 24 hours of the day (midnight to noon, and noon to midnight) both for men and women. The diameter of each circle is proportional to the number of subjects analyzed in study population.

for men, afternoon for women),[56] 1 did not find any peak (both overall sample and subgroups),[59] and 1 identified an evening peak for men, and no peak for women.[40] The very limited number of cases, and in particular the scarce data

regarding sex analysis, as well as the different results obtained, do not permit the extrapolation of any safe conclusion. This may seem apparently strange, because SCD and cardiac arrest share some, but not all, pathophysiologic underlying causes with AMI. In fact, an arrhythmic basis might be often present in SCD and cardiac arrest. For most acute cardiovascular diseases a double peak has been confirmed (8 AM and 8 PM), with the morning peak being more prevalent in comparison with the evening one. In contrast, a double peak distribution (6 AM and 8 PM) has been reported for idiopathic ventricular fibrillation[65] and ventricular tachyarrhythmias.[66] In this latter study, performed in patients with heart failure and implantable cardioverter defibrillators, first and recurrent ventricular tachyarrhythmia episodes were more common in the morning and evening with bimodal peaks from 7:00 to 10:59 AM and 6:00 to 9:59 PM Moreover, ventricular tachyarrhythmia events that occurred during morning hours were associated with a higher mortality (hazard ratio, 2.07; 95% CI, 1.14–3.77, $P = .018$), and women had a significantly higher risk of death than men (hazard ratio, 6.78 [95% CI, 1.55–29.86; $P = .011$] vs hazard ratio, 1.79 [95% CI, 0.92–3.46, $P = .086$], respectively) (interaction $P = .041$).[66] Differences by sex exist for SCD. The incidence rate ratio of SCD in young men, compared with young women, has been found to be 2 (95% CI, 1.7–2.4; $P<.91$),[67] and women have increased odds to survive at hospital discharge after SCD (OR, 1.1; 95% CI, 1.03–1.20; $P = .006$).[68] However, the topic of possible sex differences in the time of onset of arrhythmias has been investigated insufficiently and surely deserves further investigation.

AORTIC ANEURYSMS, RUPTURE, AND DISSECTION

Acute aortic dissection is a life-threatening medical emergency associated with high rates of morbidity and mortality.[69] Classification of aortic dissection is based on anatomic location: Stanford type A dissections involve the ascending aorta and type B occur distal to the left subclavian artery.[70] Results from the International Registry of Acute Aortic Dissection, consisting (at that time) of 12 international referral centers, showed that the mortality of patients with type A dissection treated by surgery was 26% versus 58% for those not receiving surgery (mainly owing to advanced age and comorbidities). Female patients tended to be older (67.9 years vs 60.6 years; $P<.001$) and had a higher mortality rate than males (33.5% vs 24.1%; $P<.001$).[69] In a recent reappraisal in the United States, the burden of mortality attributable to aortic abdominal aneurysms was more than twice the current estimates from the American Heart Association.[70] Females accounted for a disproportionately high

percentage of deaths (45%), despite constituting a low percentage of prevalent cases (21%) compared with men.[71]

The importance of sex in aortic diseases is highlighted in a series of recent studies, conducted in different countries, focusing both on abdominal and thoracic aneurysms. In all these cited studies, women were older than men.[72–77] Different results by sex have been reported for outcome, but generally worst for women.[72–77] As for abdominal aneurysms, greater frequency than men at all aneurysm diameter size intervals (<5.5 or >5.5 cm) and a 4-fold increased frequency of rupture at less than 5.5 cm in women compared with men (2.6% vs 0.6%; $P<.01$),[72] longer duration of stay (5 days vs 4 days, respectively; $P<.001$), higher readmission rate (30 days and 1 year), and higher mortality rate (30 days and 1 year),[73] significantly higher mortality rates after elective endovascular repair, but not after ruptured or elective open repair interventions,[74] a higher risk for 30-day death and major complications after intact aneurysm repair.[75] With regard to thoracic aneurysms, women were reported to have a higher 30-day mortality (7.9% vs 3.5%; $P = .058$) and reduced long-term survival (log-rank $P = .0052$).[76] Female sex was not an independent predictor of operative and late mortality for type A aneurysms.[77]

We identified 9 studies, 4 performed in Europe, 3 in Japan, 1 in Korea, and 1 in the United States, but based on an international registry (**Table 3**), accounting for more than 2300 cases.[78–86] All studies reported the number of men and women included, and 4 of them (44%) provided a separate analysis by sex (**Fig. 3**). Studies with analysis by sex accounted for 59% of the overall sample. The presence of a morning peak of onset was reported in 8 out of 9 studies (89%). As for the 4 studies with analysis by sex, 3 showed a morning peak for either men and women,[78,81,83] and 1 failed to detect any peak for women (probably owing to the very limited sample size, n = 16).[79] These studies may provide sufficient evidence that both men and women are at greatest risk of aortic aneurysms dissection and rupture during the morning hours.

Such circadian pattern of onset of aortic aneurysms dissection or rupture may depend on both unfavorable pathophysiologic mechanisms peaking at that time, and concurrent underlying condition that weakens aortic wall, for example, genetic or acquired diseases, congenital diseases of the connective tissue, or atherosclerosis.[87] Overall, the prevalence, rupture rate, complications, and mortality of aortic aneurysms differ in women compared with men, and the role of sex hormones

Table 3
Studies on circadian periodicity of rupture and/or dissection of aortic aneurysms (PubMed search 1996–2015)

Author, Year, Country	Cases (n)	M/W	Peak (Overall)	Analysis by Sex	Peak (M)	Peak (W)
Gallerani et al,[78] 1997, Italy	70	40/30	8 AM and 8 PM	Yes	8 AM and 8 PM	8 AM and 8 PM
Manfredini et al,[79] 1999, Italy	136	120/16	8 AM and 8 PM	Yes	8 AM and 8 PM	Not Significant
Kojima et al,[80] 2002, Japan	267	188/79	10 AM–12 PM	No	No analysis	No analysis
Mehta et al,[81] 2002, IRAD Registry	957	653/304	8–9 AM	Yes	8–9 AM	9–10 AM
Sumiyoshi et al,[82] 2002, Japan	312	214/98	8–11 AM and 5–7 PM	No	No analysis	No analysis
Lasica et al,[83] 2006, Serbia-Montenegro	204	136/68	9–10 AM	Yes	6 AM–12 PM	6 AM–12 PM
Killeen et al,[84] 2007, Ireland	148	124/44	8–10 AM and 3 PM	No	No analysis	No analysis
Ryu et al,[85] 2010, Korea	166	85/81	12 PM–2 PM	No	No analysis	No analysis
Seguchi et al,[86] 2015, Japan	68	41/27	8–9 AM and 5–6 PM	No	No analysis	No analysis

Per chronobiologic definition, 12 AM is intended as midnight, 12 PM as noon.
Abbreviations: M, men; W, women.

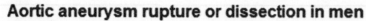

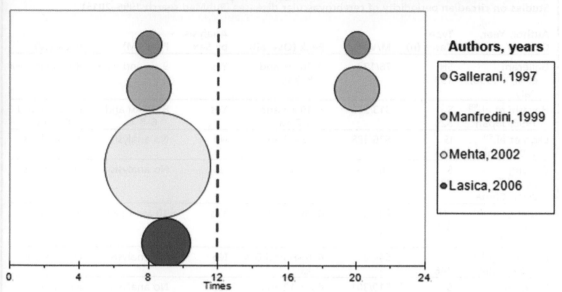

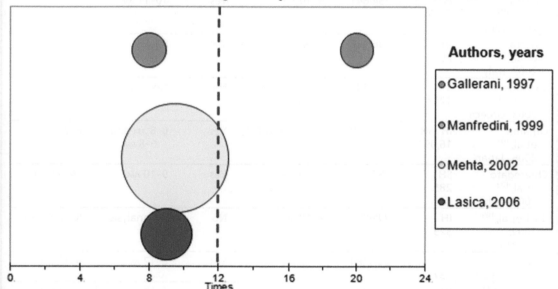

Fig. 3. Aortic aneurysms, rupture, or dissection: studies with analysis by sex. Weighted mean ratio between number of events per hour during the 24 hours of the day (midnight to noon, and noon to midnight) both for men and women. The diameter of each circle is proportional to the number of subjects analyzed in study population.

has some evidence in animals models, but need further research in humans.[88] Future research should focus also on aortic weakening processes. In this context, collagen composition in the aneurysm wall is similar in men and women, with the exception of collagen cross-linking.[89] In fact, women had more lysyl pyridinoline than men (0.14 vs 0.07; P = .005), resulting in a lower

hydroxyl pyridoline:lysyl pyridinoline ratio (3.28 vs 8.41; P = .003).[89] In contrast, less elastin is found in the non–thrombus-covered aneurysm wall in women, with a simultaneously higher level of matrix metalloproteinase-9 in women compared with men (−0.83 vs 0.09; P = .041), suggesting possible differences by sex in the elastolytic processes.[90]

Table 4
Studies on circadian periodicity of cerebrovascular diseases (PubMed search 1996–2015)

Author, Year, Country	Type Cases (n)	M/W	Peak (Overall)	Analysis by Sex	Peak (M)	Peak (W)
Gallerani et al,[97] 1996, Italy	SH 199	76/123	9–10 AM and 8–9 PM	Yes	9 AM and 9 PM	9 AM and 9 PM
Hayashi et al,[98] 1996, Japan	S 529	313/216	8–10 AM and 6–8 PM	Yes	8–10 AM and 6–8 PM	8–10 AM and 6–8 PM
Lago et al,[99] 1998, Spain	IS 914	526/388	6 AM–12 PM	No	No analysis	No analysis
Cheung et al,[100] 2001, China	S 832	465/367	6 AM–12 PM	No	No analysis	No analysis
Feigin et al,[101] 2001, Australia	SH 689	248/441	8 AM–12 PM	Yes	10 AM–12 PM	8 AM–10 PM
Bhalla et al,[102] 2002, India	S 146	94/52	4–8 AM and 0–4 PM	No	No analysis	No analysis
Stergiou et al,[103] 2002, Greece	S 811	510/301	6 AM–12 PM and 4–8 PM	No	No analysis	No analysis
Casetta et al,[104] 2002, Italy	IS 1395	754/641	9–10 AM	Yes	10–11 AM	9–11 AM
Casetta et al,[105] 2002, Italy	IH 258	136/122	8 AM	Yes	8 AM	8 AM
Spengos et al,[106] 2003, Greece	S 1253	761/492	8–10 AM and 4–6 PM	No	No analysis	No analysis
Omama et al,[107] 2006, Japan	IH -SH 16,997	9121/7876	6–8 AM and 6–8 PM	Yes	6–8 AM and 6–8 PM	6–8 PM
Chieregato et al,[108] 2007, Italy	SH 285	189/96	9–10 AM	Yes	9–10 AM	10–11 AM
Butt et al,[109] 2009, Pakistan	IH 329	249/80	8–12 AM	No	No analysis	No analysis
Turin et al,[110] 2009, Japan	IS 637	353/284	6–12 AM	Yes	6–12 AM	6–12 AM
Turin et al,[111] 2010, Japan	IH 429	186/243	6 AM–12 PM	Yes	6–12 AM	No peak
Turin et al,[112] 2012, Japan	S 1080	549/531	6 AM–12 PM	No	No analysis	No analysis
Temes et al,[113] 2012, USA	SH 251	79/172	5–11 AM	Yes	5–11 AM	5–11 AM
Fodor et al,[114] 2014, Romania	S 1083	572/511	6 AM–12 PM	No	No analysis	No analysis

Per chronobiologic definition, 12 AM is intended as midnight, 12 PM as noon.
Abbreviations: IH, intracerebral hemorrhage; IS, ischemic stroke; M, men; S, stroke; SH, subarachnoid hemorrhage; W, women.

CEREBROVASCULAR DISEASES

Stroke is the culmination of a heterogeneous group of cerebrovascular diseases that is manifested as ischemia or hemorrhage in 1 or more brain vessels.[91] Stroke has a large negative effect on the society, being the fifth leading cause of death for men and the third leading cause for women.[92] Atrial fibrillation is the most common arrhythmia that increases the risk of

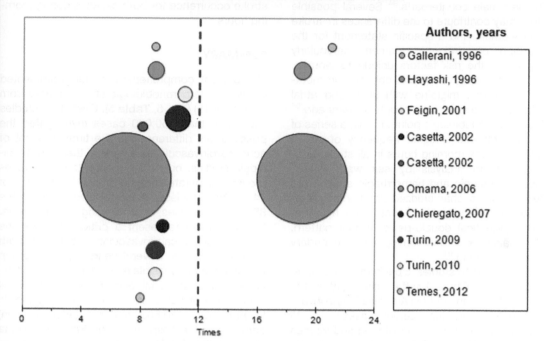

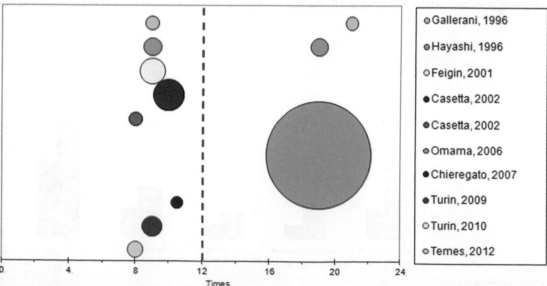

Fig. 4. Cerebrovascular accidents: studies with analysis by sex. Weighted mean ratio between number of events per hour during the 24 hours of the day (midnight to noon, and noon to midnight) both for men and women. The diameter of each circle is proportional to the number of subjects analyzed in study population.

thromboembolism and stroke.[93] Atrial fibrillation does not exhibit the same risks for women and men: in a recent review of more than 30 studies published since 1999 examining the association between sex and thromboembolic risk, 17 studies reported that female sex was a significant risk factor for stroke.[93] Women seem to have an increased risk for stroke (1.31-fold) compared with their male counterparts.[94] Several possible factors may contribute to the differences in stroke risk in women, and a specific statement for the prevention of stroke in women, particularly focusing on the risk factors unique to women, such as reproductive factors, obesity, the metabolic syndrome, migraine with aura, and atrial fibrillation, were released a couple of years ago.[95]

From a chronobiologic point of view, a series of studies confirmed a higher frequency of stroke incidence in the morning hours in all stroke subtypes, but no analysis by sex was done.[96] Although ischemic and hemorrhagic strokes are different entities, characterized by different pathophysiologic mechanisms, it has been hypothesized an identical double-peak 24-hour pattern, with a main peak in the morning and a secondary one in the evening.[91]

We identified 18 studies, 8 performed in Europe, 5 in Japan, 1 in China, 1 in the United States, 1 in India, 1 in Pakistan, and 1 in Australia (**Table 4**), accounting for more than 28,000 cases.[97–114] All studies reported the number of men and women included, and 10 of 18 (56%) provided a separate analysis by sex, accounting for 85% of the overall sample. The presence of a morning peak of stroke incidence was reported in 18 of the 18 studies (100%). As for the 10 studies with analysis by sex (**Fig. 4**), 8 showed a morning peak for men or women,[97,98,101,104,105,108,110,113] 1 showed the main peak for women in the evening,[107] and 1 found a morning peak in total sample and men, but no peak for women.[111] Similar to AMI, a sample of more than 12,000 cases of stroke in women provides discrete evidence that highest risk of stroke occurrence for both sexes is during morning hours.

SUMMARY

The present comprehensive review commented on worldwide chronobiologic studies (dated from 1996 to 2015) (**Fig. 5**, **Table 5**). Overall, 64 studies with more than 650,000 cases investigated the possible sex differences in the time of onset of acute cardiovascular diseases. In these chronobiologic studies, only a low percentage of studies provided separate analysis by sex (an average of 44%). Nevertheless, these studies included the 85% of total cases, thus allowing robust results. Morning hours represent a critical time for the onset of acute cardiovascular diseases in both men and women. Several years ago, our group investigated the possible existence of a sex difference in the seasonal and weekly patterns of occurrence of acute cardiovascular diseases.[115] In particular, 130,693 patients (45% women) admitted to the hospitals of the Emilia-Romagna region of Italy for AMI, stroke, transient ischemic attack, aortic diseases, and pulmonary embolism were investigated for monthly and daily percentage of admissions. The results confirmed the

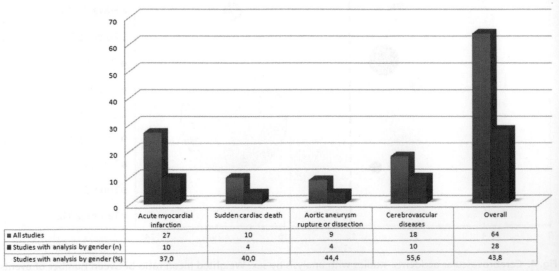

	Acute myocardial infarction	Sudden cardiac death	Aortic aneurysm rupture or dissection	Cerebrovascular diseases	Overall
■ All studies	27	10	9	18	64
■ Studies with analysis by gender (n)	10	4	4	10	28
Studies with analysis by gender (%)	37,0	40,0	44,4	55,6	43,8

Fig. 5. Comprehensive review commented on worldwide chronobiologic studies (dated from 1996 to 2015): overall studies and number (and percentage) of studies with separate analysis by sex.

Table 5
Studies on circadian periodicity of acute cardiovascular disease (1996–2015) and men/women distribution (overall)

Disease	Studies (n)	Cases (n)	M/W (n)	Studies with Analysis by Sex (n/%)	Cases in Studies with Analysis by Sex (n)	Percent of Cases in Studies with Analysis by Sex/Overall (%)	M/W in Studies with Analysis by Sex (n)	M/W in Studies with Analysis by Sex (%)
AMI	27	549,568	340,168/209,400	12/44.4	522,669	95.1	320,983/20,1093	61.4/38.6
SCD	10	71,094	40,502/30,592	4/40.0	6956	9.8	4921/2035	70.7/29.3
AARD	9	2328	1601/727	4/44.4	1367	58.7	978/389	71.5/28.5
CD	18	28,117	15,181/12,936	10/55.6	21,669	77.1	11,455/10,214	52.9/47.1
Overall	64	651,107	382,998/253,655	28/43.8	552,142	84.8	338,337/213,805	61.3/38.7

Abbreviations: AARD, aortic aneurysm rupture or dissection; AMI, acute myocardial infarction; CD, cerebrovascular diseases; M/W, men/women; SCD, sudden cardiac death.

presence of the well-known peaks of occurrence in winter, and especially in January, and on Monday, but with no differences between men and women.[115]

'Time is a gentleman,' and it makes not differences in striking men and women in a similar temporal frame. However, cardiovascular disease remains the leading cause of death in women. Even though morning is the preferred risk time for heart attack,[116] we all have to keep in mind that cardiovascular risk factors, both traditional and emerging, are different in women,[22,117] as well as the presenting signs and symptoms.[19]

ACKNOWLEDGMENTS

The authors thank Mrs Daniela Giulio and Alfredo De Giorgi, MD, for their help in producing the final art works.

REFERENCES

1. Bennett JC. Inclusion of women in clinical trials–policies for population subgroups. N Engl J Med 1993;329:288–92.
2. U.S. Food and Drug Administration. Investigational new drug applications and new drug applications. 21 CFR 312, 63 FR 6854. 1998. Available at: http://www.gpo.gov/fdsys/granule/FR-1998-02-11/98-3422. Accessed December 12, 2016.
3. Geller SE, Koch A, Pellettieri B, et al. Inclusion, analysis, and reporting of sex and race/ethnicity in clinical trials: have we made progress? J Womens Health (Larchmt) 2011;20:315–20.
4. Downing NS, Shah ND, Neiman JH, et al. Participation of the elderly, women, and minorities in pivotal trials supporting 2011-2013 U.S. Food and Drug Administration approvals. Trials 2016; 17:199.
5. Mazure CM, Jones DP. Twenty years and still counting: including women as participants and studying sex and gender in biomedical research. BMC Womens Health 2015;15:94.
6. Manfredini R, Manfredini F, Fabbian F, et al. Chronobiology of Takotsubo syndrome and myocardial infarction: analogies and differences. Heart Fail Clin 2016;12:531–42.
7. Tarquini R, Mazzoccoli G. Clock genes, metabolism and cardiovascular risk. Heart Fail Clin 2017;13(4):645–55.
8. Mistry P, Duong A, Kirshenbaum L, et al. Circadian clocks and preclinical translation. Heart Fail Clin 2017;13(4):657–72.
9. Portaluppi F, Manfredini R, Fersini C. From a static to a dynamic concept of risk: the circadian epidemiology of cardiovascular events. Chronobiol Int 1999;16:33–49.
10. Manfredini R, Boari B, Salmi R, et al. Twenty-four-hour patterns in occurrence and pathophysiology of acute cardiovascular events and ischemic heart disease. Chronobiol Int 2013;30:6–16.
11. Smolensky MH, Portaluppi F, Manfredini R, et al. Diurnal and twenty-four hour patterning of human diseases: cardiac, vascular, and respiratory diseases, conditions, and syndromes. Sleep Med Rev 2015;21:3–11.
12. Fabbian F, Bathia S, De Giorgi A, et al. Circadian periodicity of ischemic heart disease. Heart Fail Clin 2017;13(4):673–80.
13. Siddiqi HK, Bossone E, Pyeritz RE, et al. Chronobiology of acute aortic syndromes. Heart Fail Clin 2017;13(4):697–701.
14. Gallerani M, Pala M, Fedeli U. Circaseptan periodicity of cardiovascular diseases. Heart Fail Clin 2017;13(4):703–19.
15. Fantoni C, Dentali F, Ageno W. Chronobiologic aspects of venous thromboembolism. Heart Fail Clin 2017;13(4):691–6.
16. Berlin JA, Ellenberg SS. Inclusion of women in clinical trials. BMC Med 2009;7:56.
17. Mosca L, Hammond G, Mochari-Greenberger H, et al. Fifteen-year trends in awareness of heart disease in women: results of a 2012 American Heart Association national survey. Circulation 2013;127:1254–63.
18. Leifheit-Limson EC, D'Onofrio G, Daneshvar M, et al. Sex differences in cardiac risk factors, perceived risk, and health care provider discussion of risk and risk modification among young patients with acute myocardial infarction: the VIRGO Study. J Am Coll Cardiol 2015;66:1949–57.
19. Mehta LS, Beckie TM, DeVon HA, et al, on behalf of the American Heart Association Cardiovascular Disease in Women and Special Populations Committee of the Council on Clinical Cardiology, Council on Epidemiology and Prevention, Council on Cardiovascular and Stroke Nursing, and Council on Quality of Care and Outcomes Research. Acute myocardial infarction in women. A scientific statement from the American Heart Association. Circulation 2016;133:916–47.
20. McSweeney JC, Rosenfeld AG, Abel WM, et al, on behalf of the American Heart Association Cardiovascular Council on Cardiovascular and Stroke Nursing, Council on Clinical Cardiology, Council on Epidemiology and Prevention, Council on Hypertension, Council on Lifestyle and Cardiometabolic Health, and Council on Quality of Care and Outcomes Research. Preventing and experiencing ischemic heart disease as a woman: state of the science. A scientific statement from the American Heart Association. Circulation 2016;133:1302–31.
21. Kolovou G, Kolovou V, Koutelou M, et al. Atherosclerotic and non-atherosclerotic coronary heart disease in women. Curr Med Chem 2015;22:3555–64.

22. Katsiki N, Mikhailidis DP. Emerging vascular risk factors in women: any differences from men? Curr Med Chem 2015;22:3552–4.

23. Muller JE, Stone PH, Turi ZG, et al. Circadian variation in the frequency of onset of acute myocardial infarction. N Engl J Med 1985;313: 1315–22.

24. Cohen MC, Rohtla KM, Lavery CE, et al. Meta-analysis of the morning excess of acute myocardial infarction and sudden cardiac death. Am J Cardiol 1997;79:1512–5.

25. Muller JE, Tofler GH, Stone PH. Circadian variation and triggers of onset of acute cardiovascular disease. Circulation 1989;79:733–43.

26. Culic V, Eterovic D, Miric D, et al. Gender differences in triggering of acute myocardial infarction. Am J Cardiol 2000;85:753–6.

27. Kono T, Morita H, Nishina T, et al. Circadian variations of onset of acute myocardial infarction and efficacy of thrombolytic therapy. J Am Coll Cardiol 1996;27:774–8.

28. Krantz DS, Kop WJ, Gabbay FH, et al. Circadian variation of ambulatory myocardial ischemia. Triggering by daily activities and evidence for an endogenous circadian component. Circulation 1996;93:1364–71.

29. Spielberg C, Falkenhahn D, Willich SN, et al. Circadian, day-of-week, and seasonal variability in myocardial infarction: comparison between working and retired patients. Am Heart J 1996;132: 579–85.

30. Cannon CP, McCabe CH, Stone PH, et al. Circadian variation in the onset of unstable angina and non-Q-wave acute myocardial infarction (the TIMI III Registry and TIMI IIIB). Am J Cardiol 1997;79: 253–8.

31. Sayer JW, Wilkinson P, Ranjadayalan K, et al. Attenuation or absence of circadian and seasonal rhythms of acute myocardial infarction. Heart 1997;77:325–9.

32. Zhou RH, Xi B, Gao HQ, et al. Circadian and septadian variation in the occurrence of acute myocardial infarction in a Chinese population. Jpn Circ J 1998;62:190–2.

33. Kinjo K, Sato H, Sato H, et al. Circadian variation of the onset of acute myocardial infarction in the Osaka area, 1998-1999: characterization of morning and nighttime peaks. Jpn Circ J 2001;65: 617–20.

34. Yamasaki F, Seo H, Furuno T, et al. Effect of age on chronological variation of acute myocardial infarction onset: study in Japan. Clin Exp Hypertens 2002;24:1–9.

35. López Messa JB, Garmendia Leiza JR, Aguilar García MD, et al. [Cardiovascular risk factors in the circadian rhythm of acute myocardial infarction]. Rev Esp Cardiol 2004;57:850–8 [in Spanish].

36. Manfredini R, Boari B, Bressan S, et al. Influence of circadian rhythm on mortality after myocardial infarction: data from a prospective cohort of emergency calls. Am J Emerg Med 2004;22:555–9.

37. Tanaka A, Kawarabayashi T, Fukuda D, et al. Circadian variation of plaque rupture in acute myocardial infarction. Am J Cardiol 2004; 93:1–5.

38. Bhalla A, Sachdev A, Lehl SS, et al. Ageing and circadian variation in cardiovascular events. Singapore Med J 2006;47:305–8.

39. Tamura A, Watanabe T, Nagase K, et al. Circadian variation in symptomatic subacute stent thrombosis after bare metal coronary stent implantation. Am J Cardiol 2006;97:195–7.

40. Savopoulos C, Ziakas A, Hatzitolios A, et al. Circadian rhythm in sudden cardiac death: a retrospective study of 2665 cases. Angiology 2006;57:197–204.

41. Leiza JR, de Llano JM, Messa JB, et al, ARIAM Study Group. New insights into the circadian rhythm of acute myocardial infarction in subgroups. Chronobiol Int 2007;24:129–41.

42. Mahmoud KD, Lennon RJ, Ting HH, et al. Circadian variation in coronary stent thrombosis. JACC Cardiovasc Interv 2011;4:183–90.

43. Itaya H, Takagi T, Sugi K, et al. Contents of second peak in the circadian variation of acute myocardial infarction in the Japanese population. J Cardiol 2012;59:147–53.

44. Jia EZ, Xu ZX, Cai HZ, et al. Time distribution of the onset of chest pain in subjects with acute ST-elevation myocardial infarction: an eight-year, single-center study in China. PLoS One 2012;7: e32478.

45. Kanth R, Ittaman S, Rezkalla S. Circadian patterns of ST elevation myocardial infarction in the new millennium. Clin Med Res 2013;11:66–72.

46. Reavey M, Saner H, Paccaud F, et al. Exploring the periodicity of cardiovascular events in Switzerland: variation in deaths and hospitalizations across seasons, day of the week and hour of the day. Int J Cardiol 2013;168:2195–200.

47. Mogagbab O, Wiviott SD, Antman EM, et al. Relation between time of symptom onset of ST-segment elevation myocardial infarction and patient baseline characteristics: from the National Cardiovascular Registry. Clin Cardiol 2013;36: 222–7.

48. Wieringa WG, Lexis CP, Mahmoud KD, et al. Time of symptom onset and value of myocardial blush and infarct size on prognosis in patients with ST-elevation myocardial infarction. Chronobiol Int 2014;31:797–806.

49. Rallidis LS, Triantafyllis AS, Sakadakis EA, et al. Circadian pattern of symptoms onset in patients ≤35 years presenting with ST-segment elevation

acute myocardial infarction. Eur J Intern Med 2015; 26:607–10.

50. Seneviratna A, Lim GH, Devi A, et al. Circadian dependence of infarct size and acute heart failure in ST elevation myocardial infarction. PLoS One 2015;10:e0128526.

51. Fournier S, Taffé P, Radovanovic D, et al. Myocardial infarct size and mortality depend on the time of day-a large multicenter study. PLoS One 2015; 10:e0119157.

52. Mahmoud KD, Nijsten MW, Wieringa WG, et al. Independent association between symptom onset time and infarct size in patients with ST-elevation myocardial infarction undergoing primary percutaneous coronary intervention. Chronobiol Int 2015; 32:468–77.

53. Arı H, Sonmez O, Koc F, et al. Circadian rhythm of infarct size and left ventricular function evaluated with tissue doppler echocardiography in ST elevation myocardial infarction. Heart Lung Circ 2016; 25:250–6.

54. Goldstein S. The necessity of a uniform definition of sudden coronary death: witnessed death within 1 hour of the onset of acute symptoms. Am Heart J 1982;103:156–9.

55. Manfredini R, Portaluppi F, Grandi E, et al. Out-of-hospital sudden death referring to an Emergency Department. J Clin Epidemiol 1996;49: 865–8.

56. Thakur RK, Hoffmann RG, Olson DW, et al. Circadian variation in sudden cardiac death: effects of age, sex, and initial cardiac rhythm. Ann Emerg Med 1996;27:29–34.

57. Peckova M, Fahrenbruch CE, Cobb LA, et al. Circadian variations in the occurrence of cardiac arrests: initial and repeat episodes. Circulation 1998;98:31–9.

58. Arntz HR, Willich SN, Schreiber C, et al. Diurnal, weekly and seasonal variation of sudden death. Population-based analysis of 24,061 consecutive cases. Eur Heart J 2000;21:315–20.

59. Soo LH, Gray D, Young T, et al. Circadian variation in witnessed out of hospital cardiac arrest. Heart 2000;84:370–6.

60. Lateef F, Ong ME, Alfred T, et al. Circadian rhythm in cardiac arrest: the Singapore experience. Singapore Med J 2008;49:719–23.

61. Pleskot M, Hazulova R, Stritecka H, et al. The highest incidence of out-of-hospital cardiac arrest during a circadian period in survivors. Int Heart J 2008;49:183–92.

62. Kriszbacher I, Bodis J, Boncz I, et al. The time of sunrise and the number of hours with daylight may influence the diurnal rhythm of acute heart attack mortality. Int J Cardiol 2010;140:118–20.

63. Tsukada T, Ikeda T, Ishiguro H, et al. Circadian variation in out-of-hospital cardiac arrests due to

cardiac cause in a Japanese patient population. Circ J 2010;74:1880–7.

64. Nakanishi N, Nishizawa S, Kitamura Y, et al. Circadian, weekly, and seasonal mortality variations in out-of-hospital cardiac arrest in Japan: analysis from AMI-Kyoto Multicenter Risk Study database. Am J Emerg Med 2011;29:1037–43.

65. Aizawa Y, Sato M, Ohno S, et al. Circadian pattern of fibrillatory events in non-Brugada-type idiopathic ventricular fibrillation with a focus on J waves. Heart Rhythm 2014;11:2261–6.

66. Ruwald MH, Moss AJ, Zareba W, et al. Circadian distribution of ventricular tachyarrhythmias and association with mortality in the MADIT-CRT trial. J Cardiovasc Electrophysiol 2015;26:291–9.

67. Winkel BG, Risgaard B, Bjune T, et al. Gender differences in sudden cardiac death in the young –a nationwide study. BMC Cardiovasc Disord 2017; 17;19.

68. Bouguin W, Mustafich H, Marijon E, et al. Gender and survival after sudden cardiac arrest: a systematic review and meta-analysis. Resuscitation 2015; 94:55–60.

69. Hagan PG, Nienaber CA, Isselbacher EM, et al. The International Registry of Acute Aortic Dissection (IRAD): new insights into an old disease. JAMA 2000;283:897–903.

70. Daily PO, Trueblood HW, Stinson EB, et al. Management of acute aortic dissections. Ann Thorac Surg 1970;10:237–47.

71. Stuntz M. Modeling the burden of abdominal aortic aneurysm in the USA in 2013. Cardiology 2016; 135:127–31.

72. Skibba AA, Evans JR, Hopkins SP, et al. Reconsidering gender relative to risk of rupture in the contemporary management of abdominal aortic aneurysms. J Vas Surg 2015;62:1429–36.

73. Lowry D, Singh J, Mytton J, et al. Sex-related outcome inequalities in endovascular aneurysm repair. Eur J Vasc Endovasc Surg 2016;52:518–25.

74. Nevidomskyte D, Shalhub S, Singh N, et al. Influence of gender on abdominal aortic aneurysm repair in the community. Ann Vasc Surg 2017;39: 128–36.

75. Deery SE, Soden PA, Zettervall SL, et al. Sex differences in mortality and morbidity following repair of intact abdominal aortic aneurysms. J Vasc Surg 2017;65(4):1006–13.

76. Beller CJ, Farag M, Wannaku S, et al. Gender-specific differences in outcome of ascending aortic aneurysm surgery. PLoS One 2015;10:e0124461.

77. Fukui T, Tabata M, Morita S, et al. Gender differences in patients undergoing surgery for acute type A aortic dissection. J Thorac Cardiovasc Surg 2015;150:581–7.e1.

78. Gallerani M, Portaluppi F, Grandi E, et al. Circadian rhythmicity in the occurrence of spontaneous acute

dissection and rupture of thoracic aorta. J Thorac Cardiovasc Surg 1997;113:603–4.

79. Manfredini R, Portaluppi F, Zamboni P, et al. Circadian variation in spontaneous rupture of abdominal aorta. Lancet 1999;353:643–4.

80. Kojima S, Sumiyoshi M, Nakata Y, et al. Triggers and circadian distribution of the onset of acute aortic dissection. Circ J 2002;66:232–5.

81. Mehta RH, Manfredini R, Hassan F, et al. Chronobiological patterns of acute aortic dissection. Circulation 2002;106:1110–5.

82. Sumiyoshi M, Kojima S, Arima M, et al. Circadian, weekly, and seasonal variation at the onset of acute aortic dissection. Am J Cardiol 2002;89:619–23.

83. Lasica RM, Perunicic J, Mrdovic I, et al. Temporal variations at the onset of spontaneous acute aortic dissection. Int Heart J 2006;47:585–95.

84. Killeen S, Neary P, O'Sullivan M, et al. Daily diurnal variation in admissions for ruptured abdominal aortic aneurysms. World J Surg 2007; 31:1869–71.

85. Ryu HM, Lee JH, Kwon YS, et al. Examining the relationship between triggering activities and the circadian distribution of acute aortic dissection. Korean Circ J 2010;40:565–72.

86. Seguchi M, Wada H, Sakakura K, et al. Circadian variation of acute aortic dissection. Int Heart J 2015;56:324–8.

87. Manfredini R, Boari B, Gallerani M, et al. Chronobiology of rupture and dissection of aortic aneurysms. J Vasc Surg 2004;40:382–8.

88. Makrygiannis G, Courtois A, Drion P, et al. Sex differences in abdominal aortic aneurysm: the role of sex hormones. Ann Vasc Surg 2014;28:1946–58.

89. Villard C, Eriksson P, Hanemaaijer R, et al. The composition of collagen in the aneurysm wall of men and women. J Vasc Surg 2016. http://dx.doi.org/10.1016/j.jvs.2016.02.056.

90. Villard C, Eriksson P, Swedenborg J, et al. Differences in elastin and elastolytic enzymes between men and women with abdominal aortic aneurysm. Aorta (Stamford) 2014;2:179–85.

91. Manfredini R, Boari B, Smolensky MH, et al. Circadian variation in stroke onset: identical temporal pattern in ischemic and hemorrhagic events. Chronobiol Int 2005;22:417–53.

92. Mozaffarian D, Benjamin EJ, Go AS, et al. Executive summary: heart disease and stroke statistics – 2016 update. A report from the American Heart Association. Circulation 2016;133:447–54.

93. Cheng EY, Kong MH. Gender differences of thromboembolic events in atrial fibrillation. Am J Cardiol 2016;117:1021–7.

94. Wagstaff AJ, Overvad TF, Lip GY, et al. Is female sex a risk factor for stroke and thromboembolism in patients with atrial fibrillation? A systematic review and meta-analysis. QJM 2014;107:955–67.

95. Bushnell C, McCullough LD, Awad IA, et al. Guidelines for the prevention of stroke in women. A statement for healthcare professionals from the American Heart Association/American Stroke Association. Stroke 2014;45:1545–88.

96. Elliott WJ. Circadian variation in the timing of stroke onset: a meta-analysis. Stroke 1998;29:992–6.

97. Gallerani M, Portaluppi F, Maida G, et al. Circadian and circannual rhythmicity in the occurrence of subarachnoid hemorrhage. Stroke 1996;27:1793–7.

98. Hayashi S, Toyoshima H, Tanabe N, et al. Daily peaks in the incidence of sudden cardiac death and fatal stroke in Niigata Prefecture. Jpn Circ J 1996;60:193–200.

99. Lago A, Geffner D, Tembl J, et al. Circadian variation in acute ischemic stroke: a hospital-based study. Stroke 1998;29:1873–5.

100. Cheung RT, Mak W, Chan KH. Circadian variation of stroke onset in Hong Kong Chinese: a hospital-based study. Cerebrovasc Dis 2001;12:1–6.

101. Feigin VL, Anderson CS, Anderson NE, et al, Australasian Co-operative Research Group on Subarachnoid Haemorrhage Study (ACROSS) and Auckland Stroke Studies. Is there a temporal pattern in the occurrence of subarachnoid hemorrhage in the southern hemisphere? Pooled data from 3 large, population-based incidence studies in Australasia, 1981 to 1997. Stroke 2001;32:613–9.

102. Bhalla A, Singh R, Sachdev A, et al. Circadian pattern in cerebrovascular disorders. Neurol India 2002;50:526–7.

103. Stergiou GS, Vemmos KN, Pliarchopoulou KM, et al. Parallel morning and evening surge in stroke onset, blood pressure, and physical activity. Stroke 2002;33:1480–6.

104. Casetta I, Granieri E, Fallica E, et al. Patient demographic and clinical features and circadian variation in onset of ischemic stroke. Arch Neurol 2002;59:48–53.

105. Casetta I, Granieri E, Portaluppi F, et al. Circadian variability in hemorrhagic stroke. JAMA 2002;287:1266–7.

106. Spengos K, Vemmos KM, Tsivgoulis G, et al. Two-peak temporal distribution of stroke onset in Greek patients. A hospital-based study. Cerebrovasc Dis 2003;15:70–7.

107. Omama S, Yoshida Y, Ogawa A, et al. Differences in circadian variation of cerebral infarction, intracerebral hemorrhage and subarachnoid haemorrhage by situation at onset. J Neurol Neurosurg Psychiatr 2006;77:1345–9.

108. Chieregato A, Tagliaferri F, Cocciolo F, et al. Can circadian rhythms influence onset and outcome of nontraumatic subarachnoid hemorrhage? Am J Emerg Med 2007;25:728–30.

109. Butt MU, Zakaria M, Hussain HM. Circadian pattern of onset of ischaemic and haemorrhagic strokes,

and their relation with sleep/wake cycle. J Pak Med Assoc 2009;59:129–32.

110. Turin TC, Kita Y, Rumana N, et al. Morning surge in circadian periodicity of ischaemic stroke is independent of conventional risk factors status: findings from the Takashima Stroke Registry 1990-2003. Eur J Neurol 2009;16:843–51.

111. Turin TC, Kita Y, Rumana N, et al. Diurnal variation in onset of hemorrhagic stroke is independent of risk factor status: Takashima Stroke Registry. Neuroepidemiology 2010;34:25–33.

112. Turin TC, Kita Y, Rumana N, et al. Is there any circadian variation consequence on acute case fatality of stroke? Takashima Stroke Registry, Japan (1990-2003). Acta Neurol Scand 2012;125:206–12.

113. Temes RE, Bleck T, Dugar S, et al. Circadian variation in ictus by aneurysmal subarachnoid hemorrhage. Neurocrit Care 2012;16:219–23.

114. Fodor DM, Babiciu I, Perju-Dumbrava L. Circadian variation of stroke onset: a hospital-based study. Clujul Med 2014;87:242–9.

115. Manfredini R, Fabbian F, Pala M, et al. Seasonal and weekly patterns of occurrence of acute cardiovascular diseases: does a gender difference exist? J Womens Health (Larchmt) 2011;20:1663–8.

116. Blue L. When are you most likely to have a heart attack? TIME 2008. Available at: http://content.time.com/time/health/article/0, 8599, 1825044,00.html.

117. Shaw LJ, Pepine CM, Reis SE, et al. Insights from the NHLBI-Sponsored Women's Ischemia Syndrome Evaluation (WISE) Study: part I: gender differences in traditional and novel risk factors, symptom evaluation, and gender-optimized diagnostic strategies. J Am Coll Cardiol 2006;47(3 Suppl):S4–20.

Signal Transduction and Chronopharmacology of Regulation of Circadian Cardiovascular Rhythms in Animal Models of Human Hypertension

Björn Lemmer, Prof.em., Dr.med., Dr.h.c.

KEYWORDS

- Circadian rhythm • Signal transduction • Animal models of hypertension • Radiotelemetry
- Chronopharmacology

KEY POINTS

- Inbred strains of rats can be used as models of human hypertension to evaluate mechanisms of regulation of the circadian rhythms underlying hypertension.
- There is sound evidence that blood pressure and heart rate rhythms in rodents are endogenous (circadian), as shown by experiments on suprachiasmatic nuclei lesions and under free-run conditions.
- Intensive studies have been performed in 2 normotensive (Wistar Kyoto [WKY], spontaneous rat [SDR]) and 2 hypertensive rat strains (spontaneously hypertensive rat [SHR], transgenic retarded [TGR]) on the turnover of norepinephrine, on processes of signal transduction in the beta-adrenoceptor–adenylate cyclase–cyclic AMP–phosphodiesterase system and in the renin-angiotensin-aldosterone system, and on circadian rhythms in blood pressure and heart rate using radiotelemetry.
- The data obtained by these methods allowed a better understanding of the circadian phase–dependent kinetics and effects of cardiovascular active drugs (chronopharmacology) used in humans.

INTRODUCTION

Living organisms are continuously influenced by external stimuli, many of which have rhythmic patterns. Environmental rhythms in daily and seasonal patterns of light, food availability, temperature, and so forth are predictable in time and animals, including humans, have the ability to anticipate these environmental events with periodically and predictably changing internal conditions. These rhythmic patterns of anticipation have clear advantages and survival value.[1] Thus, rhythmicity is the most ubiquitous feature of nature. Rhythms are found from unicellular to complex multicellular organisms in plants, animals, and humans. The frequencies of rhythms in nature cover nearly every division of time; the most prominent rhythm studied is the circadian

Disclosure: The author has no conflict of interest.
Medical Faculty Mannheim, Institute of Experimental and Clinical Pharmacology and Toxicology, Ruprecht-Karls-University of Heidelberg, Theodor-Kutzer-Ufer 1-3, Haus 20, Mannheim 68167, Germany
E-mail address: bjoern.lemmer@medma.uni-heidelberg.de

Heart Failure Clin 13 (2017) 739–757
http://dx.doi.org/10.1016/j.hfc.2017.05.009

heartfailure.theclinics.com

(from circa dies, meaning about 24 hours) rhythm[2,3] driven by an internal "clock".

Since more than 40 years ago when I, as a naive pharmacologist, noticed that rats are night-active animals, I was fascinated by the timely organization in the sympathetic nervous system, initially studied in rats.[4,5] In this article, the experimental data on daily variation in the mechanisms of regulation of the sympathetic nervous system are compiled. These data on circadian rhythmic organization were collected when the molecular biology of circadian clocks did not yet exist.

TEMPORAL ASPECTS OF THE SYMPATHETIC NERVOUS SYSTEM

The sympathetic nervous system is part of the autonomic nervous system, which is widely distributed throughout the body and controls so-called autonomic or vegetative functions. Regulatory mechanisms of the cardiovascular system are, for example, greatly dependent on the proper functioning of the sympathetic nervous system.

The nerves of the autonomic nervous system transmit their impulses across the synapses by means of neurotransmitters. The main neurotransmitter within the sympathetic nervous system is the catecholamine norepinephrine (NE). NE is released on nerve impulse into the synaptic cleft and binds to the postsynaptic receptor. The signal transduction at the cell membrane through beta-adrenoceptors involves stimulation of adenylate cyclase (AC), leading to subsequent increased accumulation of the intracellular second messenger cyclic AMP (cAMP). A guanine nucleotide binding site (N_s) is involved in the signal transfer from the beta-adrenoceptor to the catalytic subunit of the AC. The cAMP formed is then hydrolyzed by phosphodiesterases (PDEs) to 5-adenosine monophosphate.

NOREPINEPHRINE CONTENT AND TURNOVER IN RAT HEART

The tissue concentrations of neurotransmitters may not be constant in time but can show significant daily variation. In contrast, only a small functional transmitter pool is necessary for the neuronal function of the noradrenergic neurons. This point is important because it indicates that the tissue concentration of the neurotransmitter may not reflect its functional role. Furthermore, both the starting material for the biosynthesis of NE, tyrosine, and the enzymes involved (tyrosine hydroxylase [TH], dopa-decarboxylase [DDC], dopamine-β-hydroxylase [DBH]) are present in the adrenergic nerve terminal. Thus, the

endogenous levels of a biogenic amine are just the results of the underlying mechanisms of synthesis, storage, and release. The lack of daily variation in the overall concentration of a neurotransmitter therefore may not indicate that there is no rhythmicity within the transmitter system and vice versa. In contrast with brain tissue,[6,7] no significant daily variation has been found in the endogenous NE content of the rat heart.[5] However, this does not indicate an absence of rhythmicity in neurotransmission, as could be shown in turnover experiments. Three independent methods[5] were applied in the experiments: the NE turnover was calculated either from the decline of the endogenous cardiac NE concentration after inhibition of the TH with H44/68 (D,L-α-methyl-p-tyrosine-methylester-hydrochloride) or the DBH with FLA 63 (methyl-homopiperazinyl-thiocarbonyl-disulfide) or after measuring the decline of the specific activity after injection of tracer doses of ^{3}H-(−)-NE. Independently from the method applied, the turnover of NE in the rat heart was significantly greater in the activity phase of the animals during darkness than in the resting phase during the light hours[4,5] (**Fig. 1**).

With these studies, the authors were the first to show a circadian rhythm in the turnover of a biogenic amine, NE, in a rat tissue.[4,5] Reversal of the light-dark cycle for at least 5 days before the turnover experiment also reversed the respective half-lives in the cardiac NE when the radioactive method was used,[4,5] indicating the importance of external zeitgebers for the synchronization of this rhythmic pattern. One year after our first article on a rhythm in NE turnover in the rat heart,[4] Julius Axelrod, the Nobel Prize winner, published similar data on the turnover of NE in the rat pineal gland.[8] In conclusion, although the endogenous concentration of the neurotransmitter NE in rat heart tissue does not display a circadian rhythm, the results of the turnover experiments clearly give evidence that the drive of the sympathetic nervous system in the rat heart is circadian dependent.

Additional studies on the mechanisms of regulation of the circadian rhythm in NE turnover revealed that ganglion blockade by chlorisondamine completely prevented the physiologic nightly induced increase in turnover rate in rat heart,[9,10] thus giving further evidence that the sympathetic drive is mainly responsible for the rhythm in NE turnover. Also, the beta-receptor–blocking drug propranolol, with a central depressant effect caused by its high lipophilicity, led to a prevention in the turnover increase during the dark phase (**Fig. 2**).[11]

Pharmacokinetic studies with different beta-adrenoceptor–blocking drugs (lipophilic,

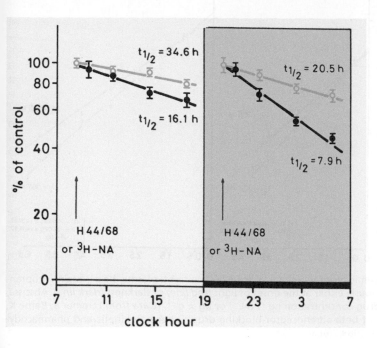

Fig. 1. Turnover of NE in rat heart determined either by injection of tracer dose of radioactively labeled NE (*blue line*) or by inhibition of the rate-limiting step in the biosynthesis of NE by the TH inhibitor H44/68 (*green line*). Both methods showed that NE half-life is significantly shorter in the dark than the light phase, indicating a higher sympathetic drive in darkness (D). (*Data from* Lemmer B, Saller R. Difference in the turnover of noradrenaline in rat heart during day and night. Naunyn Schmiedebergs Arch Pharmacol 1973;278(1):107–9; and Lemmer B, Saller R. Influence of light and darkness on the turnover of noradrenaline in the rat heart. Naunyn Schmiedebergs Arch Pharmacol 1974;282(1):75–84.)

propranolol and metoprolol; hydrophilic, atenolol and sotalol) revealed that, independent from the physicochemical property and the kind of drug elimination (lipophilic, hepatic metabolism; hydrophilic, renal excretion), all drugs showed a significantly shorter half-life in the activity phase at night than in the resting phase during daytime.[12–15] A representative experiment is shown for propranolol in **Fig. 3.**

These data clearly show that, in the activity phase of the night-active rats, elimination of β-blockers is faster than during rest, independent of the site of drug elimination (**Fig. 4**). Thus, both the kinetics and the effects of β-blockers are circadian phase dependent in rats. This dual effect makes it more difficult to estimate the relative contribution of kinetics/effects to the overall action of the drugs.

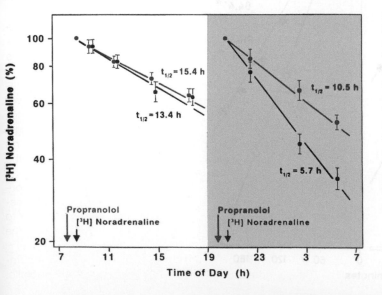

Fig. 2. Effect of beta-receptor–blocking drug propranolol (0.1 mmol/kg [−] propranolol) on the turnover of NE in rat heart. The β-blocker (*red line*) antagonized the nightly induced increase in NE turnover shown under control conditions (*blue line*). (*Data from* Lemmer B, Saller R. The effects of acute administration of propranolol and practolol on the uptake, content, release, and turnover of noradrenaline in the rat heart in vivo. Naunyn Schmiedebergs Arch Pharmacol 1974;282(1):85–96.)

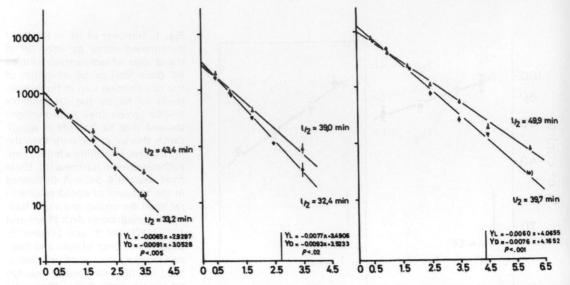

Fig. 3. Chronopharmacokinetics of racemic propranolol in rat tissue (left to right: plasma, heart, brain). Propranolol (8.89 mg/kg) was injected intravenously either at the onset of light (*red line*) or darkness (*dark line*). Abscissa, hours after drug injection; ordinate, drug concentration ng × mL^{-1} or ng × g^{-1}. (*Data from* Lemmer B, Bathe K, Lang PH, et al. Chronopharmacology of beta-adrenoceptor-blocking drugs: pharmacokinetic and pharmacodynamic studies in rats. J Am Coll Toxicol 1983;2(6):347–58.)

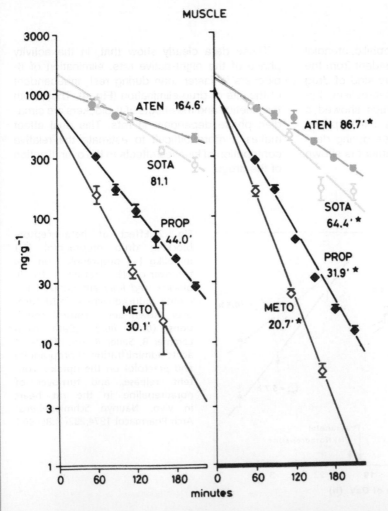

Fig. 4. Chronokinetics of 4 different beta-adrenoceptor blockers in rat muscle determined in the light (*left*) or dark (*right*) phase. (*Data from* Lemmer B, Winkler H, Ohm T, et al. Chronopharmacokinetics of beta-receptor blocking drugs of different lipophilicity (propranolol, metoprolol, sotalol, atenolol) in plasma and tissues after single and multiple dosing in the rat. Naunyn Schmiedebergs Arch Pharmacol 1985;330(1):42–9.)

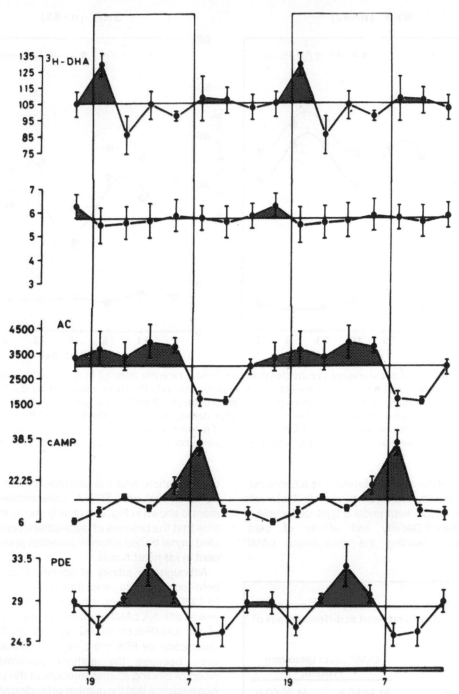

Fig. 5. Rhythm in beta-receptor–mediated signal transduction in rat heart. Shown are, from top to bottom, total beta-receptor numbers (B_{max} fmol/mg), affinity (k_d), adenylyl cyclase activity (pmol/mg/min), cAMP content (pmol/mg), and PDE activity (nmol/mg/min). Ordinate = time of day. (*Data from* Lemmer B, Lang PH, Schmidt S, et al. Evidence for circadian rhythmicity of the beta-adrenoceptor - adenylate cyclase - cAMP - phosphodiesterase system in the rat. J Cardiovasc Pharmacol 1987;10(Suppl 4):138–40.)

THE BETA-RECEPTOR EFFECTOR SYSTEM

The process of sympathetic signal transduction involves several steps that were outlined earlier.

With the advent of techniques of receptor binding assays with radioactive ligands at the end of the last century, it was possible to study the circadian phase–dependent variation of beta-adrenoceptors

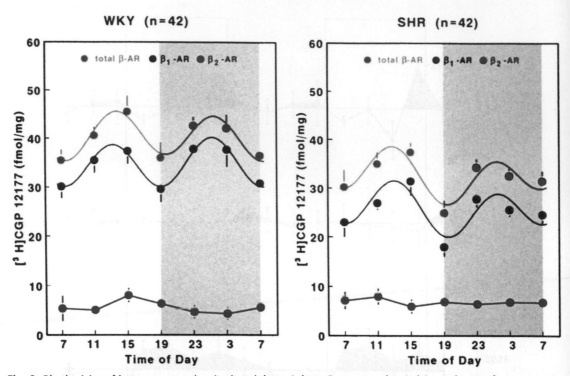

Fig. 6. Rhythmicity of beta-receptor density (total, beta-1, beta-2 receptor density) in rat heart of normotensive Wistar Kyoto (WKY) and hypertensive spontaneously hypertensive rats (SHRs) as evaluated by the hydrophilic ligand 3H- (4-[3-tertiarbutylamino-2-hydroxypropoxy-benzimidazole -2-on]) radioligand (^{3}HCGP) 12177. With this ligand a 12—hour rhythmicity in total and β_1-receptor density was found. (*Data from* Witte K, Parsa-Parsi R, Vobig M, et al. Mechanisms of the circadian regulation of β-adrenoceptor density and adenylyl cyclase activity in cardiac tissue from normotensive and spontaneously hypertensive rats. J Mol Cell Cardiol 1995;27:1195–202.)

at the level of the cell membrane. The authors performed many studies in hearts of male Wistar rats around the clock, kept under a light-dark cycle of 12:12 hours. Density and affinity of beta-adrenoceptor binding, the endogenous cAMP

Table 1
Effect of forskolin on cyclic AMP 15 minutes before sacrifice in rat heart at different times of day

Treatment	cAMP Level (pmol/mg Protein)	
	At 14:00 h	At 20:00 h
Saline	36.9 ± 1.2	49.8 ± 3.0[a]
Forskolin (5 mg/kg i.p.)	50.0 ± 4.1[b]	52.6 ± 3.7

Mean values ± standard error of the mean, n = 10.
Abbreviation: IP, intra peritoneal.
[a] From 14:00 to 20:00 h, P<.01.
[b] Saline to forskolin P<.01.
Data from Lemmer B, Bissinger H, Lang PH. Effect of forskolin on cAMP levels in rat heart at different times of day. IRCS Med Sci 1986;14:1104.

concentration, and the activities of PDE and the AC were evaluated.[16–20] A representative experiment is shown in **Fig. 5**. It clearly shows for the first time that the process of beta-adrenoceptor–mediated signal transduction is circadian phase dependent in rat heart tissue.

Although the affinity of specific binding of the beta-receptor antagonist ligand 3-dihydroalprenolol (3HDHA) does not vary with circadian time (as well as affinity), cAMP concentration and the activity of the cAMP-forming AC as well as the cAMP destruction by PDE were highly rhythmic.[20] However, because the authors performed beta-receptor binding studies throughout the year, there was evidence that the number of binding sites in cardiac tissue varied in a seasonal manner, although only to a small degree.[21] This rhythmicity was obvious only for the selective beta-1 receptor density (and consequently for total receptor density), but not for the beta-2 receptor density (**Fig. 6**), again showing circadian rhythmicity in sympathetic drive, which is mainly driven by beta-1 receptors. Pronounced circadian variations were also described in alpha-adrenoceptor and beta-adrenoceptor density in various regions of rat brain.[22,23]

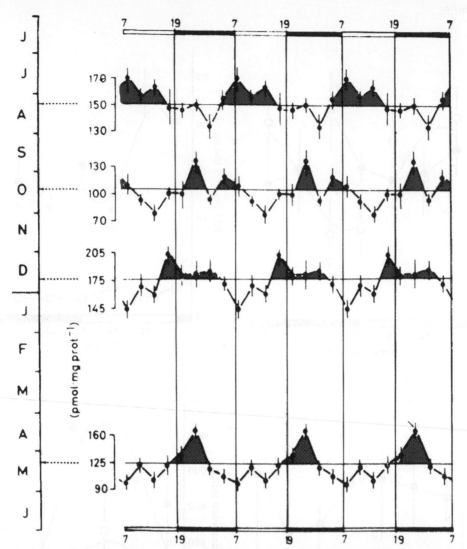

Fig. 7. Seasonal variation in cAMP concentration in rat heart tissue. Ordinate: month (there is a shift in the peak with season). All experiments were performed under 12:12 LD conditions. (*Data from* Lang PH, Bissinger H, Lemmer B. Circadian rhythm and seasonal variations in the basal cAMP content of rat heart ventricles. Chronobiol Int 1985;2(1):41–5.)

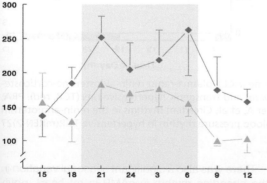

Fig. 8. Circadian rhythm in plasma NE (ordinate: pg/mL) in WKY (*black*) and SHR (*green*) rats. NE is downregulated in hypertensive rats. (*Data from* Lemmer B. Effects of music composed by Mozart and Ligeti on blood pressure and heart rate circadian rhythms in normotensive and hypertensive rats. Chronobiol Int 2008;25(6):971–86.)

Most interestingly, the peak in cAMP concentration in rat heart did not occur when basal AC activity was high as has been expected. In contrast, in this experiment the peak in cAMP activity coincided with the trough in basal AC activity, In contrast, a correlation between the rhythm in cAMP level and the PDE activity was found: the trough value in cAMP activity coincided with the peak value in low-affinity PDE activity (see **Fig. 5**). This finding gives some evidence that the rhythmic changes in basal cAMP are under a greater influence of the rhythmic changes in PDE than in AC.

Furthermore, this observation could indicate that the degree of stimulation of cAMP is better when basal AC activity is low. This hypothesis was tested again using forskolin, which can directly activate the catalytic unit of the AC

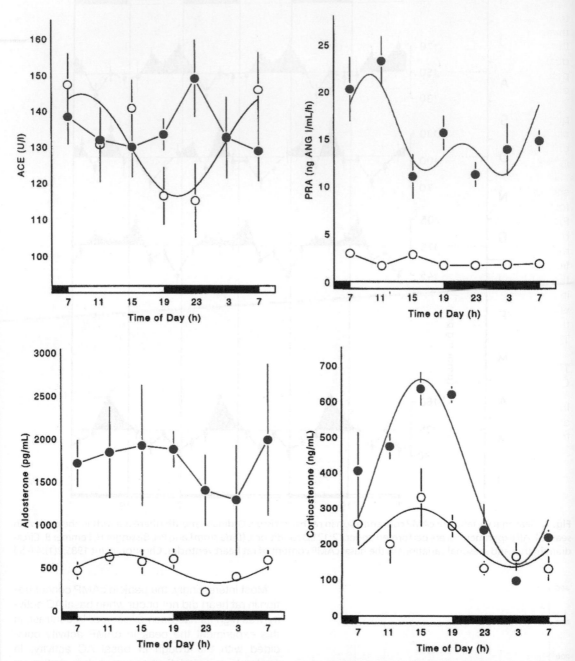

Fig. 9. Circadian rhythm in the angiotensin-converting enzyme (ACE)–plasma-renin-renin-aldosterone-corticosterone system in normotensive spontaneous dwarf rat (SDR; *blue*) and transgenic hypertensive rats (TGR, *red*). PRA, plama renin activity. (*Data from* Lemmer B, Witte K, Schanzer A, et al. Circadian rhythms in the renin-angiotensin system and adrenal steroids may contribute to the inverse blood pressure rhythm in hypertensive TGR(mREN-2)27 rats. Chronobiol Int 2000;17(5):645–58.)

system. **Table 1** shows that the cAMP level in rat heart in this experiment is again circadian phase dependent; in addition it supports the notion that the lower the basal level in cAMP, the more pronounced the stimulatory effect of forskolin. Thus, the degree of AC stimulation is negatively correlated with the unstimulated level of AC.

There was also a significant seasonal variation in the circadian rhythm in cAMP in rat heart, obviously free run, although the animals were always kept under constant light/dark (LD) conditions (**Fig. 7**).

Because the authors studied different strains of rats, normotensive as well as hypertensive, signal transduction processes were investigated in these strains in order to get information about the extent to which disturbance in signal transduction could be correlated with the kind of hypertension, as well as its effect on rhythm disturbances.

In normotensive sprague-dawley (SPD) rats, plasma NE concentration showed a significant circadian rhythm with a peak value in the middle of the dark phase (**Fig. 8**), indicating a maximum in the sympathetic drive.

In hypertensive rats (spontaneously hypertensive rat [SHR]), significant lower NE values were found throughout the 24 hours of a day (see **Fig. 8**), obviously caused by a counter-regulation by the increased blood pressure (BP); in addition, rhythmicity was nearly abolished. A downregulation of the rate-limiting step in NE formation by the TH[24] and the NE transporter was also found in transgenic growth retarded (TGR) compared with normotensive SPD rats.[25] Rhythmicity in these two important enzymes was reduced in TGR.

THE RENIN-ANGIOTENSIN-ALDOSTERONE-CORTICOSTERONE SYSTEM

In addition, the circadian rhythm in the renin-angiotensin-aldosterone system was greatly distorted and NE plasma concentration downregulated

in transgenic rats[26,27] (**Fig. 9**), giving additional evidence that, in secondary hypertension, rhythmic organization at the hormonal level is also affected.

THE NITRIC OXIDE SYSTEM

The nitric oxide (NO) system plays an additional role in the regulation of the vascular bed, so the authors also studied this system.[28,29] At a young age of 5 weeks, both normotensive and transgenic hypertensive rats showed a significant daily rhythm in NO excretion with a pronounced peak at night (**Fig. 10**). However, at a slightly older age of 11 weeks, NO excretion was already reduced in both strains, but with a much more pronounced loss of NO in TGR (see **Fig. 10**). These data indicate that vascular regulation via NO is age dependent, and that vascular reactivity is better at a younger age and is reduced by aging. Most important, the loss in NO leading to a decrease in vascular reactivity is more evident in the hypertensive rat strain.

There is also a gender-specific difference in NO; optical density of Western blot in thoracic aortae is significantly lower in male than female SHR rats, together with a reduction in renal NO excretion.[30,31] In hypertensive patients, there is sound evidence that nitrate excretion is not only lower than in healthy subjects but the circadian rhythm is also abolished.[32–34]

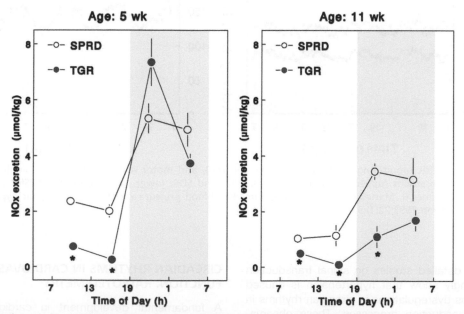

Fig. 10. Daily variation in NO excretion in normotensive SDR and hypertensive TGR rats at 2 different days after birth. SPRD, sprague-dawley rat. (*Data from* Borgonio A, Witte K, Stahrenberg R, et al. Influence of circadian time, ageing, and hypertension on the urinary excretion of nitric oxide metabolites in rats. Mech Ageing Dev 1999;111(1):23–37; and Globig S, Witte K, Lemmer B. Urinary excretion of nitric oxide, cyclic GMP, and catecholamines during rest and activity period in transgenic hypertensive rats. Chronobiol Int 1999;16(3):305–14.)

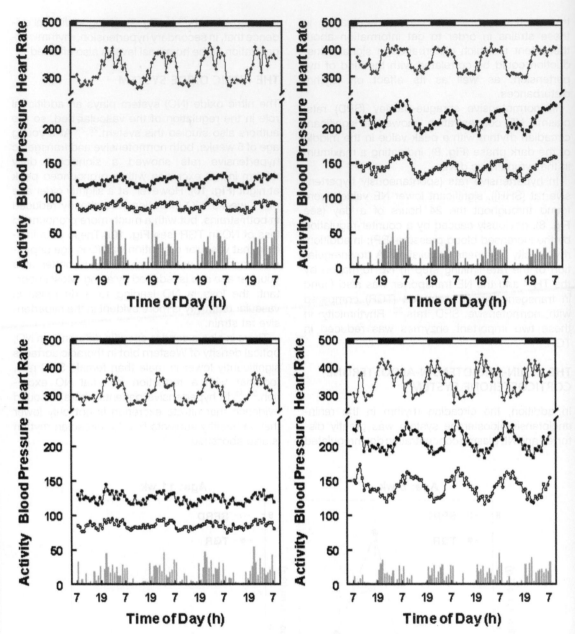

Fig. 11. Telemetric monitoring of BP (*black, blue*), HR (*red*), and motor activity (*green*) in a single rat of 4 different inbred strains (upper part normotensives, WKY and SDR; lower part hypertensives, SHR and TGR). (*Data from* Lemmer B, Mattes A, Bohm M, et al. Circadian blood pressure variation in transgenic hypertensive rats. Hypertension 1993;22(1):97–101.)

These detailed studies on signal transduction convincingly show that hypertension is caused by various dysregulations in circadian rhythms in signal transduction processes. These observations also support the notion that several different drugs using different mechanisms of action are useful and effective to treat BP hypertension in humans.

CIRCADIAN RHYTHMS IN CARDIOVASCULAR FUNCTION: RADIOTELEMETRY

A fundamental development in cardiovascular research was achieved by the introduction of radiotelemetry by DataSciences, which allowed clinicians to monitor BP, heart rate (HR), motility (MA), and additional functions in unrestrained, freely

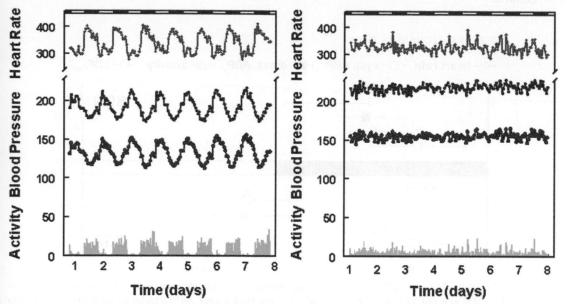

Fig. 12. Effect of SCN lesion on circadian profiles in BP, HR, and MA in a single transgenic rat compared with control conditions (*left*). All rhythms are abolished by the SCN lesioning but BP remains high. diast, diastolic; syst, systolic. (*Data from* Witte K, Schnecko A, Buijs RM, et al. Effects of SCN-lesions on circadian blood pressure rhythm in normotensive and transgenic hypertensive rats. Chronobiol Int 1998;15:135–45.)

Sprague-Dawley Rat

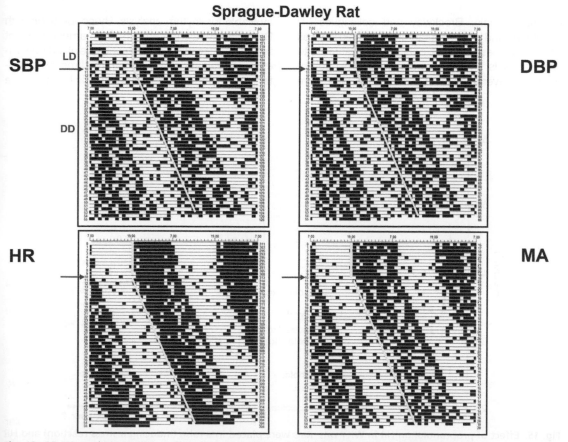

Fig. 13. BP, HR, and MA in SDR under control conditions (L/D = 12:12 hours) and after release in free-run in total darkness (DD). All rhythms persist but with an increase in half-life (*yellow line*). (*Data from* Lemmer B. The importance of circadian rhythms on drug response in hypertension and coronary heart disease–from mice and man. Pharmacol Ther 2006;111(3):629–51.)

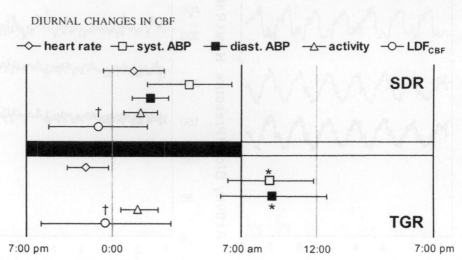

Fig. 14. Cerebral blood flow (CBF) in transgenic hypertensive rats (TGR) compared with normotensive SDR. Although BP in TGR was out of phase, CBF still peaked in the dark phase. ABP, arterial blood pressure; DD, total darkness; LDF CBF, laser-doppler flowmetry. (*Data from* Wauschkuhn CA, Witte K, Gorbey S, et al. Circadian periodicity of cerebral blood flow revealed by laser-Doppler flowmetry in awake rats: relation to blood pressure and activity. Am J Physiol Heart Circ Physiol 2005;289(4):H1662–8.)

moving animals. Brockway and colleagues[35,36] developed and later manufactured and sold devices (Data Sciences Inc) that could be implanted into small animals and used radiotelemetry to collect data for several days or weeks and then were

available for rhythm analysis. By cooperation with Brian Brockway, the authors were among the first to test and use this modern technique of radiotelemetry for evaluation of circadian rhythms in normotensive, hypertensive, and transgenic hypertensive

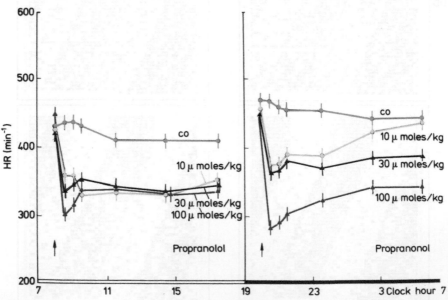

Fig. 15. Effect of propranolol on HR in WKY rats. Rats were placed in a tube (inducing a stress reaction) and HR was monitored by the electrocardiogram from the rats' feet. Thus effects of propranolol were caused by reducing this stress reaction. (*Data from* Lemmer B, Winkler H, Ohm T, et al. Chronopharmacokinetics of beta-receptor blocking drugs of different lipophilicity (propranolol, metoprolol, sotalol, atenolol) in plasma and tissues after single and multiple dosing in the rat. Naunyn Schmiedebergs Arch Pharmacol 1985;330(1):42–9.)

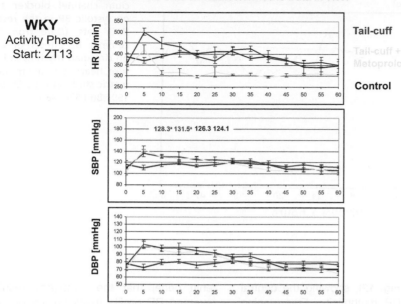

Fig. 16. Effect of tail-cuff measurement on BP and HR in SHR. Data were obtained either by radiotelemetry (*black line*) or in a tail-cuff device (*violet*), additionally, rats under tail cuff were treated with the β-blocker metoprolol (*yellow*), which abolished the tail cuff–induced stress reaction on HR, leaving the effects on BP unchanged. [a] Tel versus Tailcuff P<.001. DBP, diastolic BP; SBP, systolic BP; ZT, zeitgeber time. (*Data from* Lemmer B. Superiority of radiotelemetry over the tail-cuff method in evaluating control and drug-induced data in cardiovascular functions. Biol Rhythm Res 2016;47:919–25.)

rats[37–41] (**Fig. 11**). This development was important because continuous, undisturbed measurements of BP data for several days or weeks was not possible in humans. Thus, these animals could be used as models for human normotension and hypertension in order to evaluate drug effects on the circadian rhythm of BP and HR in humans.[39,42] These animal studies greatly stimulated a better understanding of the chronopharmacologic observations in humans.[34,43,44] Most important, it could also be shown that the rhythms in HR and BP in these strains were abolished by suprachiasmatic nuclei

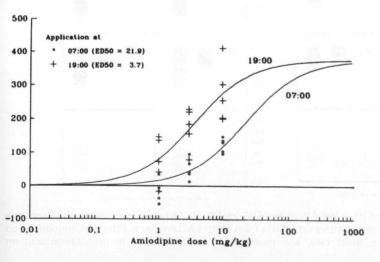

Fig. 17. Dose-response curve of amlodipine applied in the light or the dark span to normotensive WKY rats. At night the BP decrease was already observed at a lower dose, indicating higher sensitivity of the cardiovascular system to amlodipine. ED50, 50% effective dose. (*Data from* Mattes A, Lemmer B. Effects of amlodipine on circadian rhythms in blood pressure, heart rate, and motility: a telemetric study in rats. Chronobiol Int 1991;8(6):526–38.)

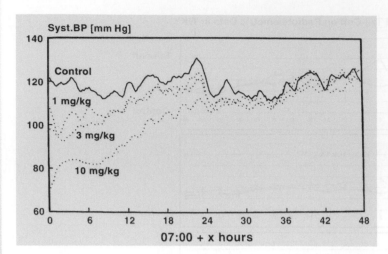

Fig. 18. Dose dependency of calcium channel blocker amlodipine on systolic BP in the rest phase of WKY rats. (*Data from* Mattes A, Lemmer B. Effects of amlodipine on circadian rhythms in blood pressure, heart rate, and motility: a telemetric study in rats. Chronobiol Int 1991;8(6):526–38.)

(SCN) lesions[45,46] (**Fig. 12**), showing the central regulation of the BP rhythmicity. Free-running rhythms in HR and BP were also shown under total darkness[47] (**Fig. 13**). **Fig. 11** shows the circadian rhythms in BP and HR of 2 normotensive (SPD, Wistar Kyoto [WKY]) and 2 hypertensive (SHR, TGR) rat strains.

In addition, BP was out of phase in TGR compared with spontaneous dwarf rat (SDR), and cerebral blood flow was still in phase with the normal BP and HR rhythm[48] (**Fig. 14**).

For the first time, the authors showed in a transgenic rat strain (TGR, bearing an additional mouse renin gene) that the transgene resulted in a reversed BP profile (peak values during rest at daytime) compared with the rhythms in HR and motility[40,49] (see **Figs. 11** and **14**). Thus, this strain of rats was addressed as an animal model of human secondary hypertension,[49] showing an abolition or even a reversed circadian BP rhythm peaking in the rest phase of both species.

In conclusion, the data obtained after SCN lesions as well as under free-run conditions clearly show that circadian rhythms in BP and HR are endogenous; that is, they are under the control of the biological clock.

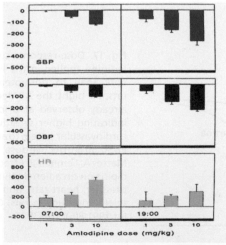
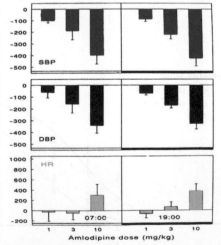

Fig. 19. Effect of amlodipine on BP and HR in WKY (*left*) and SHR (*right*) rats. Hypertensive rats are more sensitive to the calcium channel blocker than normotensive rats. (*Data from* Mattes A, Lemmer B. Effects of amlodipine on circadian rhythms in blood pressure, heart rate, and motility: a telemetric study in rats. Chronobiol Int 1991;8(6):526–38.)

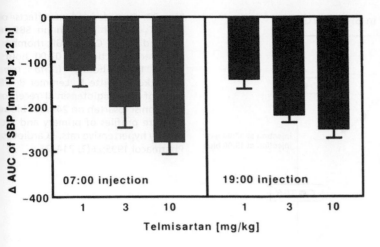

Fig. 20. Effect of the AT_1-receptor blocker telmisartan on BP in SHR. A dose dependency was found both in the rest as well in the activity period. Thus, its effectiveness is independent from the time of application in hypertension. AUC, area under the curve. (*Data from* Pummer S, Lemmer B. Dose-dependent effects of telmisartan on circadian rhythm in blood pressure and heart rate in spontaneously hypertensive rats (SHR). Dtsch Med Wochenschr 2000;125(Suppl 3):S39.)

CHRONOPHARMACOLOGY OF ANTIHYPERTENSIVE DRUGS

In these inbred strains of rat, HR, but more obviously circadian BP regulation, was greatly strain dependent, mainly concerning amplitude.

These animal models of human normal and hypertensive BP rhythms were used intensively in chronopharmacologic experiments, evaluating the circadian phase–dependent effects of various antihypertensive drugs[50–52] (ie, α-blockers,[53,54] β-blockers,[55] angiotensin-converting enzyme inhibitors,[56] Angiotensin 1 (AT1)-receptor blockers,[57] calcium channel blockers).[37,39] The

following examples are presented to show that the time of day of drug application can have pronounced impact on the drug effects.

Beta-receptor blockers reduce the sympathetic drive, mainly acting on HR. However, under unstressed conditions in vivo there is no obvious effect of β-blockers on HR in rats (**Fig. 15**): only if the sympathetic tone is increased (eg, by stress reaction) are β-blockers effective (see **Fig. 15**; **Fig. 16**).

Calcium channel blockers are among the drugs of first choice in the treatment of human hypertension. The authors studied the effect of amlodipine both in normotensive and in hypertensive rats by radiotelemetry. In SHR, amlodipine showed similar

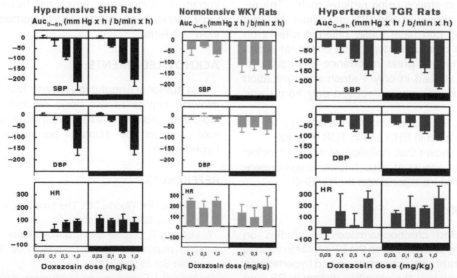

Fig. 21. Dose-dependent effects of doxazosin on BP and HR in 3 strains of rats. Although no dose dependency was found in the normotensive rat strain, doxazosin was equally effective in light and in dark in SHR, but more effective on BP in the transgenic strain. (*Data from* Lemmer B. Genetic aspects of chronobiologic rhythms in cardiovascular disease. In: Zehender M, Breithardt G, Just H, editors. From molecule to men - molecular basis of congenital cardiovascular disorders. Darmstadt (Germany): Steinkopff Verlag; 2000. p. 201–13.)

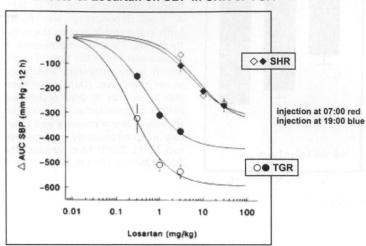

Effects of Losartan on SBP in SHR or TGR

injection at 07:00 red
injection at 19:00 blue

Fig. 22. Dose-dependent effects of the AT$_1$-blocker losartan on SBP in SHR and in TGR. Circle, TGR; rhombus, SHR; red, injection at 07:00 hours; blue, 19:00 hours. (Data from Schnecko A, Witte K, Lemmer B. Effects of the angiotensin II receptor antagonist losartan on 24-hour blood pressure profiles of primary and secondary hypertensive rats. J Cardiovasc Pharmacol 1995;26(2):214–21.)

dose-response curves in light and in dark (**Figs. 17–19**), whereas in normotensive rats amlodipine was more effective at night. This finding indicates that the rhythmic cardiovascular setting of BP regulation is strain dependent.

AT$_1$-receptor blockers are now drugs of first choice in the treatment of hypertension and have nearly no side effects. The authors studied, as a representative of this group, telmisartan in SHR animals[58] (**Fig. 20**).

The alpha-receptor–blocking drug doxazosin was studied for its effects on BP and HR of 3 different rat strains using radiotelemetry. The results are shown in **Fig. 21** and show that the same drug can have totally different effects on BP in light or in dark, depending on the rat strain. This finding is of great importance when drug effects are studied in only 1 strain and evaluation of the drug efficacy is deduced only from these data.

The AT$_1$ antagonist losartan was studied for the BP profile both in SHR and in TGR (**Fig. 22**).

Fig. 22 shows that inhibition of the AT$_1$ blocker by losartan occurs at a much lower drug concentration in the transgenic rats than in SHR.

SUMMARY

The detailed chronopharmacologic studies on signal transduction and on the BP profile in various strains of rats with normotension and hypertension clearly show that the circadian rhythm in BP (and not only in HR) is under the control of the biological clock: SCN lesions abolished the rhythm and, under free-run conditions, the circadian rhythms in BP and HR persisted but with a longer half-life.

Moreover, investigations on the rhythms in the beta-receptor–AC-cAMP-PDE-system and in the renin-angiotensin-aldosterone and NO systems showed that hypertension leads to a much more pronounced disturbance at the biochemical and hormonal levels of mechanisms of vascular regulation than had been shown earlier. That this can affect the antihypertensive efficacy of drugs used in the treatment of human hypertension is also shown in the chronopharmacologic experiments performed with various drugs that greatly differ in their mechanisms of action, as well as having an impact on dosing time, which has been convincingly shown in clinical studies in humans (for review see Refs.[50,59,60]).

ACKNOWLEDGMENTS

The author is grateful to Roberto Manfredini for allowing him to review basic chronopharmacologic data obtained within the last 4 decades in animal models of human normotension and hypertension.

REFERENCES

1. Strubbe JH, Woods SC. The timing of meals. Psychol Rev 2004;111(1):128–41.
2. Halberg F, Stephens AN. Susceptibility to ouabain and physiologic circadian periodicity. Proc Minn Acad Sci 1959;27:139–43.
3. Aschoff J. Exogenous and endogenous components in circadian rhythms. Cold Spring Harb Symp Quant Biol 1960;25:11–28.
4. Lemmer B, Saller R. Difference in the turnover of noradrenaline in rat heart during day and night.

Naunyn Schmiedebergs Arch Pharmacol 1973; 278(1):107–9.

5. Lemmer B, Saller R. Influence of light and darkness on the turnover of noradrenaline in the rat heart. Naunyn Schmiedebergs Arch Pharmacol 1974; 282(1):75–84.

6. Kung W, Chappuis-Arndt E, Wirz-Justice A. Variations of monoamine levels in 18 rat brain regions in relation to the oestrus cycle. Experientia 1975;31:722.

7. Kafka MS, Wirz-Justice A, Naber D, et al. Circadian rhythms in rat brain neurotransmitter receptors. Fed Proc 1983;42:2796–801.

8. Brownstein M, Axelrod J. Pineal gland: 24-hour rhythm in norepinephrine turnover. Science 1974; 184:163–5.

9. Lemmer B, Charrier A. Diurnal rhythm in the cardiac turnover of noradrenaline: effects of chlorisond-amine and of alpha- and beta-blocking drugs. Chronopharmacology. Oxford (United Kingdom): Pergamon Press; 1979. p. 149–58.

10. Lemmer B, Charrier A. Antagonism by chlorisond-amine and propranolol, but not by atenolol, of the circadian phase-dependent phentolamine-induced changes in the cardiac noradrenaline turnover in the rat. Naunyn Schmiedebergs Arch Pharmacol 1980;313(3):205–12.

11. Lemmer B, Saller R. The effects of acute administration of propranolol and practolol on the uptake, content, release, and turnover of noradrenaline in the rat heart in vivo. Naunyn Schmiedebergs Arch Pharmacol 1974;282(1):85–96.

12. Lemmer B, Bathe K. Stereospecific and circadian-phase-dependent kinetic behavior of d,l-, l-, and d-propranolol in plasma, heart, and brain of light–dark-synchronized rats. J Cardiovasc Pharmacol 1982;4(4):635–44.

13. Lemmer B, Bathe K, Lang PH, et al. Chronopharmacology of beta-adrenoceptor-blocking drugs: pharmacokinetic and pharmacodynamic studies in rats. J Am Coll Toxicol 1983;2(6):347–58.

14. Lemmer B, Winkler H, Fink M. Comparative pharmacokinetics of propranolol, metoprolol and atenolol after single and multiple dosing in the rat. Naunyn Schmiedebergs Arch Pharmacol 1983;322(Suppl): R 9 [abstract: 33].

15. Lemmer B, Winkler H, Ohm T, et al. Chronopharmacokinetics of beta-receptor blocking drugs of different lipophilicity (propranolol, metoprolol, sota-lol, atenolol) in plasma and tissues after single and multiple dosing in the rat. Naunyn Schmiedebergs Arch Pharmacol 1985;330(1):42–9.

16. Lang PH, Lemmer B. Kinetics of 3H-DHA binding to rat heart membranes and circadian rhythm in sympathic tone. Naunyn Schmiedebergs Arch Pharmacol 1982;319(Suppl):R 68.

17. Lang PH, Bissinger H, Lemmer B. Circadian rhythm in cAMP content and in the activities of basal adenylate cyclase and phosphodiesterase in rat heart ventricles. Annu Rev Chronopharmacol 1984; 1:219–22.

18. Lemmer B, Lang PH. Circadian-phase-dependency in 3H-dihydroalprenolol binding to rat heart ventricular membranes. Chronobiol Int 1984;1:217–23.

19. Lang PH, Bissinger H, Lemmer B. Circadian rhythm and seasonal variations in the basal cAMP content of rat heart ventricles. Chronobiol Int 1985;2(1):41–5.

20. Lemmer B, Lang PH, Schmidt S, et al. Evidence for circadian rhythmicity of the beta-adrenoceptor - adenylate cyclase - cAMP - phosphodiesterase system in the rat. J Cardiovasc Pharmacol 1987;10(Suppl 4):138–40.

21. Witte K, Parsa-Parsi R, Vobig M, et al. Mechanisms of the circadian regulation of β-adrenoceptor density and adenylyl cyclase activity in cardiac tissue from normotensive and spontaneously hypertensive rats. J Mol Cell Cardiol 1995;27:1195–202.

22. Wirz-Justice A, Kafka MS, Naber D, et al. Circadian rhythms in rat brain alpha- and beta-adrenergic receptors are modified by chronic imipramine. Life Sci 1980;27:341–7.

23. Kafka MS, Wirz-Justice A, Naber D. Circadian and seasonal rhythms in alpha- and beta-adrenergic receptors in the rat brain. Brain Res 1981;207:409–19.

24. Schiffer S, Enzminger H, Hauptfleisch S, et al. Day-night differences in catecholamine turnover and tyrosine-hydroxylase mRNA in normotensive Sprague-Dawley (SPRD) and hypertensive TGR(mREN2)27 rats. Chronobiol Int 2001;18(6): 1186–7.

25. Lemmer B, Schiffer S, Witte K, et al. Inverse blood pressure rhythm of transgenic hypertensive TGR(mREN2)27 rats: role of norepinephrine and expression of tyrosine-hydroxylase and reuptake1-transporter. Chronobiol Int 2005;22(3):473–88.

26. Lemmer B, Witte K, Schanzer A, et al. Circadian rhythms in the renin-angiotensin system and adrenal steroids may contribute to the inverse blood pressure rhythm in hypertensive TGR(mREN-2)27 rats. Chronobiol Int 2000;17(5):645–58.

27. Hauptfleisch S, Enzminger H, Schiffer S, et al. An overexpressed renin-angiotensin-system and its impact on the circadian clock. Chronobiol Int 2001; 18:1114–5.

28. Borgonio A, Witte K, Stahrenberg R, et al. Influence of circadian time, ageing, and hypertension on the urinary excretion of nitric oxide metabolites in rats. Mech Ageing Dev 1999;111(1):23–37.

29. Globig S, Witte K, Lemmer B. Urinary excretion of nitric oxide, cyclic GMP, and catecholamines during rest and activity period in transgenic hypertensive rats. Chronobiol Int 1999;16(3):305–14.

30. Lemmer B, Meier K, Gorbey S. Effects on blood pressure, nitric oxide urinary excretion and on eNOS protein expression by nebivolol and

metoprolol in spontaneously-hypertensive rats. Am J Hypertens 2004;17(5 Pt 2):115c/P-226.

31. Meier K, Lemmer B. Blood pressure and heart rate after metoprolol or nebivolol and effects on nitric oxide urinary excretion in spontaneously hypertensive rats with and without I-NAME. Z Kardiol 2004; 93(Suppl 3):P1320.

32. Bode-Boger SM, Boger RH, Kielstein JT, et al. Role of endogenous nitric oxide in circadian blood pressure regulation in healthy humans and in patients with hypertension or atherosclerosis. J Investig Med 2000;48(2):125–32.

33. Hartig V, Lemmer B. Gender-related circadian variations in blood pressure, plasma catecholamines and urinary excretion of nitric oxide and cGMP. Naunyn Schmiedebergs Arch Pharmacol 2003;367(Suppl 1):R 113 [abstract: 438].

34. Lemmer B. The importance of biological rhythms in drug treatment of hypertension and sex-dependent modifications. Chronophysiol Ther 2012;2:9–18.

35. Brockway BP, Mills PA, Azar SH. A new method for continuous chronic measurement and recording of blood pressure, heart rate and activity in the rat via radio-telemetry. Clin Exp Hypertens A 1991;13(5):885–95.

36. Lange J, Brockway B, Azar S. Telemetric monitoring of laboratory animals: an advanced technique that has come of age. Lab Anim 1991;20:28–33.

37. Mattes A, Lemmer B. Effects of amlodipine on circadian rhythms in blood pressure, heart rate, and motility: a telemetric study in rats. Chronobiol Int 1991;8(6):526–38.

38. Lemmer B, Mattes A, Boese S. 24-hour blood pressure profiles in normotensive and hypertensive rats and dose-dependent effects of the calcium-channel blocker amlodipine. J Interdiscipl Cycle Res 1992;23:232–4.

39. Lemmer B, Mattes A, Bose S. Dose-dependent effects of amlodipine on 24-hour rhythms in blood pressure and heart rate in the normotensive and hypertensive rat. Am J Hypertens 1992;5:110 A.

40. Lemmer B, Mattes A, Bohm M, et al. Circadian blood pressure variation in transgenic hypertensive rats. Hypertension 1993;22(1):97–101.

41. Lemmer B, Witte K, Minors D, et al. Circadian rhythms of heart rate and blood pressure in four strains of rat: differences due to, and separate from, locomotor activity. Biol Rhythm Res 1995;26:493–504.

42. Lemmer B. Chronopharmacology: time, a key in drug treatment. Ann Biol Clin 1994;52:1–7.

43. Lemmer B, editor. Chronopharmacology - cellular and biochemical interactions. New York: Marcel Dekker; 1989.

44. Redfern P, Lemmer B, editors. Physiology and pharmacology of biological rhythms, vol. 125. Berlin (Heidelberg): Springer Berlin; 1997.

45. Witte K, Schnecko A, Buijs R, et al. Circadian rhythms in blood pressure and heart rate in SCN-lesioned and unlesioned transgenic hypertensive rats. Biol Rhythm Res 1995;26:458–9.

46. Witte K, Schnecko A, Buijs RM, et al. Effects of SCN-lesions on circadian blood pressure rhythm in normotensive and transgenic hypertensive rats. Chronobiol Int 1998;15:135–45.

47. Witte K, Lemmer B. Free-running rhythms in blood pressure and heart rate in normotensive and transgenic hypertensive rats. Chronobiol Int 1995;12(4):237–47.

48. Wauschkuhn CA, Witte K, Gorbey S, et al. Circadian periodicity of cerebral blood flow revealed by laser-Doppler flowmetry in awake rats: relation to blood pressure and activity. Am J Physiol Heart Circ Physiol 2005;289(4):H1662–8.

49. Lemmer B, Mattes A, Ganten D. Transgen-hypertensive (TGR[mRen-2]27) Ratten als Modell der sekundären Hypertonie. Nieren- und Hochdruckkrankheiten 1993;22:219–20.

50. Lemmer B. The importance of circadian rhythms on drug response in hypertension and coronary heart disease–from mice and man. Pharmacol Ther 2006;111(3):629–51.

51. Lemmer B. Chronopharmacology of hypertension. Paper presented at: New York Academy of Sciences, 'Time-Dependent Structure and Control of Arterial Blood Pressure'. Ferrara, Italy, 1995.

52. Lemmer B, Witte K, Schanzer A, et al. Circadian regulation of blood pressure mechanisms and therapeutic implications. Am J Hypertens 1995;8(4 P1 2):23 A.

53. Lemmer B, Boese S, Mattes A. Wirkung von Doxazosin auf circadiane Rhythmen im Blutdruck normotensiver und hypertensiver Ratten. Z Kardiol 1993; 82(Suppl 1):139/457.

54. Lemmer B. Genetic aspects of chronobiologic rhythms in cardiovascular disease. In: Zehender M, Breithardt G, Just H, editors. From molecule to men - molecular basis of congenital cardiovascular disorders. Darmstadt (Germany): Steinkopff Verlag; 2000. p. 201–13.

55. Mattes A, Lemmer B. Telemetric registrations on the effects of atenolol and amlodipine on circadian rhythms in blood pressure and heart rate of the rat. J Interdiscipl Cycle Res 1991;22:154.

56. Schnecko A, Witte K, Schanzer A, et al. Circadian rhythm in plasma renin and converting enzyme activity, cortocosterone and aldosterone concentration in normotensive Sprague-Dawley and transgenic hypertensive rats. Biol Rhythm Res 1995;26:442.

57. Schnecko A, Witte K, Lemmer B. Effects of the angiotensin II receptor antagonist losartan on 24-hour blood pressure profiles of primary and secondary hypertensive rats. J Cardiovasc Pharmacol 1995;26(2):214–21.

58. Pummer S, Lemmer B. Dose-dependent effects of telmisartan on circadian rhythm in blood pressure and heart rate in spontaneously hypertensive rats (SHR). Dtsch Med Wochenschr 2000;125(Suppl 3):S39.

59. Lemmer B. Chronobiology and chronopharmacology of hypertension: importance of timing of dosing. In: White WB, editor. Blood pressure monitoring in cardiovascular medicine and therapeutics. 2nd edition. Totowa (NJ): Humana Press; 2007. p. 410–35.

60. Lemmer B. Chronopharmakologie. 4th edition. Stuttgart (Germany): Wiss. Verlagsges; 2012.

Bedtime Blood Pressure Chronotherapy Significantly Improves Hypertension Management

Ramón C. Hermida, PhD[a],*, Diana E. Ayala, MD, MPH, PhD[a],
José R. Fernández, PhD[a], Artemio Mojón, PhD[a],
Juan J. Crespo, MD, PhD[a,b], María T. Ríos, MD, PhD[a,c],
Michael H. Smolensky, PhD[d]

KEYWORDS

- Hypertension chronotherapy • Asleep blood pressure • Cardiovascular risk
- Ambulatory blood pressure monitoring • Hygia project • Diabetes • Chronic kidney disease
- Resistant hypertension

KEY POINTS

- Consistent evidence of numerous studies substantiates the asleep blood pressure (BP) mean derived from ambulatory BP monitoring (ABPM) is both an independent and a stronger predictor of cardiovascular disease (CVD) risk than are daytime clinic BP measurements or the ABPM-determined awake or 24-hour BP means.
- Cost-effective adequate control of sleep-time BP is of marked clinical relevance.
- Ingestion time, according to circadian rhythms, of hypertension medications of 6 different classes and their combinations significantly improves BP control, particularly sleep-time BP, and reduces adverse effects.
- Recent findings authenticate therapeutic reduction of the sleep-time BP by a bedtime hypertension treatment strategy entailing the entire daily dose of ≥1 hypertension medications significantly reduces not only CVD risk but also progression toward new-onset type 2 diabetes and renal disease.

Disclosure Statement: The authors have nothing to disclose.
Sources of Support: Research supported by unrestricted grants from Instituto de Salud Carlos III, Ministerio de Economía y Competitividad, Spanish Government (PI14-00205); Ministerio de Ciencia e Innovación, Spanish Government (SAF2006-6254-FEDER; SAF2009-7028-FEDER); Consellería de Economía e Industria, Xunta de Galicia (09CSA018322PR); European Research Development Fund and Consellería de Cultura, Educación e Ordenación Universitaria, Xunta de Galicia (CN2012/251; CN2012/260; GPC2014/078); Atlantic Research Center for Information and Communication Technologies (AtlantTIC); and Vicerrectorado de Investigación, University of Vigo.
[a] Bioengineering & Chronobiology Laboratories, Atlantic Research Center for Information and Communication Technologies (AtlantTIC), E.I. Telecomunicación, University of Vigo, Campus Universitario, Pontevedra, Vigo 36310, Spain; [b] Centro de Salud de Bembrive, Estructura de Gestión Integrada de Vigo, Servicio Galego de Saúde (SERGAS), Vigo, Spain; [c] Centro de Salud de A Doblada, Estructura de Gestión Integrada de Vigo, Servicio Galego de Saúde (SERGAS), Vigo, Spain; [d] Department of Biomedical Engineering, Cockrell School of Engineering, The University of Texas at Austin, Austin, TX, USA
* Corresponding author.
E-mail address: rhermida@uvigo.es

INTRODUCTION

Blood pressure (BP) exhibits a mostly predictable 24-hour pattern as the culmination of the inter-relationship of many 24-hour cyclic biological, behavioral, and environmental determinants: (1) endogenous circadian (~24-hour) variation in neuroendocrine, endothelial, vasoactive peptide and opioid, and hemodynamic parameters (eg, plasma noradrenaline and adrenaline [autonomic nervous system, ANS], atrial natriuretic and calcitonin gene-related peptides, and renin, angiotensin, and aldosterone [renin-angiotensin-aldosterone system, RAAS]); (2) rest-activity–associated changes in behavior such as activity routine and level, fluid and stimulant (eg, caffeine) consumption, meal timings and content, emotional and mental stress, and posture; (3) day-night divergence in ambient light intensity and spectrum, temperature, humidity, and noise.[1–4] The normally lower BP during nighttime sleep relative to daytime wakefulness thus repre-sents the simultaneous influence of several predicable-in-time behavioral and environmental cycles combined with circadian rhythm stage-dependent alterations, most prominently the decline of sympathetic and increase of vagal tone, elevation of atrial natriuretic and calcitonin gene-related vasoactive peptides, and depression of the RAAS during the first half of the rest span followed by progressive activation during the second half of rest until peaking in the morning.[2,4–7]

Only ambulatory BP monitoring (ABPM) properly describes and quantifies the BP 24-hour variation. The findings of multiple ABPM studies consistently document strong association between the abnormal physiologic feature of blunted sleep-time relative BP decline (non-dipper/riser BP patterning) and the increased incidence of fatal and nonfatal cardiovascular disease (CVD) events, not only in hypertensive[8–13] but also in normotensive individuals.[14] Furthermore, various independent prospective studies demonstrate CVD events are better predicted by the ABPM-derived asleep than either the awake or 24-hour BP means or conventional daytime office BP measurements (OBPM).[10–13,15–20] Accordingly, there is great clinical interest of how to best tailor treatment to achieve the novel therapeutic goals of normalizing asleep BP and sleep-time relative BP decline (percent decrease in mean BP during nighttime sleep relative to the mean BP during awake-time activity) to the usual dipper pattern, which as a consequence protects against CVD and other events.[12,13,21] Thus, the purpose of this review is to present the latest findings pertaining to bedtime hypertension chronotherapy: the judicious scheduling of conventional BP-lowering medications in accord with circadian rhythm de-terminants, as a simple and cost-effective means to both regularize these abnormal characteristics of the 24-hour BP pattern and reduce CVD, stroke, renal, metabolic, and other risks.

INGESTION-TIME DIFFERENCES IN PHARMACODYNAMICS OF HYPERTENSION MEDICATIONS

The pharmacokinetics (PK) of hypertension medi-cations are significantly influenced by the well-documented circadian rhythms in gastric pH, transport, and emptying; gastrointestinal motility; biliary function; glomerular filtration; hepatic enzyme activity; and organ (duodenum, liver, and kidney) blood flow.[22–24] Statistically and clinically significant ingestion time (more specifically, circa-dian stage) differences in the pharmacodynamics (PD) of hypertension medications,[25–31] that is, therapeutic modulation of the features of the 24-hour BP pattern and risk to adverse effects, can result not only from circadian rhythm dependencies of their PK but also from their circulating active free fraction plus receptor number/confor-mation and second messengers/signaling path-ways of drug-targeted sites, for example, blood vessel, heart, and kidney tissue, and ANS and RAAS.[25,26,32] However, ingestion-time differences in the therapeutic and adverse effects of BP-reducing medications need not be solely depen-dent upon PK because the timing of peak and trough drug blood concentrations relative to the staging of the many underlying circadian rhythms that give rise to the unique 24-hour BP pattern may be more important.[3,4]

Two common mistakes made in the design and conduct of chronopharmacology–, ingestion-time differences of the PK and PD of medications due to biological rhythm influences, and chrono-therapy trials of BP-lowering agents are (1) failure to require as a key inclusion criterion only subjects who have a life routine of diurnal activity alter-nating with nighttime sleep as confirmed by diary entries, and (2) selection of treatment times ac-cording to clock hour rather than meaningful bio-logical markers of circadian stage, for example, upon morning awakening and at bedtime for par-ticipants adhering to a consistent diurnal wake and nocturnal sleep routine. Such an approach takes into account individual differences in exact activity onset (awakening from repose) and activity offset (bedtime), as consistently done in the au-thors' prospective trials.[28] Another frequent error is reliance solely upon daytime OBPM. Qualifica-tion of subjects for medication trials when relying on clinical cuff methods alone can be misleading because of probable incorporation of individuals with masked normotension (also termed isolated-office hypertension, ie, elevated clinic BP but normal out-of-office BP validated by ABPM)[33] and exclusion of otherwise high-risk patients with masked normotension (normal OBPM and elevated ABPM, mainly during nighttime sleep).[17,33] In addition, reliance upon daytime OBPM and/or at-home awake-time BP self-measurements precludes evaluation of effects of different therapies and their dosing times on the most pertinent and highly significant prognostic characteristics of the 24-hour BP pattern: the asleep BP mean and sleep-time relative BP decline. Accordingly, the legitimate means of researching and quantifying ingestion time (circadian rhythm–dependent) differences in the PD of BP medications is through trials that incorporate 24-hour or longer ABPM to enable assessment of therapeutic outcomes in terms of reductions of both the awake and the asleep BP means individually derived by taking into consideration the actual activity and sleep spans of each participant. Thus, this review focuses almost exclusively on trials that (1) entail 24-hour or longer patient ABPM assessment and (2) report therapeutic effects of different medication timings upon both the actual awake *and* the asleep systolic blood pressure (SBP) and diastolic blood pressure (DBP) means of patients, with the clock times of the commencement and conclusion of the awake and asleep spans based on actual diary or activity monitoring of each participant rather the preassumed or software default ones that are often the case in such investigations.

Numerous prospective randomized clinical trials clearly verify the nature and extent of the desired effects upon the 24-hour BP pattern exerted by angiotensin-converting enzyme inhibitors (ACEIs):

angiotensin-II receptor blockers (ARBs), calcium-channel blockers (CCBs), α-blockers, β-blockers, and diuretics differ, often substantially, according to treatment time. Moreover, patient tolerance, in terms of adverse effects, to some classes of these hypertension therapies is greatly improved when ingested alone or in combination at bedtime rather than upon awakening from sleep.[25–31]

Angiotensin-Converting Enzyme Inhibitor Monotherapy

A substantial series of studies demonstrates the ACEIs of benazepril, captopril, enalapril, imidapril, lisinopril, perindopril, quinapril, ramipril, spirapril, trandolapril, and zofenopril, as a class and independent of medication terminal half-life, when routinely ingested in the evening or at bedtime in comparison to upon morning awakening: (1) exerts significantly better BP-lowering effects upon the asleep than awake BP means (for extensive review see Ref.[28]); (2) better converts the 24-hour BP profile toward or into the normal dipping one; and/or (3) improves patient tolerance to therapy.[25–31]

An illustrative example is provided by the clinical trial of Hermida and Ayala[34] entailing 115 previously untreated hypertensive patients who were randomized to either upon-wakening or bedtime 5-mg ramipril monotherapy and assessed by 48-hour ABPM before and after 6 weeks of therapy. Although ingestion time shows no differential effect on the daytime OBPM values or 48-hour and awake SBP/DBP means, the bedtime schedule, compared with the morning treatment schedule, results in very significant larger reduction of the asleep SBP/DBP means (−13.5/−11.5 vs −4.5/−4.1 mm Hg; P<.001 between groups). **Fig. 1**, which depicts the differential ingestion time–dependent effects of ramipril on SBP, reveals peak BP-lowering effects is achieved more rapidly

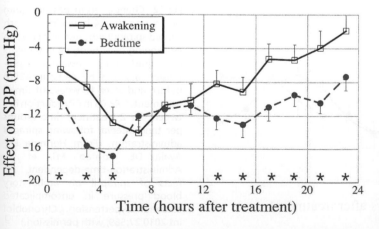

Fig. 1. Changes from baseline (mm Hg) during the 24 hours in SBP with 5 mg/d ramipril ingested either upon awakening or at bedtime in patients with grade 1 to 2 essential hypertension assessed by 48-hour ABPM before and after 6 weeks of timed treatment. * P<.05 in BP reduction between the 2 treatment-time groups per time interval following ramipril administration. (*Modified from* Hermida RC, Ayala DE. Chronotherapy with the angiotensin-converting enzyme inhibitor ramipril in essential hypertension: improved blood pressure control with bedtime dosing. Hypertension 2009;54:44; with permission.)

with the bedtime than upon morning awakening treatment schedule, giving rise to significantly greater therapeutic efficacy during the initial 6 hours after drug administration. Moreover, the BP-lowering effect duration is shorter when ramipril is ingested upon awakening than at bedtime, resulting in BP reduction with bedtime ramipril administration being significantly greater during the last 12 hours of the 24-hour dosing interval.[34]

The findings of another study by Hermida and colleagues[35] using an identical investigative protocol and involving 165 previously untreated hypertensive patients demonstrate the differential treatment-time effects of ACEIs upon the 24-hour BP profile are independent of medication half-life. Treatment with the long (~40-hour) terminal plasma half-life ACEI spirapril in a 6-mg once-daily dose for 12 weeks in patients randomized to bedtime, compared with upon-awakening, dosing better decreases the asleep SBP/DBP means (−12.8/−8.6 vs −5.7/−4.6 mm Hg; P<.001 between treatment-time groups) and enhances the sleep-time relative BP decline toward normal dipper pattern.[35] When ingested in the morning, spirapril loses its BP-lowering efficacy shortly after attaining its peak effect, ~3 hours after dosing (**Fig. 2**). In contrast, when ingested at bedtime, maximum BP-lowering effect is maintained for the ensuing 8-hour span, thus showing greater efficacy, relative to morning administration, during this time span. Thus, the efficacy of spirapril, like ramipril, is significantly greater during the last half, particularly the last 4 hours, of the 24-hour dosing interval with bedtime, as compared with upon awakening, administration (see **Fig. 2**).[35] The findings for zofenopril (30 mg once daily for 1 month) in a study of 33 previously untreated hypertensive patients are similar: bedtime, compared with awakening, dosing of zofenopril better

reduces the asleep BP mean and increases from 51.5% to 84.8% (P<.001) the proportion of patients with controlled ambulatory BP.[36]

Angiotensin-II Receptor Blockers Monotherapy

Prospective clinical trials with irbesartan, olmesartan, telmisartan, and valsartan also corroborate significant ingestion-time differences in therapeutic effects independent of medication terminal half-life.[25–31] As found for ACEIs, choice of treatment time with various ARBs exerts no differential reduction of the awake SBP/DBP means; however, reduction of the asleep SBP/DBP means is more profound by the bedtime than morning therapeutic regimen, thereby significantly decreasing the prevalence from baseline of non-dipping.[37–44] Importantly, bedtime, but not upon-waking time, ingestion of valsartan,[40] candesartan,[45,46] and olmesartan,[47] also significantly reduces urinary albumin excretion, a measure of renal hemodynamics and abnormality, which correlates strongly with extent of decrease in the asleep BP mean and increase in the sleep-time relative BP decline,[40] and in one study improvement of baroreflex sensitivity.[46]

Hermida and colleagues[40] were the first to assess the efficacy of valsartan monotherapy (160 mg once daily for 12 weeks) when ingested either upon awakening or at bedtime in a randomized trial involving 90 hypertensive patients. When valsartan is ingested at bedtime, attenuation of the asleep SBP/DBP means is significantly greater than the awake SBP/DBP means (−17.9/−13.3 vs −12.0/−9.8 mm Hg, respectively; P = .009/.015). Consequently, the bedtime treatment schedule results in a highly significant average increase by 6% in the sleep-time relative BP decline,

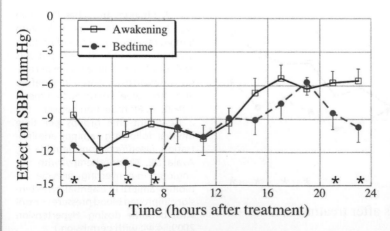

Fig. 2. Changes from baseline (mm Hg) during the 24 hours in SBP with 6 mg/d spirapril ingested either upon awakening or at bedtime in patients with grade 1 to 2 essential hypertension assessed by 48-hour ABPM before and after 12 weeks of timed treatment. * P<.05 in BP reduction between the 2 treatment-time groups per time interval following spirapril administration. (*From* Hermida RC, Ayala DE, Fontao MJ, et al. Administration-time-dependent effects of spirapril on ambulatory blood pressure in uncomplicated essential hypertension. Chronobiol Int 2010;27:569; with permission.)

which translates into 73% reduction from baseline in the number of non-dipper patients.[40] These results are corroborated by 2 subsequent independent prospective trials, one involving elderly hypertensive patients,[41] who as a group are prone to greater blunting of sleep-time relative BP decline than younger hypertensive patients,[48] and the second involving non-dipper hypertensive patients.[39,42] The composite findings of all these trials entailing valsartan again show reduction of the asleep SBP/DBP mean is significantly greater when valsartan is ingested at bedtime than upon awakening (−18.4/−12.6 vs −12.4/−8.9 mm Hg, respectively; P<.001 between treatment-time groups). The differential effects of the 160 mg/d valsartan dose on SBP according to the circadian time of drug ingestion are shown in **Fig. 3**. Significant SBP lowering throughout the entire 24-hour dosing interval is achieved independent of medication ingestion time; however, SBP reduction is significantly greater during the first 10 hours following treatment when valsartan is ingested at bedtime. The greater reduction of the asleep SBP/DBP means by a bedtime than morning schedule with a higher 320 mg/d dose of valsartan is also documented in a recent investigator-promoted independent study on hypertensive patients with sleep apnea,[49] but not in an industry-promoted trial limited by faulty study design, that is, selection of treatment times according to clock hour plus improper reliance upon daytime and nighttime BP means determined by using the same respective fixed clock-hour spans for all participants, instead of the most pertinent individualized and properly representative awake and asleep means.[50]

Of particular interest is the fact that telmisartan, even though having a terminal plasma half-life greater than 24 hours, also exerts significant ingestion-time differences in therapeutic effects.[43] A total of 215 grade 1 to 2 essential hypertensive patients were randomized to 12 weeks of 80 mg/d telmisartan monotherapy dosed either consistently upon awakening or at bedtime. Significant and comparable lowering of the OBPM- and ABPM-derived 48-hour and awake SBP/DBP means from baseline is achieved by the 2 treatment strategies. However, bedtime, relative to morning, treatment achieves significantly greater attenuation of the asleep SBP/DBP means (−13.8/−9.7 vs −8.3/−6.4 mm Hg; P<.001 between treatment-time groups). Thus, when telmisartan is ingested upon awakening, the sleep-time relative SBP/DBP decline is actually slightly decreased toward the non-dipping pattern (−1.6/−1.0; P = .010/.157), whereas when ingested at bedtime, it is significantly enhanced toward normal (3.1/3.9; P<.001), thereby reducing the prevalence from baseline of the abnormal non-dipper BP pattern by 76% (P<.001).[43] **Fig. 4** shows the differential effects of telmisartan on ambulatory BP relative to its administration time. Despite the long half-life of telmisartan, when taken in the morning upon awakening, compared with at bedtime, its BP-lowering efficacy is progressively lost to a greater extent, commencing 16 hours after ingestion. Consequently, BP reduction is significantly greater during the last 8 hours of the dosing interval when the medication is administered routinely at bedtime (see **Fig. 4**). These differential ingestion-time effects can be largely explained in terms of when, during the 24 hours, highest and lowest telmisartan concentrations are attained relative to the sleep-time activation of the RAAS circadian rhythm. The same explanation applies to the differential effects of ACEIs when ingested

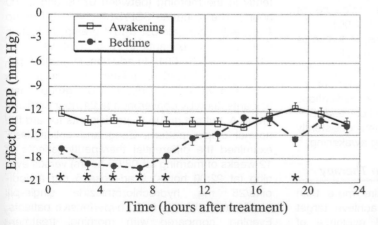

Time (hours after treatment)

Fig. 3. Changes from baseline (mm Hg) during the 24 hours in SBP with 160 mg/d valsartan ingested either upon awakening or at bedtime in patients with grade 1 to 2 essential hypertension assessed by 48-hours ABPM before and after 12 weeks of timed treatment. * P<.05 in BP reduction between the 2 treatment-time groups per time interval following valsartan administration. (*Modified from* Hermida RC, Ayala DE, Smolensky MH, et al. Chronotherapy with conventional blood pressure medications improves management of hypertension and reduces cardiovascular and stroke risks. Hypertens Res 2016;39:284; with permission.)

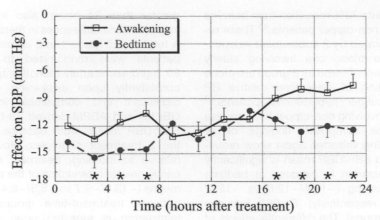

Fig. 4. Changes from baseline (mm Hg) during the 24 hours in SBP with 80 mg/d telmisartan ingested either upon awakening or at bedtime in patients with grade 1 to 2 essential hypertension assessed by 48-hour ABPM before and after 12 weeks of timed treatment. * $P<.05$ in BP reduction between the 2 treatment-time groups per time interval following telmisartan administration. (*Modified from* Hermida RC, Ayala DE, Smolensky MH, et al. Chronotherapy with conventional blood pressure medications improves management of hypertension and reduces cardiovascular and stroke risks. Hypertens Res 2016;39:283; with permission.)

in the morning upon awakening versus at bedtime, as discussed in the previous section.

Other Hypertension Monotherapies

Prospective clinical trials involving amlodipine, cilnidipine, diltiazem, isradipine, nifedipine, nisoldipine, and nitrendipine indicate dihydropyridine CCBs generally reduce BP homogeneously throughout the 24 hours, whether routinely ingested in the morning or evening.[28] However, dosing time can be a determinant of risk for drug-associated adverse effects. The findings of a randomized by treatment time study by Hermida and colleagues[51,52] of 238 previously untreated hypertensive patients revealed 8-week bedtime, compared with upon-awakening, 30-mg once-daily nifedipine gastrointestinal therapeutic system (GITS) monotherapy significantly reduces the incidence of peripheral edema, from 13% to 1% ($P<.001$).

Other hypertension monotherapies, including α-blocker doxazosin,[53] β-blockers carvedilol[54] and nebivolol,[55] and loop-diuretic torasemide,[56] also evidence significant administration-time differences in beneficial effect. All these medications exert enhanced asleep BP reduction and BP-lowering effect of longer duration when consistently taken at bedtime than upon morning awakening.

Fixed Combination Hypertension Therapy

Most hypertensive patients require more than one BP-lowering medication to achieve target BP goals.[57] Despite substantial evidence of treatment-time differences in effects of hypertension monotherapies, only a limited number of

studies have trialed combination medications at different times of the day.[28]

Middeke and colleagues[58] reported the once-daily 25 mg captopril/12.5 mg hydrochlorothiazide combination therapy (13 hypertensive men for 3 weeks) slightly better reduces the nighttime BP mean when ingested at 20:00 hours and significantly more effectively ($P<.01$) reduces daytime BP when taken at 08:00 hours. Meng and colleagues[59] randomized 40 hypertensive patients uncontrolled by either amlodipine or fosinopril monotherapy into 2 groups for 4 weeks of combination therapy with both medications. Group A patients routinely took 5 mg amlodipine in the morning (between 07:00 and 08:00 hours) and 10 mg fosinopril at bedtime, and group B patients always took the 2 medications together consistently in the morning (between 07:00 and 08:00 hours). The nighttime SBP/DBP means of group A patients show almost 3-fold greater reduction than group B patients ($-22.4/-17.4$ vs $-7.6/-6.3$ mm Hg, $P<.001$). In addition, in group A patients, the sleep-time relative BP decline is increased, whereas it is decreased in group B participants, thereby converting the 24-hour profile of group A, but not group B, participants toward the normal dipper pattern. Zeng and colleagues[60] examined the differential therapeutic effects of 12 weeks of morning (at 08:00 hours) versus evening (at 22:00 hours) fixed-dose 5 mg amlodipine/25 mg hydrochlorothiazide single-pill combination therapy in 80 hypertensive patients. Evening, compared with morning, treatment significantly better reduces the nighttime BP mean, resulting in 3-fold lesser proportion of patients with non-dipper BP patterning (25% vs 8%; P<.001). Hoshino and colleagues,[47] in a small sample study of 31 hypertensive patients, compared the BP-lowering effect of bedtime versus morning amlodipine/olmesartan combination therapy, with titration of doses on a per-patient basis ranging from 2.5 to 10 mg of amlodipine and 20 to 40 mg of olmesartan. The bedtime, relative to the morning, regimen more effectively reduces nighttime BP in non-dipper but not dipper patients, and it more effectively reduces urinary albumin/creatinine ratio (42.5 ± 59.9 mg/g vs 75.3 ± 26.4 mg/g; P = .044), thereby inferring the bedtime scheduling of this combination therapy exerts significantly better renoprotection.

In a much larger and more comprehensive combination therapy study, Hermida and colleagues[61] randomly assigned 203 hypertensive patients to 1 of 4 different 160 mg valsartan/5 mg amlodipine regimens for 12 weeks: both medications taken together upon awakening, both taken together at bedtime, or either one of them ingested upon awakening and the other at bedtime. Ingestion of both medications together at bedtime best reduces the asleep SBP/DBP means and in so doing significantly increases the sleep-time relative BP decline toward the normal dipper pattern (P<.001). Finally, Hermida and colleagues[62] evaluated 204 hypertensive patients with uncontrolled ambulatory BP according to published ABPM criteria[33,57] after initial randomization to 160 mg/d valsartan monotherapy either upon awakening or at bedtime for 12 weeks. Hydrochlorothiazide (12.5 mg) was added and administered as a single-pill combination formulation with valsartan, with patients adhering to the same original awakening or bedtime treatment-time schedule for an additional 12 weeks. The bedtime, relative to upon awakening, combination therapy better reduces the asleep means of SBP (20.1 mm Hg vs 16.0 mm Hg, P = .015) and pulse pressure, that is, SBP/DBP, a measure of arterial tree compliance (6.5 mm Hg vs 4.0 mm Hg, P = .007), and significantly reduces non-dipper BP pattern, from 59% of patients at baseline to 23% at study conclusion (P<.001).

BEDTIME CHRONOTHERAPY FOR DIFFICULT TO CONTROL AND COMPLICATED HYPERTENSION
Resistant Hypertension

Resistant hypertension (RH) constitutes a clear illustration of the clinical relevance of a chronotherapeutic strategy that takes into account circadian changes in the physiology and biochemistry of BP control and regulation. RH patients are at considerably greater risk for renal disease and insufficiency and CVD and stroke events than are patients whose BP is well controlled by medication.[19,63] According to present criteria,[63] hypertension is designated as resistant to treatment when lifestyle measures plus therapeutic doses of ≥3 prescription BP-lowering medications, one preferably a diuretic unless contraindicated, fails to reduce SBP and DBP to OBPM threshold values,[63] a definition the authors contend lacks validity,[33] as later discussed. Current RH therapeutic strategies, which are far too often unsuccessful, either comprise prescription of additional medications or exchange of ≥1 of them for others in an attempt to improve synergic BP-reducing effects.[57,63] Based upon the information presented in the preceding sections, which clearly substantiates enhancement of BP-lowering efficacy by the bedtime treatment schedule, it is logical to question whether RH patients are said to be "resistant" to therapy because it is prescribed for ingestion at the wrong, morning, rather than right, bedtime (ie, circadian stage) when most effective.[28,64–68]

One cross-sectional study conducted by Hermida and colleagues[64] of 700 RH patients who were assessed by 48-hour ABPM reports the proportion of patients with controlled ambulatory BP (awake and asleep SBP/DBP means below current diagnostic thresholds) is 2-fold greater in those who ingest the entire daily dose of ≥1 hypertension medications routinely at bedtime than in those who ingest all medications upon awakening. In addition, the prevalence of non-dipping is significantly lower in patients taking ≥1 medications at bedtime than in those taking all of them on awakening, respectively, 57% versus 82%.[64] A larger identically designed cross-sectional study of 1794 RH patients evaluated by 48-hour ABPM also documents control of ambulatory BP among those ingesting the entire daily dose of ≥1 medications at bedtime is significantly higher (than among those ingesting all medications upon awakening [31.9% vs 23.1%; P<.001]).[66] Moreover, the bedtime, versus upon awakening, treatment schedule better lowers the asleep SBP/DBP means (by 9.7/4.4 mm Hg, P<.001), resulting in significantly greater (by 5.8%; P<.001) sleep-time relative BP decline and consequently significantly lower prevalence of non-dipper BP patterning (40% vs 83%, respectively; P<.001).

Another even larger trial by Hermida and colleagues,[67] also entailing 48-hour ABPM, assessed the role of treatment-time regimen on 24-hour BP patterning of 2899 RH patients enrolled in the ongoing large multicenter outcomes Hygia Project.[21] The Hygia Project, comprising patients of primary care centers of Galicia (Northwest Spain), is a prospective investigation of the prognostic value of ABPM and treatment-time strategy on BP control and CVD and other risks. ABPM is done upon recruitment and at least annually thereafter, always for 48 hours to achieve confidence of findings and with diary recording of time of retiring to bed at night and awakening in the morning to enable accurate calculation of the awake and asleep SBP and DBP means. Of the total cohort of 2899 RH patients, 1084 consistently took all their hypertension medications upon awakening (awakening regimen), 1436 others took the entire daily dose of $\geq$1 of them at bedtime (bedtime chronotherapy regimen), and the remaining 379 patients took equally divided doses of $\geq$1 medications twice daily, upon awakening and at bedtime (twice daily regimen). The bedtime chronotherapy regimen, compared with the awakening and twice daily ones, achieves significantly higher prevalence of properly controlled ambulatory BP, best reduces the asleep SBP/DBP means, and best enhances the sleep-time relative BP decline, resulting in lowest prevalence of non-dipping (54.4% vs 80.5% and 77.3%, respectively; P<.001 for comparison between the 3 treatment strategies).[67]

The findings and conclusions of these cross-sectional RH studies were prospectively validated in a randomized trial that examined the role of treatment time, without increase in the number of prescribed medications, on ambulatory BP pattern and control of 250 true RH patients, defined by uncontrolled awake and/or asleep ambulatory BP means when ingesting all 3 prescribed BP-lowering medications upon awakening.[65] Participants were randomly assigned to 1 of 2 groups according to treatment strategy: (1) Group A: exchange of 1 of the 3 medications for a new one, and retaining the same upon-awakening administration schedule; and (2) Group B: also exchange of 1 of the 3 medications for a new one, and administrating it always at bedtime. Forty-eight-hour ABPM studies conducted before and after 12 weeks of the new therapeutic schemes reveals for group A no change in ambulatory BP from baseline and slight increase in non-dipping prevalence, from 79% at baseline to 86% at study conclusion (P = .131); for group B significant reduction in ambulatory 48-hour SBP/DBP means ($-9.4/-6.0$ mm Hg; P<.001), with greater decrease of the asleep than awake BP mean, so the proportion of patients displaying the dipper pattern increases from only 16% at baseline to 57% at study conclusion (P<.001).[65] Finally, the findings of a recent small study of 27 RH patients by another group[69] are consistent with those of the above-cited studies. Shifting all nondiuretic hypertension medications from morning to evening not only significantly reduces the nighttime BP

(P = .005) but also enhances the sleep-time relative BP decline toward the more dipper pattern.

Collectively, the findings of the above-reviewed studies verify a bedtime hypertension therapy regimen that entails the full daily dose of $\geq$1 medication for RH, which ought to be established properly by around-the-clock ABPM, is the therapeutic scheme of choice.[33,70] Moreover, together the findings additionally indicate the current definition of RH is invalid and must be modified to take into account the major deterministic variable of circadian time of treatment; accordingly, a patient should be categorized as resistant to treatment *only* if his/her ABPM-determined awake and/or (preferably) asleep SBP/DBP means are greater than the reference diagnostic thresholds[33,57] when at least one of the prescribed $\geq$3 hypertension medications of different classes, ideally including a diuretic unless contraindicated, is ingested in full daily dose at bedtime.[33]

Chronic Kidney Disease

The prevalence of hypertension is elevated in chronic kidney disease (CKD), increasing with diminishing estimated glomerular filtration rate (eGFR), and according to one report being as high as 86% in end-stage renal disease.[71] Elevated asleep BP (sleep-time hypertension) and non-dipper BP pattern are highly prevalent in CKD.[72–75] Mojón and colleagues,[75] using 48-hour ABPM to assess 10,271 hypertensive participants enrolled in the ongoing Hygia Project, reports (1) prevalence of non-dipper BP patterning is much greater in CKD than in absence of CKD (60.6% vs 43.2%, respectively; P<.001 between groups); (2) prevalence of riser BP patterning (sleep-time relative SBP decline <0) is more than 2-fold higher in CKD than in absence of CKD (17.6% vs 7.1%, respectively; P<.001), and (3), perhaps most importantly, among CKD participants with uncontrolled BP, 90.7% evidence sleep-time hypertension. These collective findings motivate the testing of chronotherapeutic interventions for CKD, as reviewed in later discussion, to improve the management of high BP, curtail disease progression, and reduce CVD and stroke risk of these exceedingly vulnerable patients.

The impact of treatment-time regimen on ambulatory BP patterning and control in CKD, defined according to current criteria of eGFR less than 60 mL/min/1.73 m^2 or albuminuria (albumin/creatinine ratio $\geq$30 mg/gCr), or both, at least twice within a 3-month span,[76] was recently investigated by Crespo and colleagues.[74] Among the 2659 evaluated hypertensive participants of the Hygia Project with CKD, 1446 ingested all their prescribed BP-lowering medications upon awakening and 1213 others ingested the entire daily dose of ≥1 of them at bedtime. Among the latter, 359 patients took all such medications at bedtime, whereas 854 took the complete daily dose of some of them upon awakening and the rest of them at bedtime. Patients managed with either one of the bedtime chronotherapy regimens, relative to those managed with the conventional upon-awakening one, evidenced significantly better: (1) reduction of the asleep SBP/DBP means, (2) enhancement of the sleep-time relative BP decline ($P<.001$), and (3) attenuation of non-dipping prevalence (68.3% in those managed conventionally vs 54.2% and 47.9%, respectively, in those managed by the ≥1 and all-medications bedtime chronotherapy regimens; $P<.001$ between groups). Moreover, the prevalence of riser BP patterning is significantly lower in participants ingesting ≥1 (15.7%) or all (10.6%) hypertension medications at bedtime rather than all of them upon awakening (21.5%; $P<.001$ between groups). Finally, patients ingesting all their medications at bedtime show significantly higher prevalence of controlled ambulatory BP ($P<.001$) that is achieved by significantly fewer BP-lowering medications ($P<.001$) compared with patients of the other treatment cohorts and who evidenced inferior BP control.[74]

Minutolo and colleagues,[77] who evaluated a rather small sample of 32 uncontrolled non-dipper CKD patients, reports significant reduction of the nighttime BP mean, with consequent decreased urinary albumin excretion, after shifting the administration of one BP-lowering medication from morning to evening. Another study entailing 151 black participants enrolled in the African American Study of Kidney Disease with controlled clinic and awake BP differs somewhat.[78] This study compared the effects on nocturnal SBP (improperly defined according to an identical fixed clock-hour span across all participants) of either shifting to bedtime an already prescribed once-a-day hypertension medication or adding at bedtime a new low-dose one. Both strategies decrease nocturnal SBP, but not significantly ($P = .08$), prompting the investigators to conclude bedtime chronotherapy might be of limited advantage in reducing nighttime BP in hypertensive African American and/or CKD patients. However, as earlier discussed, failure to detect statistical significance could be due to faulty study design, that is, failure to assess changes in the actual asleep SBP mean based on data truly representative of the sleep period of each participant rather than an assumed, and most likely poorly representative, common nighttime span defined by a priori selected clock-time. Indeed, confirmation of the expected better effect of bedtime chronotherapy, relative to conventional morning-time therapy, for black African persons is reported in a Nigerian study of 165 high-BP presumably diurnally active patients randomized to 12 weeks of either morning (at 10:00 hours) or evening (at 22:00 hours) hypertension treatment. The evening therapeutic strategy, in comparison to the conventional morning one, results in significantly greater reduction not only of BP but also of left ventricular mass ($P<.001$).[79] Finally, a recent study of 60 non-dipper Chinese CKD patients asserts bedtime, relative to morning-time, valsartan (per patient doses ranging from 80 to 320 mg) therapy for 1 year achieves significantly greater reduction not only of nighttime BP and left ventricular mass, as in the Nigeria study,[79] but also of albuminuria (P always $<.05$).[80] Because of the very high prevalence of abnormal 24-hour BP profiling in CKD, that is, sleep-time hypertension and non-dipping and rising BP patterning, plus documented better effects of a bedtime hypertension regimen on asleep BP regulation,[25–31] as documented by most of the above reviewed studies, bedtime treatment is now recommended as the preferred strategy to manage hypertension in CKD patients.[29,33]

Diabetes

There is strong association between diabetes and elevated risk of end-organ damage, stroke, and CVD morbidity and mortality. In addition, non-dipping and sleep-time hypertension are highly prevalent in patients with diabetes.[81–83] Ayala and colleagues[82] compared features of the ambulatory BP pattern of 2954 hypertensive patients with type 2 diabetes and 9811 hypertensive patients without diabetes enrolled in the Hygia Project. Prevalence of non-dipping is significantly higher in those with than without diabetes (62.1 vs 45.9%; $P<.001$); however, prevalence of riser BP patterning constitutes the most profound difference between groups (19.9 vs 8.1% in patients with and without diabetes, respectively; $P<.001$). In addition, 89.2% of the uncontrolled hypertensive patients with diabetes in this cohort evidence sleep-time hypertension. Despite the very high prevalence of sleep-time hypertension and non-dipper and riser patterns, only a small number of investigations have explored the impact of hypertension treatment time on BP regulation and control in persons with diabetes.

A crossover design investigation by Tofé and García[84] evaluated the ambulatory BP response of 40 type 2 diabetes hypertensive patients to 40 mg/d olmesartan when taken for 8 weeks either always upon awakening or at bedtime. The bedtime treatment approach results in both significantly greater reduction of nighttime SBP (-16.2 vs -11.8; $P = .007$) and increase in sleep-time relative SBP decline (7.4 vs 2.2%; $P<.001$). Rossen and colleagues[85] also used a crossover design to explore the effect of changing the administration time of hypertension medications in 41 patients with type 2 diabetes, finding the bedtime in comparison to morning treatment regimen results in significant reduction of the nighttime SBP mean (7.5 mm Hg, $P<.001$) with nonsignificant reduction of the daytime SBP mean (1.3 mm Hg, $P = .336$). Moyá and colleagues[83] evaluated the differential beneficial effects of hypertension treatment-time regimen on ambulatory BP patterning of 2429 hypertensive participants with type 2 diabetes participants of the Hygia Project. Among them, 1176 took all BP-lowering medications upon awakening and 1253 took the entire daily dose of ≥ 1 medications at bedtime: 336 patients taking all hypertension medications at bedtime and the other 917 patients taking the entire daily dose of some of them upon awakening and the others at bedtime. Ingestion of ≥ 1 medications at bedtime, compared with ingestion of all of them upon awakening, significantly better reduces the asleep SBP/DBP means and better normalizes the sleep-time relative BP decline. Thus, the prevalence of non-dipping is significantly higher when all hypertension medications are taken upon awakening (68.6%) than when ≥ 1 (55.8%) or all of them (49.7%; $P<.001$ between groups) are taken at bedtime. The bedtime treatment group, relative to all the other ones, also shows significantly higher prevalence of properly controlled ambulatory BP ($P<.001$) that is achieved by a significantly lesser number of hypertension medications ($P<.001$).[83]

Finally, Suzuki and Aizawa[86] provide an example of the misleading conclusions that commonly result from poorly conceptualized protocols when applied to assessing chronotherapeutic interventions. These investigators randomized 34 already treated hypertensive patients with type 2 diabetes into 3 valsartan (160 mg) therapy groups defined by the ingestion of the following: the entire daily dose following breakfast or dinner, or twice daily, that is, one-half the daily dose (80 mg) in the morning and other half (80 mg) in the evening. The investigators report no significant between-group difference in the reduction of OBPM or home self-measured BP. Findings of this and several other studies of administration-time differences in therapeutic effect of hypertension medications that rely solely upon daytime OBPM and/or

wake-time home BP measurements are of little, if any, practical utility for many reasons. First, "white-coat" and "masking" effects may compromise the representativeness of OBPM, whereas inconsistent technique of self-assessment and poor patient compliance may compromise accuracy of home BP data. Second, choice of dosing times is based on clock time, rather than biological (circadian) time relative to the individual patient sleep-wake routine. Third, and most important, the investigative protocol of these studies fail to collect data throughout the entire 24 hours to reliably derive the clinically meaningful characteristics of the 24-hour BP profile proven to be closely linked with CVD risk, that is, the asleep SBP mean and sleep-time relative SBP decline. Thus, the findings of improperly conceptualized protocols, as illustrated by this example, are not only useless but misleading and detrimental by adding confusion, uncertainty, and unfounded controversy to the medical literature and patient care.

Non-Dipper Hypertension

Patients diagnosed with RH,[64–69] CKD,[74,77,78,80] and type 2 diabetes[83–85] have high prevalence of non-dipping, as reviewed in the several preceding sections. In addition, several chronotherapy trials have specifically researched control of the asleep BP and/or increase of the sleep-time relative BP decline (dipping) of non-dipper hypertensive patients.

The first such bedtime chronotherapy trial entailing non-dipping hypertensive patients was conducted by Hermida and colleagues.[39] It involved 148 individuals randomized to 160 mg/d valsartan either upon awakening or at bedtime who were assessed by 48-hour ABPM both before and after 12 weeks of timed therapy. Significant substantial lowering from baseline of the 48-hour SBP/DBP means ($P<.001$) is ingestion-time independent (upon awakening treatment: $-13.1/-8.4$ vs at bedtime treatment: $-14.6/-10.1$ mm Hg; $P>.126$ for treatment-time effect). However, reduction of the asleep SBP/DBP means is significantly greater when valsartan is consistently taken at bedtime than conventionally upon awakening ($-21.1/$ -13.9 vs $-12.5/-8.3$ mm Hg, respectively; $P<.001$ between treatment-time groups), resulting in significant enhancement of the sleep-time relative BP decline and with 75% of the patients reverting to the normal dipper BP pattern. In addition, the bedtime chronotherapy strategy not only significantly increases the proportion of patients with controlled ambulatory BP but significantly decreases urinary albumin excretion.[40] An extension of this valsartan trial to include a total of 200 non-dipper hypertensive patients yields similar favorable results of the bedtime chronotherapy strategy relative to the traditional morning one, that is, more aggressive reduction of the asleep BP mean plus improved normalization of the sleep-time relative BP decline.[42]

A prospective, double-blind, placebo-controlled study by Qiu and colleagues[87] of 121 treated non-dipper hypertensive patients randomized to evening (at 22:00 hours) 12.5 mg captopril or placebo indicates the ACEI treatment strategy both significantly reduces nighttime BP and restores normal BP dipping in 70% of patients. The study, however, lacks a morning-time treatment comparison group to properly evaluate the findings. Another trial by Takeda and colleagues[88] involved 71 Japanese hypertensive patients, approximately half of them non-dippers, who had been ingesting long-acting once-daily BP-lowering medications in the morning. Shifting therapy for the 35 non-dipper patients from morning to bedtime results in a slight increase of the daytime SBP/DBP means (+5/+3 mm Hg; $P<.02$) and marked decrease in the nighttime ones ($-13/-6$ mm Hg, $P<.001$), thereby enhancing the sleep-time relative SBP decline from 2.6% to 15.5% ($P<.001$). Finally, Farah and colleagues[89] investigated the role of treatment time on BP patterning of 60 non-dipper hypertensive patients randomly assigned to continue to take their prescribed BP-lowering medications upon awakening or shift their administration to bedtime. Investigators verified significant reduction in the nighttime BP mean among patients transferred to the bedtime therapy schedule, with 86% of them showing controlled ambulatory BP.

SUMMARY

The goal of all hypertension treatment strategies is reduction of SBP and DBP as a means of preventing end-organ injury and decreasing CVD, stroke, renal disease, and other life-threatening risks. Early outcome trials, based solely on daytime OBPM, report prevention of CVD events by BP-lowering treatment is consistent and, to a certain extent, independent of class of prescribed hypertension medications. However, such findings are based primarily on outcome trials that have involved the customary morning-time treatment schedule to target correction of only the daytime OBPM level as opposed to correction of features, mainly the asleep SBP mean and sleep-time relative SBP decline, of the 24-hour BP pattern known to be much more strongly associated with CVD risk. The diagnostic approaches and treatment strategies that today dominate the clinical practice of medicine unfortunately disregard the facts that (1) correlation between BP and CVD risk is far stronger for the ABPM-derived asleep SBP mean and sleep-time relative SBP decline than the daytime OBPM[10–20]; and (2) BP-lowering efficacy and other beneficial effects on the daily BP pattern of 6 different classes of hypertension medications and their combinations exhibit statistically and clinically significant awakening versus bedtime treatment differences.[25–31]

Prospective long-term outcomes trials that incorporate periodic, annual, or more frequent, ABPM assessments and simultaneous diary recording of bed and wake times, to accurately and reliably ascertain the asleep and wake-time BP level and dipping status, as done in the completed MAPEC (Monitorización Ambulatoria para Predicción de Eventos Cardiovasculares, ie, ABPM for prediction of cardiovascular events) study[12–14,17–19,90–94] and currently ongoing Hygia Project,[21] are needed to confirm the highly significant independent prognostic value of the sleep-time BP plus the beneficial effects (reduced risk of CVD events and target tissue and organ injury) and safety of the enhanced sleep-time BP reduction by bedtime hypertension chronotherapy with conventional medications.[95,96] In the interim, the authors recommend this bedtime treatment strategy be adopted for management of persons with predominant sleep-time hypertension or non-dipper BP patterning as assessed by around-the-clock ABPM; this includes, but it is not limited to, the elderly and those diagnosed with elevated asleep BP due to diabetes, CKD, obstructive sleep apnea, history of past CVD events, or resistance to pharmacotherapy when timed upon awakening.[33,97,98]

REFERENCES

1. Hermida RC, Ayala DE, Portaluppi F. Circadian variation of blood pressure: the basis for the chronotherapy of hypertension. Adv Drug Deliv Rev 2007; 59:904–22.
2. Portaluppi F, Tiseo R, Smolensky MH, et al. Circadian rhythms and cardiovascular health. Sleep Med Rev 2012;16:151–66.
3. Fabbian F, Smolensky MH, Tiseo R, et al. Dipper and non-dipper blood pressure 24-hour patterns: circadian rhythm-dependent physiologic and pathophysiologic mechanisms. Chronobiol Int 2013;30:17–30.
4. Smolensky MH, Hermida RC, Portaluppi F. Circadian mechanisms of 24-hour blood pressure regulation and patterning. Sleep Med Rev 2017;33:4–16.
5. Angeli A, Gatti G, Masera R. Chronobiology of the hypothalamic-pituitary-adrenal and renin-angiotensin-

aldosterone systems. In: Touitou Y, Haus E, editors. Biologic rhythms in clinical and laboratory medicine. Berlin: Springer-Verlag; 1992. p. 292–314.

6. Sothern RB, Vesely DL, Kanabrocki EL, et al. Temporal (circadian) and functional relationship between atrial natriuretic peptides and blood pressure. Chronobiol Int 1995;12:106–20.

7. Smolensky MH, Hermida RC, Castriotta RJ, et al. Role of sleep-wake cycle on blood pressure circadian rhythms and hypertension. Sleep Med 2007;8: 668–80.

8. Verdecchia P, Porcellati C, Schillaci G, et al. Ambulatory blood pressure: an independent predictor of prognosis in essential hypertension. Hypertension 1994;24:793–801.

9. Ohkubo T, Hozawa A, Yamaguchi J, et al. Prognostic significance of the nocturnal decline in blood pressure in individuals with and without high 24-h blood pressure: the Ohasama study. J Hypertens 2002;20:2183–9.

10. Dolan E, Stanton A, Thijs L, et al. Superiority of ambulatory over clinic blood pressure measurement in predicting mortality: the Dublin outcome study. Hypertension 2005;46:156–61.

11. Boggia J, Li Y, Thijs L, et al. Prognostic accuracy of day versus night ambulatory blood pressure: a cohort study. Lancet 2007;370:1219–29.

12. Hermida RC, Ayala DE, Mojón A, et al. Decreasing sleep-time blood pressure determined by ambulatory monitoring reduces cardiovascular risk. J Am Coll Cardiol 2011;58:1165–73.

13. Hermida RC, Ayala DE, Fernández JR, et al. Sleep-time blood pressure: prognostic value and relevance as a therapeutic target for cardiovascular risk reduction. Chronobiol Int 2013;30:68–86.

14. Hermida RC, Ayala DE, Mojón A, et al. Blunted sleep-time relative blood pressure decline increases cardiovascular risk independent of blood pressure level – The "normotensive non-dipper" paradox. Chronobiol Int 2013;30:87–98.

15. Ben-Dov IZ, Kark JD, Ben-Ishay D, et al. Predictors of all-cause mortality in clinical ambulatory monitoring. Unique aspects of blood pressure during sleep. Hypertension 2007;49:1235–41.

16. Fagard RH, Celis H, Thijs L, et al. Daytime and nighttime blood pressure as predictors of death and cause-specific cardiovascular events in hypertension. Hypertension 2008;51:55–61.

17. Hermida RC, Ayala DE, Mojón A, et al. Sleep-time blood pressure and the prognostic value of isolated-office and masked hypertension. Am J Hypertens 2012;25:297–305.

18. Hermida RC, Ayala DE, Mojón A, et al. Sleep-time blood pressure as a therapeutic target for cardiovascular risk reduction in type 2 diabetes. Am J Hypertens 2012;25:325–34.

19. Ayala DE, Hermida RC, Mojón A, et al. Cardiovascular risk of resistant hypertension: dependence on

treatment-time regimen of blood pressure-lowering medications. Chronobiol Int 2013;30:340–52.

20. Roush GC, Fagard RH, Salles GF, et al. Prognostic impact from clinic, daytime, and nighttime systolic blood pressure in 9 cohorts on 13,844 patients with hypertension. J Hypertens 2014;32:2332–40.

21. Hermida RC. Sleep-time ambulatory blood pressure as a prognostic marker of vascular and other risks and therapeutic target for prevention by hypertension chronotherapy: rationale and design of the Hygia Project. Chronobiol Int 2016;33:906–36.

22. Bélanger PM, Bruguerolle B, Labrecque G. Rhythms in pharmacokinetics: absorption, distribution, metabolism. In: Redfern PH, Lemmer B, editors. Physiology and pharmacology of biological rhythms. Handbook of experimental pharmacology series, vol. 125. Berlin: Springer-Verlag; 1997. p. 177–204.

23. Labrecque G, Beauchamp D. Rhythms and pharmacokinetics. In: Redfern P, editor. Chronotherapeutics. London: Pharmaceutical Press; 2003. p. 75–110.

24. Okyar A, Dressler C, Hanafy A, et al. Circadian variations in exsorptive transport: In-situ intestinal perfusion data and in-vivo relevance. Chronobiol Int 2012;29:443–53.

25. Hermida RC, Ayala DE, Calvo C, et al. Chronotherapy of hypertension: administration-time dependent effects of treatment on the circadian pattern of blood pressure. Adv Drug Deliv Rev 2007;59:923–39.

26. Smolensky MH, Hermida RC, Ayala DE, et al. Administration-time-dependent effect of blood pressure-lowering medications: basis for the chronotherapy of hypertension. Blood Press Monit 2010;15:173–80.

27. Hermida RC, Ayala DE, Fernández JR, et al. Circadian rhythms in blood pressure regulation and optimization of hypertension treatment with ACE inhibitor and ARB medications. Am J Hypertens 2011;24:383–91.

28. Hermida RC, Ayala DE, Fernández JR, et al. Administration-time-differences in effects of hypertension medications on ambulatory blood pressure regulation. Chronobiol Int 2013;30:280–314.

29. Hermida RC, Ayala DE, Smolensky MH, et al. Chronotherapy improves blood pressure control and reduces vascular risk in CKD. Nat Rev Nephrol 2013;9:358–68.

30. Smolensky MH, Hermida RC, Ayala DE, et al. Bedtime hypertension chronotherapy: concepts and patient outcomes. Curr Pharm Des 2015;21:773–90.

31. Hermida RC, Ayala DE, Smolensky MH, et al. Chronotherapy with conventional blood pressure medications improves management of hypertension and reduces cardiovascular and stroke risks. Hypertens Res 2016;39:277–92.

32. Witte K, Lemmer B. Rhythms and pharmacodynamics. In: Redfern P, editor. Chronotherapeutics. London: Pharmaceutical Press; 2003. p. 111–26.

33. Hermida RC, Smolensky MH, Ayala DE, et al. 2013 ambulatory blood pressure monitoring recommendations for the diagnosis of adult hypertension, assessment of cardiovascular and other hypertension-associated risk, and attainment of therapeutic goals. Joint recommendations from the International Society for Chronobiology (ISC), American Association of Medical Chronobiology and Chronotherapeutics (AAMCC), Spanish Society of Applied Chronobiology, Chronotherapy, and Vascular Risk (SECAC), Spanish Society of Atherosclerosis (SEA), and Romanian Society of Internal Medicine (RSIM). Chronobiol Int 2013;30:355–410.

34. Hermida RC, Ayala DE. Chronotherapy with the angiotensin-converting enzyme inhibitor ramipril in essential hypertension: improved blood pressure control with bedtime dosing. Hypertension 2009; 54:40–6.

35. Hermida RC, Ayala DE, Fontao MJ, et al. Administration-time-dependent effects of spirapril on ambulatory blood pressure in uncomplicated essential hypertension. Chronobiol Int 2010;27:560–74.

36. Balan H, Popescu E, Angelescu G. Comparing different treatment schedules of Zomen (zofenopril). Rom J Intern Med 2011;49:75–84.

37. Pechère-Bertschi A, Nussberger J, Decosterd L, et al. Renal response to the angiotensin II receptor subtype 1 antagonist irbesartan versus enalapril in hypertensive patients. J Hypertens 1988;16:385–93.

38. Hermida RC, Calvo C, Ayala DE, et al. Administration-time-dependent effects of valsartan on ambulatory blood pressure in hypertensive subjects. Hypertension 2003;42:283–90.

39. Hermida RC, Calvo C, Ayala DE, et al. Treatment of non-dipper hypertension with bedtime administration of valsartan. J Hypertens 2005;23:1913–22.

40. Hermida RC, Calvo C, Ayala DE, et al. Decrease in urinary albumin excretion associated to the normalization of nocturnal blood pressure in hypertensive subjects. Hypertension 2005;46:960–8.

41. Hermida RC, Calvo C, Ayala DE, et al. Administration time-dependent effects of valsartan on ambulatory blood pressure in elderly hypertensive subjects. Chronobiol Int 2005;22:755–76.

42. Hermida RC, Ayala DE, Calvo C. Optimal timing of antihypertensive dosing: focus on valsartan. Ther Clin Risk Manag 2007;3:119–31.

43. Hermida RC, Ayala DE, Fernández JR, et al. Comparison of the efficacy of morning versus evening administration of telmisartan in essential hypertension. Hypertension 2007;50:715–22.

44. Hermida RC, Ayala DE, Chayán L, et al. Administration-time-dependent effects of olmesartan on the ambulatory blood pressure of essential hypertension patients. Chronobiol Int 2009;26:61–79.

45. Kario K, Hoshide S, Shimizu M, et al. Effects of dosing time of angiotensin II receptor blockade titrated by self-measured blood pressure recordings on cardiorenal protection in hypertensives: the Japan Morning Surge-Target Organ Protection (J-TOP) study. J Hypertens 2010;28:1574–83.

46. Eguchi K, Shimizu M, Hoshide S, et al. A bedtime dose of ARB was better than a morning dose in improving baroreflex sensitivity and urinary albumin excretion–the J-TOP study. Clin Exp Hypertens 2012;34:488–92.

47. Hoshino A, Nakamura T, Matsubara H. The bedtime administration ameliorates blood pressure variability and reduces urinary albumin excretion in amlodipine-olmesartan combination therapy. Clin Exp Hypertens 2010;32:416–22.

48. Hermida RC, Ayala DE, Crespo JJ, et al. Influence of age and hypertension treatment-time on ambulatory blood pressure in hypertensive patients. Chronobiol Int 2013;30:176–91.

49. Kasiakogias A, Tsioufis C, Thomopoulos C, et al. Evening versus morning dosing of antihypertensive drugs in hypertensive patients with sleep apnoea: a cross-over study. J Hypertens 2015;33:393–400.

50. Zappe DH, Crikelair N, Kandra A, et al. Time of administration important? Morning versus evening dosing of valsartan. J Hypertens 2015;33:385–92.

51. Hermida RC, Calvo C, Ayala DE, et al. Dose- and administration-time-dependent effects of nifedipine GITS on ambulatory blood pressure in hypertensive subjects. Chronobiol Int 2007;24:471–93.

52. Hermida RC, Ayala DE, Mojon A, et al. Chronotherapy with nifedipine GITS in hypertensive patients: improved efficacy and safety with bedtime dosing. Am J Hypertens 2008;21:948–54.

53. Hermida RC, Calvo C, Ayala DE, et al. Administration-time-dependent effects of doxazosin GITS on ambulatory blood pressure of hypertensive subjects. Chronobiol Int 2004;21:277–96.

54. Koga H, Hayashi J, Yamamoto M, et al. Prevention of morning surge of hypertension by the evening administration of carvedilol. Jap Med Ass J 2005; 48:398–403.

55. Hermida RC, Calvo C, Ayala DE, et al. Administration time-dependent effects of nebivolol on the diurnal/nocturnal blood pressure ratio in hypertensive patients. J Hypertens 2006;24(Suppl 4):S89.

56. Hermida RC, Ayala DE, Mojón A, et al. Comparison of the effects on ambulatory blood pressure of awakening versus bedtime administration of torasemide in essential hypertension. Chronobiol Int 2008;25: 950–70.

57. Mancia G, Fagard R, Narkiewicz K, et al. 2013 ESH/ESC Guidelines for the management of arterial hypertension: the Task Force for the management of arterial hypertension of the European Society of Hypertension (ESH) and of the European Society of Cardiology (ESC). J Hypertens 2013;31: 1281–357.

58. Middeke M, Kluglich M, Holzgreve H. Chronopharmacology of captopril plus hydrochlorothiazide in hypertension: morning versus evening dosing. Chronobiol Int 1991;8:506–10.

59. Meng Y, Zhang Z, Liang X, et al. Effects of combination therapy with amlodipine and fosinopril administered at different times on blood pressure and circadian blood pressure pattern in patients with essential hypertension. Acta Cardiol 2010;65:309–14.

60. Zeng J, Jia M, Ran H, et al. Fixed-combination of amlodipine and diuretic chronotherapy in the treatment of essential hypertension: improved blood pressure control with bedtime dosing–a multicenter, open-label randomized study. Hypertens Res 2011; 34:767–72.

61. Hermida RC, Ayala DE, Fontao MJ, et al. Chronotherapy with valsartan/amlodipine combination in essential hypertension: improved blood pressure control with bedtime dosing. Chronobiol Int 2010; 27:1287–303.

62. Hermida RC, Ayala DE, Mojón A, et al. Chronotherapy with valsartan/hydrochlorothiazide combination in essential hypertension: improved sleep-time blood pressure control with bedtime dosing. Chronobiol Int 2011;28:601–10.

63. Calhoun DA, Jones D, Textor S, et al. Resistant hypertension: diagnosis, evaluation, and treatment. A scientific statement from the American Heart Association Professional Education Committee of the Council for High Blood Pressure Research. Hypertension 2008;51:1403–19.

64. Hermida RC, Ayala DE, Calvo C, et al. Effects of the time of day of antihypertensive treatment on the ambulatory blood pressure pattern of patients with resistant hypertension. Hypertension 2005;46: 1053–9.

65. Hermida RC, Ayala DE, Fernández JR, et al. Chronotherapy improves blood pressure control and reverts the nondipper pattern in patients with resistant hypertension. Hypertension 2008;51:69–76.

66. Hermida RC, Ayala DE, Mojón A, et al. Effects of time of antihypertensive treatment on ambulatory blood pressure and clinical characteristics of subjects with resistant hypertension. Am J Hypertens 2010;23:432–9.

67. Hermida RC, Ríos MT, Crespo JJ, et al. Treatment-time regimen of hypertension medications significantly affects ambulatory blood pressure and clinical characteristics of patients with resistant hypertension. Chronobiol Int 2013;30:192–206.

68. Ríos MT, Domínguez-Sardiña M, Ayala DE, et al. Prevalence and clinical characteristics of isolated-office and true resistant hypertension determined by ambulatory blood pressure monitoring. Chronobiol Int 2013;30:207–20.

69. Almirall J, Comas L, Martínez-Ocaña JC, et al. Effects of chronotherapy on blood pressure control in non-dipper patients with refractory hypertension. Nephrol Dial Transplant 2012;27:1855–9.

70. Niskikawa T, Omura M, Saito J, et al. The possibility of resistant hypertension during the treatment of hypertensive patients. Hypertens Res 2013;36:924–9.

71. Agarwal R, Nissenson AR, Battle D, et al. Prevalence, treatment, and control of hypertension in chronic hemodialysis patients in the United States. Am J Med 2003;115:291–7.

72. Davidson MB, Hix JK, Vidt DG, et al. Association of impaired diurnal blood pressure variation with a subsequent decline in glomerular filtration rate. Arch Intern Med 2006;166:846–52.

73. Pogue V, Rahman M, Lipkowitz M, et al. Disparate estimates of hypertension control from ambulatory and clinic blood pressure measurements in hypertensive kidney disease. Hypertension 2009;53: 20–7.

74. Crespo JJ, Piñeiro L, Otero A, et al. Administration-time-dependent effects of hypertension treatment on ambulatory blood pressure in patients with chronic kidney disease. Chronobiol Int 2013;30: 159–75.

75. Mojón A, Ayala DE, Piñeiro L, et al. Comparison of ambulatory blood pressure parameters of hypertensive patients with and without chronic kidney disease. Chronobiol Int 2013;30:145–58.

76. Kidney Disease: Improving Global Outcomes (KDIGO) CKD Work Group. KDIGO 2012 clinical practice guideline for the evaluation and management of chronic kidney disease. Kidney Int Suppl 2013;3:1–150.

77. Minutolo R, Gabbai FB, Borrelli S, et al. Changing the timing of antihypertensive therapy to reduce nocturnal blood pressure in CKD: an 8-week uncontrolled trial. Am J Kidney Dis 2007;50:908–17.

78. Rahman M, Greene T, Phillips RA, et al. A trial of 2 strategies to reduce nocturnal blood pressure in blacks with chronic kidney disease. Hypertension 2013;61:82–8.

79. Okeahialam B, Ohihoin E, Ajuluchukwu J. Chronotherapy in Nigerian hypertensives. Ther Adv Cardiovasc Dis 2011;5:113–8.

80. Wang C, Zhang J, Liu X, et al. Effect of valsartan with bedtime dosing on chronic kidney disease patients with nondipping blood pressure pattern. J Clin Hypertens (Greenwich) 2013;15:48–54.

81. Cuspidi C, Meani S, Lonati L, et al. Short-term reproducibility of a non-dipping pattern in type 2 diabetic hypertensive patients. J Hypertens 2006;24:647–53.

82. Ayala DE, Moyá A, Crespo JJ, et al. Circadian pattern of ambulatory blood pressure in hypertensive patients with and without type 2 diabetes. Chronobiol Int 2013;30:99–115.

83. Moyá A, Crespo JJ, Ayala DE, et al. Effects of time-of-day of hypertension treatment on ambulatory blood pressure and clinical characteristics of

patients with type 2 diabetes. Chronobiol Int 2013; 30:116–31.

84. Tofé S, García B. 24-hour and nighttime blood pressures in type 2 diabetic hypertensive patients following morning or evening administration of olmesartan. J Clin Hypertens (Greenwhich) 2009;11: 426–31.

85. Rossen NB, Knudsen ST, Fleischer J, et al. Targeting nocturnal hypertension in type 2 diabetes mellitus. Hypertension 2014;64:1080–7.

86. Suzuki K, Aizawa Y. Evaluation of dosing time-related anti-hypertensive efficacy of valsartan in patients with type 2 diabetes. Clin Exp Hypertens 2011;33:56–62.

87. Qiu YG, Zhu JH, Tao QM, et al. Captopril administered at night restores the diurnal blood pressure rhythm in adequately controlled, nondipping hypertensives. Cardiovasc Drugs Ther 2005;19:189–95.

88. Takeda A, Toda T, Fujii T, et al. Bedtime administration of long-acting antihypertensive drugs restores normal nocturnal blood pressure fall in nondippers with essential hypertension. Clin Exp Nephrol 2009;13:467–72.

89. Farah R, Makhoul N, Arraf Z, et al. Switching therapy to bedtime for uncontrolled hypertension with a nondipping pattern: a prospective randomized-controlled study. Blood Press Monit 2013;18:227–31.

90. Hermida RC, Ayala DE, Mojón A, et al. Influence of circadian time of hypertension treatment on cardiovascular risk: results of the MAPEC study. Chronobiol Int 2010;27:1629–51.

91. Hermida RC, Ayala DE, Mojón A, et al. Influence of time of day of blood pressure-lowering treatment on cardiovascular risk in hypertensive patients with type 2 diabetes. Diabetes Care 2011;34:1270–6.

92. Hermida RC, Ayala DE, Mojón A, et al. Bedtime dosing of antihypertensive medications reduces cardiovascular risk in CKD. J Am Soc Nephrol 2011;22: 2313–21.

93. Hermida RC, Ayala DE, Mojón A, et al. Prognostic marker of type 2 diabetes and therapeutic target for prevention. Diabetologia 2016;59:244–54.

94. Hermida RC, Ayala DE, Mojón A, et al. Bedtime ingestion of hypertension medications reduces the risk of new-onset type 2 diabetes: a randomised controlled trial. Diabetologia 2016;59: 255–65.

95. Hermida RC, Ayala DE, Smolensky MH, et al. Sleep-time blood pressure: unique sensitive prognostic marker of vascular risk and therapeutic target for prevention. Sleep Med Rev 2017;33:17–27.

96. Manfredini R, Fabbian F. A pill at bedtime, and your heart is fine? Bedtime hypertension chronotherapy: an opportune and advantageous inexpensive treatment strategy. Sleep Med Rev 2017;33:1–3.

97. Hermida RC, Smolensky MH, Ayala DE, et al. Ambulatory blood pressure monitoring (ABPM) as the reference standard for diagnosis of hypertension and assessment of vascular risk in adults. Chronobiol Int 2015;32:1329–42.

98. Smolensky MH, Ayala DE, Hermida RC. Ambulatory blood pressure monitoring (ABPM) as THE reference standard to confirm diagnosis of hypertension in adults: recommendation of the 2015 U.S. Preventive Services Task Force (USPSTF). Chronobiol Int 2015;32:1320–2.

Bedtime Chronotherapy with Conventional Hypertension Medications to Target Increased Asleep Blood Pressure Results in Markedly Better *Chrono*prevention of Cardiovascular and Other Risks than Customary On-awakening Therapy

Michael H. Smolensky, PhD[a],*, Ramón C. Hermida, PhD[b],
Diana E. Ayala, MD, MPH, PhD[b], Artemio Mojón, PhD[b],
José R. Fernández, PhD[b]

KEYWORDS

- Prevention • Cardiovascular risk • Ambulatory blood pressure monitoring
- Hypertension chronotherapy • Asleep blood pressure • MAPEC Study • Diabetes
- Resistant hypertension

KEY POINTS

- There are three bases for bedtime hypertension chronotherapy (BHCT) as superior prevention against cardiovascular disease (CVD).
- The first is the correlation between blood pressure (BP) and risk for target organ and vascular injury plus CVD events is greater for ambulatory BP monitoring (ABPM) than office BP measurements (OBPM).

Continued

Disclosure: The authors have nothing to disclose.
Sources of Support: The MAPEC Study and subsequent ongoing Hygia Project are independent investigator-promoted trials supported by unrestricted grants from Instituto de Salud Carlos III, Ministerio de Economía y Competitividad, Spanish Government (PI14-00205); Ministerio de Ciencia e Innovación, Spanish Government (SAF2006-6254-FEDER; SAF2009-7028-FEDER); Consellería de Economía e Industria, Xunta de Galicia (09CSA018322PR); European Research Development Fund and Consellería de Cultura, Educación e Ordenación Universitaria, Xunta de Galicia (CN2012/251; CN2012/260; GPC2014/078); Atlantic Research Center for Information and Communication Technologies (AtlantTIC); and Vicerrectorado de Investigación, University of Vigo.
Conflicts of Interest: None of the authors have conflicts of interests to declare.
[a] Department of Biomedical Engineering, Cockrell School of Engineering, The University of Texas at Austin, 1 University Station C0800, Austin, TX 78712-0238, USA; [b] Bioengineering & Chronobiology Laboratories, Atlantic Research Center for Information and Communication Technologies (AtlantTIC), University of Vigo, 36310 Vigo, Spain
* Corresponding author.
E-mail address: Michael.H.Smolensky@uth.tmc.edu

Heart Failure Clin 13 (2017) 775–792
http://dx.doi.org/10.1016/j.hfc.2017.05.011
1551-7136/17/© 2017 Elsevier Inc. All rights reserved.

heartfailure.theclinics.com

Continued

- The second is the asleep BP mean is an independent and stronger predictor of CVD risk than the daytime OBPM and ABPM-derived awake and 24-hour BP means.
- The third is the MAPEC (Ambulatory Blood Pressure Monitoring for Prediction of Cardiovascular Events) trial, which showed, with confirmation by others, targeting asleep BP by BHCT entailing one or more conventional medications versus usual on-awakening therapy reduces total CVD events by 61% and major events (CVD death, myocardial infarction, ischemic and hemorrhagic stroke) by 67%.
- BHCT thus offers the most cost-effective *chrono*prevention against adverse CVD outcomes in regular and vulnerable renal, diabetic, and resistant hypertensive patients.

INTRODUCTION

The most routine procedure of clinical practice is measurement of systolic blood pressure (SBP) and diastolic blood pressure (DBP), either to detect newly developed arterial hypertension or assess attainment of treatment goals of previously diagnosed hypertensive patients. This emphasis on BP assessment is intended for cardiovascular disease (CVD) risk reduction and future adverse outcomes and incidents prevention. However, of fundamental relevance to both clinicians, in terms of providing optimal care, and patients, in terms of preserving health and wellbeing, is the following question: are the limited number of office BP measurements (OBPM) made at one specific time of the day representative of BP status throughout the 24 hours and of CVD risk? A primary driver of modern medical practice is the concept of homeostasis; relative constancy of the milieu intérieur (internal environment) and thus biological indicators of health and disease. Accordingly, it is assumed that it is of little or no importance when, during the 24 hours or other time domains, diagnostic tests such as OBPM are done and medications are taken. However, a multitude of publications prove that the biology of human beings, as a heritable trait, is organized in a predictable-in-time fashion that is expressed as endogenous circadian (~24 hours) and other periods; for example, menstrual and annual rhythms.[1–3] Twenty-four-hour bioperiodicities, whose stagings (eg, peaks and troughs) are synchronized internally as a circadian time structure as well as externally to the environmental and social time structure primarily by the person's activity in light/sleep in darkness daily routine,[4,5] are especially relevant to medicine, because not only do they influence the findings of diagnostic tests but also the response to curative interventions. This is especially relevant to risk for hypertension and CVD events as shown by the great many research investigations of BP chronobiology (rhythm determinants of SBP and DBP 24-hour patterns)[6–9] and BP chronotherapy (rhythm determinants of hypertension medication effects according to timing: morning on

awakening versus bedtime)[10–17] as subsequently reviewed relative to the now well-demonstrated impact on CVD risk and prevention,[18–20] which the authors prefer to term chronoprevention to highlight the critical importance of biological time to clinical practice and prevention research.

This article first discusses the particular features of the SBP and DBP circadian rhythms, assessable only by around-the-clock ambulatory BP monitoring (ABPM), which is of the greatest importance in making the differential diagnosis of hypertension versus normotension. In this regard, this article presents evidence for the ABPM-derived asleep SBP mean as the most sensitive and independent prognostic indicator of patient CVD risk. In addition, this article reviews the findings of pertinent outcomes trials that show the attenuation of the asleep BP, most effectively achieved by bedtime scheduling of conventional hypertension medications, best chronoreduces and chronoprevents adverse CVD and other outcomes.[18–22]

AROUND-THE-CLOCK AMBULATORY BLOOD PRESSURE MONITORING VERSUS OFFICE BLOOD PRESSURE MONITORING IN THE DIAGNOSIS OF HYPERTENSION

The diagnosis of hypertension and clinical decisions regarding its treatment are typically based on a limited number of specific time-of-day OBPM that may or may not be supplemented by occasional at-home and at-work wake-time patient self-assessments, thought to be representative of the SBP and DBP both during the day and night,[23] but in reality are not.[24,25] Thus, such casual OBPM, even when complemented by home BP measurements (HBPM), disregard the mostly predictable 24-hour patterning of SBP and DBP, which in diurnally active normotensive and uncomplicated hypertensive persons is characterized by (1) striking morning BP increase, (2) two daytime peaks (the first ~2–3 hours after awakening and the second early evening), (3) small midafternoon nadir, and (4) 10% to 20% decline during sleep relative to the wake-time mean, with the magnitude of decline greater for SBP than DBP.[6,26–28] This temporal variation is representative of many deterministic 24-hour cyclic phenomena: rest-activity–associated changes in behavior, including activity routine and level; fluid and stimulant (eg, caffeine) consumption; meal timings and content; emotional and mental stress; posture; external day-night divergence in ambient light intensity and spectrum, temperature, humidity, and noise; and (of most importance) endogenous circadian rhythms in neuroendocrine, endothelial, vasoactive peptide and opioid, and hemodynamic parameters, such as plasma noradrenaline and adrenaline (autonomic nervous system [ANS]); atrial natriuretic and calcitonin gene–related peptides; and renin, angiotensin, and aldosterone (renin-angiotensin-aldosterone system [RAAS]).[6–9]

The usually higher awake BP primarily stems from the high-amplitude circadian rhythms of both sympathetic tone, which peaks during the daytime, as shown by the highest concentrations of plasma noradrenaline and adrenaline after morning awakening and initial hours of the diurnal activity span,[29] and elements of the RAAS (prorenin, plasma renin activity, angiotensin-converting enzyme, angiotensin I and II, and aldosterone), which peak between the middle and later hours of nighttime sleep.[30] The normally lower BP during nighttime sleep relative to daytime wakefulness arises from several simultaneous circadian stage–dependent factors. These include, most prominently, attenuated sympathetic and increased vagal tone of the ANS, increased concentration and activity of atrial natriuretic and calcitonin gene–related vasoactive peptide systems, and suppressed RAAS state during the first half of the rest span followed by progressive activation thereafter until morning peak activity. Predictable-in-time behavioral and environmental cycles further contribute to the BP 24-hour pattern of higher diurnal and lower nocturnal values.[6–9,30–35]

The sleep-time BP and sleep-time BP decline (dipping status) are important clinical biomarkers of CVD risk that can be ascertained only by around-the-clock ABPM, a diagnostic tool that allows thorough description and quantification of all aspects of the BP 24-hour variation. Numerous published outcome trials and meta-analyses substantiate the correlation between BP level and target organ injury and CVD events risk is much higher for ABPM-obtained parameters, particularly sleep-time BP, than it is for daytime OBPM.[36–46] The decrease of BP during sleep from its wake-time level is commonly quantified by the sleep-time relative BP decline; that is, percentage decrease in mean BP during nighttime sleep relative to mean BP during wake-time activity. Although the conventional practice is to designate individuals as dippers when the sleep-time relative SBP decline is greater than or equal to 10% and as nondippers when less than 10%, the preferred and more precise categorization is extreme dippers (decline $\geq$20%), dippers (decline $\geq$10%), nondippers (decline <10%), and risers (decline <0%; ie, asleep SBP mean > awake SBP mean).[23,24] The dipper pattern is perceived as the norm, being the most common; however, prevalence of the nondipper and riser patterns is much greater than recognized, even in the absence of sleep disorders; for example, as great as 65% to 81% in cohorts of elderly,[47] type 2 diabetes,[48] chronic kidney disease (CKD),[49] and resistant hypertension patients.[50]

In summary, ABPM is the only method of determining the wake-time, sleep-time, and 24-hour BP features and patterns. Furthermore, it is now the preferred manner of accurately diagnosing hypertension, assessing intervention strategies, and predicting patient CVD risk.[24,25] In this regard, we emphasize two critically important points. Accurate differential diagnosis of hypertension from normotension and assessment of BP dipping pattern are confounded when using nonrepresentative ABPM software–generated default daytime and nighttime means rather than truly representative asleep and wake SBP and DBP means calculated from patient bed and rise times. Abnormal sleep-time BP and sleep-time BP decline, as discussed later, are the most sensitive predictors of CVD and other hypertension-associated risks; thus, the primary goal of curative interventions ought to be their normalization, which, based on findings of outcomes trials and meta-analyses, is best achieved by the simple and low-cost hypertension chronotherapeutic strategy that consists of scheduling at bedtime one or more conventional BP-lowering medications in accord with circadian rhythm requirements to enhance effects.[10–22,42,45]

SLEEP-TIME BLOOD PRESSURE: INDEPENDENT PROGNOSTIC MARKER OF CARDIOVASCULAR DISEASE RISK

Specific features of the 24-hour BP pattern determined by ABPM have been explored as biomarkers or mediators of target tissue injury and triggers of, and risk factors for, CVD events (angina pectoris, severe arrhythmias, myocardial infarction, cardiac arrest, heart failure emergencies, pulmonary embolism, sudden cardiac death) and cerebrovascular events (ischemic and hemorrhagic stroke).[7,42,51–53] Numerous studies consistently substantiate strong association between the abnormal physiologic feature of blunted sleep-time relative BP decline (nondipper/riser 24-hour BP patterns) and increased incidence of fatal and nonfatal CVD events, not only in hypertensive[37,39,42,52,54–57] but in normotensive individuals.[58] Furthermore, various independent prospective investigations show that CVD events are better predicted by the ABPM-ascertained asleep than the awake and 24-hour BP means or daytime OBPM.[39,42–46,52,53,56,57,59–61]

Verdecchia and colleagues[37] conducted one of the first prospective studies of the relationship between several features of the 24-hour ambulatory BP pattern, determined only by a single around-the-clock ABPM at baseline, on patient recruitment, and subsequent CVD morbidity during a short, 3.2-year average, follow-up. The investigators found that nondipper compared with dipper hypertensive patients experienced nearly 3-fold more adverse CVD events. Ohkubo and colleagues[54] also performed a population-based evaluation of the prognostic value of a single baseline 24-hour ABPM, finding in their average 9.2-year-per-patient follow-up a 31% increase in CVD mortality per 5% blunting of the sleep-time relative SBP decline in hypertensive patients. Of particular clinical relevance is their finding of no difference in hazard ratio (HR) of CVD mortality between dipper hypertensives (HR = 2.37) and non-dipper normotensives (HR = 2.16).[54] Dolan and colleagues[39] additionally examined whether a single baseline 24-hour ABPM better forecasted CVD mortality than daytime OBPM in their median 8.4-year follow-up of 5292 initially untreated hypertensive patients, finding the nighttime BP mean to be the strongest predictor of such outcome. Furthermore, Ingelsson and colleagues[55] explored whether, in elderly men, nondipping BP 24-hour patterning and increased nighttime DBP mean are indicative of incident congestive heart failure (CHF). After inclusion of the 24-hour SBP and DBP means as covariates, in addition to BP-lowering treatment and established risk factors for CHF, nondipping and nighttime DBP remained significant predictors of this heart condition, thus implicating the nondipping BP pattern and nighttime hypertension as key deterministic risk factors for CHF.

Published meta-analyses also confirm the crucial importance of the sleep-time BP in predicting CVD risk and events. Fagard and colleagues,[60] for example, conducted a meta-analysis of the BP data from four prospective European studies, representing 3468 hypertensive patients. Daytime and nighttime SBP means predicted all-cause and CVD mortality, coronary heart disease, and stroke, independent of OBPM and all potential confounding variables. However, when these same ABPM-derived daytime and nighttime BP means were entered simultaneously into survival models, the nighttime SBP mean predicted all outcomes, whereas the daytime SBP mean contributed no further prognostic precision, rendering nighttime SBP as the only independent marker of CVD outcome. The most recent meta-analysis, which incorporated data from nine cohorts of 13,844 total hypertension patients, concluded on the basis of a series of separate single-variable analyses that increases in clinic SBP as well as ABPM-derived awake and asleep SBP means are all significantly associated with increased risk; however, when all three SBP measurements were simultaneous included into the same survival model, only the asleep SBP mean emerged as an independent predictor of CVD events.[46]

Overall, these and other such prospective studies as well as meta-analyses of past conducted trials show that increased sleep-time BP constitutes the most significant CVD risk factor, independent of daytime OBPM or ambulatory awake and 24-hour BP means. Nonetheless, the findings and conclusions of most previous ABPM studies may be imprecise because of inherent limitations of their investigative methods,[62,63] thereby leading to profound inaccuracies and inconsistencies of the prognostic value of the various ABPM-derived variables, but mainly the awake and asleep SBP/DBP means. All previous trials addressing the merit of ABPM relative to OBPM to determine CVD risk, except the subsequently discussed MAPEC (Monitorización Ambulatoria para Predicción de Eventos Cardiovasculares; ie, ambulatory blood pressure monitoring for prediction of cardiovascular events) study[18–22,42,44,45,52,57,58,64,65] only relied on a single low-reproducible[66] 24-hour ABPM evaluation per participant conducted at study inclusion. Such a study design is unsound because it presumes that all features of the baseline-determined ambulatory BP and pattern are maintained without alteration throughout the many years of follow-up despite aging, development of target organ damage and concomitant morbidity, and institution or modification of BP-lowering therapy.[47] Additional limitations of most previous ABPM studies are (1) frequent use of author-declared or ABPM-software programmed default arbitrarily fixed clock hours to define the start and end times of diurnal activity, resulting in the generation of nonrepresentative and inaccurate daytime and nighttime BP means because they are calculated without taking into account differences between participants in commencement and termination of their rest and activity spans; (2) analysis of the prognostic value of dipping status and nighttime (rather than the actual asleep) BP mean without proper adjustment for the daytime (or more preferably the actual awake) BP mean; and (3) lack of systematic and multiple ABPM evaluation of patients over time in all previously reported long-term follow-up studies, which precludes the opportunity to explore potential reduction by hypertension therapy for CVD risk through modification of the most sensitive prognostic parameters (ie, increase of the sleep-time relative BP decline toward the more normal dipper patterning or, more specifically, reduction of the asleep BP mean). Incorporation of periodic, at least annual, ABPM patient assessment during follow-up, as in the MAPEC study, clearly establishes that features of the 24-hour BP pattern change over time and that therapeutic reduction of the asleep BP mean plus increase of the sleep-time relative BP decline toward the normal dipping pattern lessen not only CVD risk[18–20,42,44,45,52,57] but progression toward new-onset type 2 diabetes.[21,22]

THE MAPEC OUTCOMES TRIAL: VERIFICATION OF THE CRUCIAL IMPORTANCE OF ASLEEP BLOOD PRESSURE AS THE MOST SENSITIVE PREDICTOR OF PATIENT CARDIOVASCULAR DISEASE RISK

The MAPEC study was designed as a prospective, randomized, open-label, blinded end point trial to test the hypothesis that bedtime hypertension chronotherapy entailing one or more conventional BP-lowering pharmacologic agents exerts better ambulatory BP control and CVD risk reduction than customary/standard therapy of all such medications ingested on morning awakening. Complete details of the rationale and design of the MAPEC study are reported elsewhere[18–22,42,52] Briefly, 3344 (1718 male/1626 female) individuals with baseline ABPM ranging from normotension to sustained hypertension were prospectively followed for a median duration of 5.6 years. Hypertensive participants at baseline were randomized to two treatment strategies: all prescribed conventional hypertension medications ingested on awakening or complete daily dose of one or more of them ingested at bedtime. The treatment protocol did not allow division of any prescribed once-a-day medications as a split dose (ie, half taken on morning arising and half at bedtime). At baseline and thereafter annually, or more frequently after doctor-ordered change in therapy either to improve ambulatory BP control or avert

sleep-time hypotension using dedicated software for individualized evaluation,[67,68] ABPM and wrist actigraphy (to determine per-patient commencement and termination of diurnal activity and nocturnal rest to accurately derive awake and asleep BP means[69]) were simultaneously conducted for 48 consecutive hours. Registered events included all-cause mortality, myocardial infarction, angina pectoris, coronary revascularization, CHF, lower-extremity acute arterial occlusion, retinal artery thrombotic occlusion, hemorrhagic and ischemic stroke, and transient ischemic attack. The primary outcome study end point was total CVD morbidity and mortality, which included all the events listed earlier.

Cox regression survival analysis of each potential prognostic BP parameter analyzed individually, fully adjusted by the significant influential characteristics of sex, age, type 2 diabetes, anemia, CKD, and hypertension treatment time, indicates that the HR of total CVD events is greater with progressively higher sleep-time SBP mean and lower sleep-time relative SBP decline; that is, more nondipper/riser BP patterning (**Fig. 1**A). The asleep SBP mean is thus the most significant predictor of total CVD events (per standard deviation [SD] increase in asleep SBP mean; HR = 1.51; 95% confidence interval [CI], [1.39–1.65]; P<.001; see **Fig. 1**A).[42,52] Moreover, joint analysis of the multiple BP parameters potentially capable of contributing to CVD risk confirms the conclusions of earlier conducted studies[39,43,46] that OBPM do not independently predict CVD morbidity and mortality when the outcomes model is adjusted by the asleep BP mean (HR = 1.44 [1.30–160], P<.001, per SD increase in asleep SBP and HR = 1.09 [0.97–1.23], P = .123, per SD increase in clinic SBP; **Fig. 1**B). The best Cox regression fully adjusted model includes only the asleep SBP mean (HR = 1.43 [1.29–1.58], P<.001) and sleep-time relative SBP decline (HR = 0.88 [0.78–0.98], P = .023; see **Fig. 1**B). Most notably, when the awake SBP mean is adjusted by the asleep SBP mean, only the latter significantly predicts CVD outcomes (HR = 1.67 [1.45–1.92], P<.001, per SD increase in asleep SBP mean; HR = 0.88; [0.75–1.02], P = .094, per SD increase in awake SBP mean; see **Fig. 1**B).[42,52]

To further investigate the clinical relevance of the asleep BP mean on CVD risk, MAPEC study participants were divided into eight nonoverlapping cohorts according to BP level; that is, normal or increased based on established ABPM thresholds of 135/85 mm Hg for the awake SBP/DBP means, 120/70 mm Hg for the asleep SBP/DBP means, and 140/90 mm Hg for the clinic SBP/DBP measurements,[23,24] at their final ABPM evaluation, either

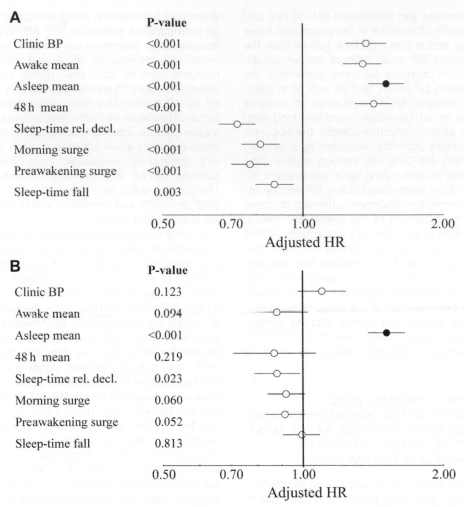

Fig. 1. Adjusted HR (95% confidence interval [CI]) of total CVD events per standard deviation (SD) increase in baseline clinic and ambulatory SBP in the MAPEC study. (*A*) Each tested parameter evaluated separately. (*B*) Results adjusted by asleep SBP mean. Adjustments were applied for sex, age, type 2 diabetes, anemia, CKD, and hypertension treatment time. All medications on awakening versus full daily dose of one or more medications at bedtime. The sleep-time relative BP decline (rel. decl.), an index of BP dipping, is defined as percentage decline in BP during nighttime sleep relative to the mean BP during daytime activity, and calculated as ([awake BP mean – asleep BP mean]/awake BP mean) × 100. The morning BP surge was calculated as the difference between the average BP during the initial 2 hours after the wake-up time (ie, morning BP) and the hourly BP average centered on the lowest BP reading during nighttime sleep (ie, lowest sleep BP). The preawakening BP surge was calculated as the difference between the average BP during the initial 2 hours after morning wake-up time and the average BP during the 2 hours before morning wake-up time. The sleep-time decrease was calculated as the difference between the average BP during the 2 hours just before going to bed and the hourly average centered on the lowest BP reading during nighttime sleep.

before the documented CVD incident in event individuals or latest assessment in nonevent individuals. The results of these analyses, which are summarized in **Fig. 2**, reveal that CVD risk is significantly higher in all four patient cohorts having an increased asleep BP mean, regardless of whether the daytime OBPM or ABPM-derived awake BP mean is normal or increased, than in the other four patient cohorts having a normal sleep-time BP mean. In summary, the asleep BP mean, but not the OBPM or

ABPM-derived awake BP means, constitutes a highly significant sensitive and independent prognostic marker of CVD morbidity and mortality.[42,52]

Sleep-time Blood Pressure: Key Therapeutic Target for Cardiovascular Disease Risk Reduction

Unlike the design of other ABPM-based studies reviewed earlier, the MAPEC study, in which

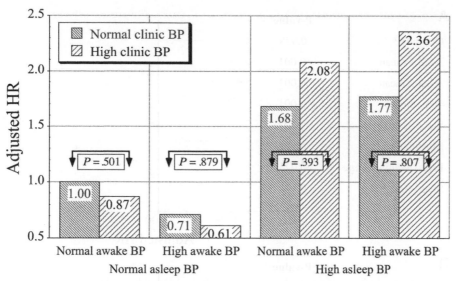

Fig. 2. Adjusted HR of total CVD events in the MAPEC study. Participants were categorized into groups, both according to daytime OBPM level (normal or high) and ABPM-derived awake and asleep SBP and DBP means (normal or high). The SBP/DBP obtained by OBPM were considered normal if less than 140/90 mm Hg and high otherwise. The ABPM-derived awake SBP/DBP means were considered normal if less than 135/85 mm Hg and high otherwise, and the asleep SBP/DBP means were considered normal if less than 120/70 mm Hg and high otherwise. Adjustments were applied for sex, age, type 2 diabetes, CKD, sleep duration, and hypertension treatment time. All medications on awakening versus full daily dose of one or more medications at bedtime. (*Data from* Hermida RC, Smolensky MH, Ayala DE, et al. 2013 ambulatory blood pressure monitoring recommendations for the diagnosis of adult hypertension, assessment of cardiovascular and other hypertension-associated risk, and attainment of therapeutic goals. Joint recommendations from the International Society for Chronobiology (ISC), American Association of Medical Chronobiology and Chronotherapeutics (AAMCC), Spanish Society of Applied Chronobiology, Chronotherapy, and Vascular Risk (SECAC), Spanish Society of Atherosclerosis (SEA), and Romanian Society of Internal Medicine (RSIM). Chronobiol Int 2013;30:355–410.)

participants were repeatedly assessed by periodic 48-hour ABPM, permitted prospective evaluation of the impact of changes in OBPM as well as ABPM-derived features of the BP 24-hour pattern on CVD risk during the median 5.6-year follow-up. Progressive treatment-induced lowering of the awake, asleep, and 48-hour BP means, but not OBPM, when each variable is analyzed individually reveals association with significantly decreased CVD risk (**Fig. 3A**). Nonetheless, among all the tested ambulatory parameters and also OBPM, reduction from baseline in the asleep SBP/DBP means is by far the most significant predictor of event-free survival during follow-up.[42,52] Changes during follow-up in morning BP surge, preawakening BP surge, and nighttime BP decrease were not significantly associated with modification of CVD risk, although, as depicted in **Fig. 3A**, progressive increase during follow-up in the sleep-time relative SBP decline toward the normal dipper pattern was significantly associated with increased event-free survival. However, the most noteworthy finding of the Cox regression analysis arises when, in the same time-dependent model, treatment-induced

changes during follow-up in the asleep and awake BP means are jointly included. As shown in **Fig. 3B**, this analysis indicates that progressive attenuation of the asleep SBP mean is significantly associated with decreased CVD risk (adjusted HR = 0.67 [0.55–0.81], P<.001, per SD reduction in asleep SBP mean), whereas progressive reduction in the awake SBP mean is not (adjusted HR = 1.00 [0.86–1.18], P = .958, per SD decrease in awake SBP mean during follow-up). Overall, the best fully adjusted time-dependent Cox regression model includes only the progressive attenuation of the asleep SBP mean (HR = 0.76 [0.68–0.85], P<.001, per SD reduction in asleep SBP mean) and increase in the sleep-time relative SBP decline (HR = 0.84 [0.72–0.99], P = .038, per SD increase in sleep-time relative SBP decline during follow-up; see **Fig. 3B**).

Fig. 4 categorizes into quintiles, for the entire MAPEC study patient population, the relationship between CVD risk and achieved asleep SBP mean at the final ABPM evaluation per participant; that is, either just before a documented CVD event in event subjects or latest assessment

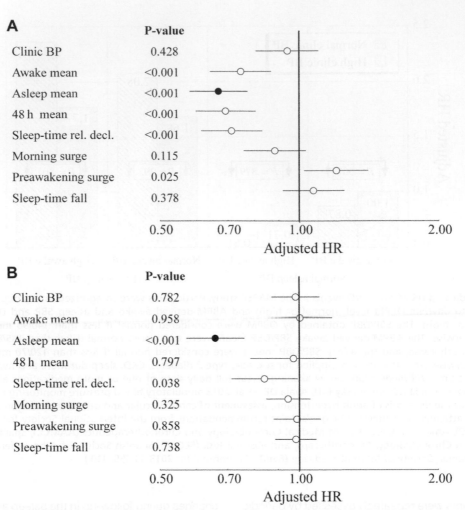

Fig. 3. Adjusted HR (95% CI) of total CVD events per SD change during follow-up in clinic and ambulatory SBP in the MAPEC study. (*A*) Each tested parameter evaluated separately. (*B*) Results adjusted by asleep SBP mean. Adjustments were applied for sex, age, type 2 diabetes, anemia, CKD, baseline BP, and hypertension treatment time. All medications on awakening versus full daily dose of one or more medications at bedtime. The sleep-time relative BP deline (rel. decl.), an index of BP dipping, is defined as the percentage decline in BP during nighttime sleep relative to the mean BP during daytime activity, and calculated as ([awake BP mean – asleep BP mean]/awake BP mean) × 100. The morning BP surge was calculated as the difference between the average BP during the initial 2 hours after the wake-up time (ie, morning BP) and the hourly BP average centered on the lowest BP reading during nighttime sleep (ie, lowest sleep BP). The preawakening BP surge was calculated as the difference between the average BP during the 2 hours after the wake-up time and the average BP during the 2 hours just before the wake-up time. The sleep-time decrease was calculated as the difference between the average BP during the 2 hours before going to bed and the hourly average centered on the lowest BP reading during nighttime sleep.

in nonevent individuals. Panel A of **Fig. 4**, which provides the HR adjusted by the significant influential variables of sex, age, type 2 diabetes, anemia, CKD, and hypertension treatment time, shows the highly significant attenuation of CVD risk with medication-achieved progressive lowering of the asleep SBP mean across all quintiles. The risk of CVD events is lowest for participants with an achieved asleep SBP mean less

than 100.3 mm Hg, with the average asleep SBP mean of 93.8 ± 5.8 mm Hg for individuals of the first quintile. Panel B of **Fig. 4** presents the HR further adjusted by the awake SBP mean. Comparison of the upper and lower panels of **Fig. 4** clearly substantiates the lack of any significant influence of the awake SBP mean on the documented highly prognostic merit of the asleep SBP mean.

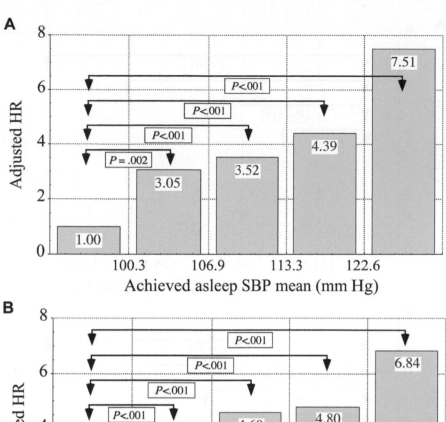

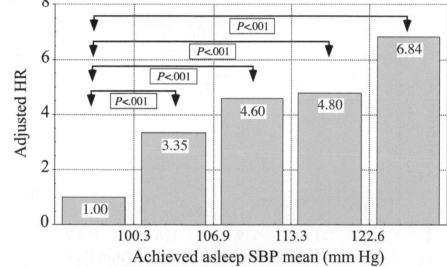

Fig. 4. Adjusted HR of total CVD events in the MAPEC study as a function of the achieved ABPM-derived asleep SBP mean at the final evaluation per participant, either before the documented CVD event in event subjects or latest assessment in nonevent individuals (*A*). The studied population was divided into five classes of equal size (quintiles). Adjustments were applied for the same variables as in **Fig. 1**. (*B*) The HRs further adjusted by the awake SBP mean.

The relationship between the HR of total CVD events (adjusted by sex, age, type 2 diabetes, anemia, CKD, and hypertension treatment time) and achieved awake SBP mean at the final evaluation per participant, as previously defined, is shown in **Fig. 5**A. The adjusted HR was only slightly larger in the last two compared with the first three quintiles; that is, when the attained awake SBP mean is less than 126 mm Hg. **Fig. 5**B, showing the HR of total CVD events for the achieved awake SBP mean further adjusted by the asleep SBP mean, reveals that the small increase in risk for participants of the last two quintiles is caused solely by the expected increased asleep SBP when awake SBP is also very high.

In conclusion, **Figs. 3–5** document the progressively diminished sleep SBP mean (but not the daytime OBPM or ABPM-derived awake means) that is the most highly significant independent prognostic marker of reduced CVD morbidity and mortality risk. It therefore constitutes a novel therapeutic target for CVD chronoprevention and prolongation of patient CVD event–free interval.[42,52]

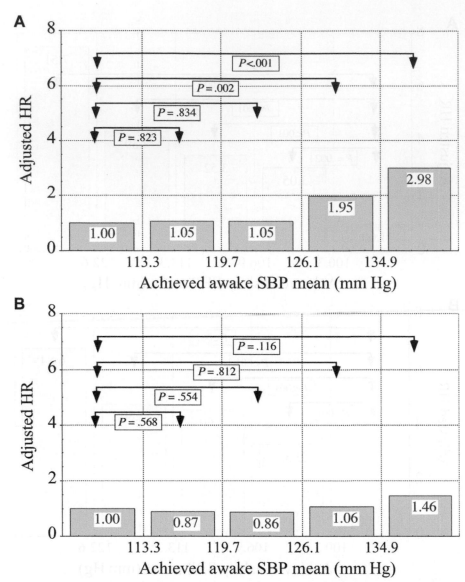

Fig. 5. Adjusted HR of total CVD events in the MAPEC study as a function of the achieved ABPM-derived awake SBP mean at the final evaluation per participant, either before the documented CVD event in event subjects or latest assessment in nonevent individuals (*A*). The studied population was divided into five classes of equal size (quintiles). Adjustments were applied for the same variables as in **Fig. 1**. (*B*) The HRs further adjusted by the asleep SBP mean.

Evidence that the Chronoprevention of Cardiovascular Disease Events is Best Achieved by Bedtime Hypertension Chronotherapy

Many published clinical trials document reduction of the asleep BP and increase of the sleep-time relative BP decline toward the normal 24-hour pattern by conventional hypertension medications of six different classes (angiotensin-converting enzyme inhibitors [ACEIs], angiotensin-II receptor blockers [ARBs], calcium-channel blockers [CCBs], α-blockers, β-blockers, and diuretics) and their combinations are greatly improved when routinely ingested at bedtime rather than on awakening, as is customary.[10–17] For example, because the high-amplitude RAAS circadian rhythm activates during sleep, bedtime versus morning dosing of conventional long-acting ACEIs and ARBs reduces the asleep BP means to a much greater extent than the awake BP means, with the additional benefit, independent of drug terminal half-life, of more efficiently converting the previously abnormal nondipper 24-hour BP pattern toward or into the more normal phenotype.[12,13] Based on review of the findings from completed long-term outcomes trials, the key question is addressed here of whether the previously described bedtime hypertension chronotherapeutic approach, which better normalizes the sleep-time BP and sleep-time relative BP decline than the usually recommended on-awakening one, constitutes a significant advance; ie, is it much more protective against nonfatal and fatal CVD events of hypertensive persons, and does it thereby embody a unique circadian rhythm–dependent chronoprevention strategy?.

Heart Outcomes Prevention Evaluation Trial

The Heart Outcomes Prevention Evaluation (HOPE) trial tested in a high-risk CVD cohort of 9297 patients 55 years of age or older whether adding the ACEI ramipril or placebo to an existing BP-lowering, cholesterol-reducing, or other preventive intervention significantly reduces CVD and stroke events.[70] Patients were additionally randomized to either vitamin E or placebo. Although the HOPE trial publication[70] fails to specify the dosing time of the placebo and ACEI therapies, oral presentations by the principal investigators at hypertension meetings and an associated publication state that they were ingested at bedtime.[71] The results of this trial established that add-on ramipril, relative to placebo, as bedtime therapy significantly reduced the primary outcome variables of death from CVD causes and new-onset myocardial infarction and stroke plus the secondary ones of death from any cause, revascularization procedures, cardiac events, complications of diabetes, and hospitalizations for CHF.[70] Surprisingly, this highly significant reduction in the adverse CVD outcomes by the ramipril versus placebo bedtime treatment arms was associated with only very minor (average 3/2 mm Hg) reduction of SBP/DBP based on traditional daytime OBPM. A subsequently published around-the-clock ABPM follow-up substudy of a small cohort of 38 HOPE participants more accurately portrays the BP-lowering effect of the bedtime ramipril strategy. The nighttime SBP/DBP levels were profoundly lowered, by an average 17/8 mm Hg (*P*<.001 compared with placebo), and this translated into a significant increase, by 8%, of the sleep-time relative BP decline.[71] Thus, the results of this small bedtime ramipril ABPM investigation are consistent with those of the several other larger investigations entailing a bedtime ACEI

strategy to manage hypertension.[12,13,72,73] However, because the HOPE trial failed to include a comparator morning ramipril treatment arm, it is not feasible to test the hypothesis that bedtime hypertension chronotherapy with a conventional medication best reduces CVD risk.

Syst-Eur and Syst-China Trials

The Syst-Eur and Syst-China CVD outcome trials investigated whether dihydropyridine CCB nitrendipine versus placebo evening therapy reduces stroke and other CVD complications in elderly patients with isolated systolic hypertension diagnosed on the sole basis of daytime OBPM.[74,75] The apparent rationale for choosing an evening-time regimen seems to be the assumed reduced risk of medication-induced peripheral edema and related patient withdrawals with this versus a morning CCB dosing time, an assumption verified by studies later conducted by Hermida and colleagues.[76,77] In the Syst-Eur trial, 4695 patients were randomized to either a nitrendipine or placebo evening treatment regimen; after two years of follow-up, CCB relative to placebo treatment reduced the primary end point of stroke by 42% (*P* = .003), CVD mortality by 27% (*P* = .07), and total CVD morbid events by 31% (*P*<.001).[74] The almost identical protocol of the Syst-China trial entailing 2394 patients found after three years of follow-up that evening nitrendipine compared with evening placebo therapy reduced total stroke events by 38% (*P* = .01), total mortality by 39% (*P* = .003), CVD mortality by 39% (*P* = .003), stroke mortality by 58% (*P* = .02), and total CVD events by 37% (*P* = .004).[75] Similar to the HOPE trial, the Syst-Eur and Syst-China trials did not include an active CCB morning-time treatment arm to enable comparative assessment of effects on CVD risk.

Controlled-onset Extended-release Verapamil Investigation of Cardiovascular Endpoints Trial

The Controlled-onset Extended-release Verapamil Investigation of Cardiovascular Endpoints (CONVINCE) trial was designed to explore whether initial treatment with 180 mg of the unique controlled-onset extended-release (COER) verapamil product, specifically formulated for bedtime ingestion so as to achieve peak serum medication concentration on morning arising and initial hours of diurnal activity when BP is assumed to rapidly increase from its reduced sleep-time level and assumedly act as a trigger of angina pectoris, myocardial infarct, and stroke, is equivalent to morning treatment with either 50 mg of the beta-agonist atenolol or 12.5 mg of the diuretic hydro-chlorothiazide in preventing as primary outcomes myocardial infarction, stroke, and CVD death.[78] Bedtime ingestion of COER-verapamil significantly reduces morning BP but exerts only limited effect on asleep BP, as documented in a randomized trial showing 2-fold greater reduction in the awake than asleep SBP/DBP means.[79] The CONVINCE trial was prematurely terminated two years earlier than planned by the sponsoring pharmaceutical company purely for commercial reasons. At the conclusion of the abbreviated three-year follow-up period, there were no significant differences in the number of primary outcome events between the two tested treatment strategies. Thus, the CONVINCE trial failed to substantiate any of the protective CVD benefits that were theorized to result through the specific attenuation of morning BP, including its rapid increase on commencement of daytime activity. An unanticipated undesired consequence of the COER-verapamil bedtime treatment strategy, which exerts strongest BP-lowering effect on wake-time BP but less effect on sleep-time BP, is increased prevalence of the higher CVD risk nondipper BP pattern.

MAPEC Study

The investigations reviewed earlier entailing evening therapeutic strategies for the hypertension medications of ramipril, nitrendipine, and COER-verapamil lacked a comparator awakening-time treatment arm; thus, they cannot be considered proper chronotherapy outcome trials. Nonetheless, it is of interest that Roush and colleagues,[80] who compared the results of the studies summarized earlier in which the tested active hypertension medications were systematically ingested in the evening/bedtime with those of 170 other clinical trials included in an earlier meta-analysis in which the investigated hypertension medications were ingested daily in the morning,[81] found significantly (48%) better attenuation ($P = .008$) in the relative risk of CVD events when BP-lowering medication was consistently taken at bedtime rather than morning.[80]

As previously discussed, the MAPEC study constitutes the first prospective trial specifically designed and conducted to completion to test the hypothesis that bedtime hypertension chronotherapy that focuses specifically on reduction of the asleep BP mean and increase of the sleep-time relative BP decline better reduces CVD and stroke risk than standard morning-time therapy.[18–20,42,44,45,52,57,58,64,65] After a median follow-up of 5.6 years, hypertensive patients randomized to ingest the full daily dose of one or

more BP-lowering medications at bedtime, compared with those randomized to ingest all prescribed hypertension medications on awakening, showed, as expected based on the many previously conducted morning versus bedtime treatment-time investigations,[10–17] significantly lower asleep BP mean, higher sleep-time relative BP decline, reduced prevalence of nondipping BP (34% vs 62%, $P<.001$), and higher prevalence of properly controlled ambulatory BP (62 vs 53%, $P<.001$). However, more germane to the major theme of this article are the findings that bedtime, compared with on-awakening, therapy resulted in significantly lower adjusted HR of total CVD events (HR = 0.39 [0.29–0.51], $P<.001$) as well as major CVD events: a composite of CVD death, myocardial infarction, and ischemic and hemorrhagic stroke (HR = 0.33 [0.19–0.55], $P<.001$).[18] Patients randomized to treatment on awakening, no matter the classes of prescribed BP-lowering medications, showed substantially greater CVD risk. However, greatest benefits were observed for bedtime, compared with awakening, treatment when the medication class was an ARB (HR = 0.29 [0.17–0.51], $P<.001$ or CCB (HR = 0.46 [0.31–0.69], $P<.001$)[64]; however, patients randomized to take an ARB at bedtime, compared with any other class of medication, with or without additional BP-lowering agents, experienced significantly lower HR of CVD events ($P<.017$).[64]

Thus, the MAPEC study not only validates the asleep SBP mean as the most significant independent ABPM-derived prognostic marker of CVD morbidity and mortality,[42,44,45,52,53] as earlier discussed, a finding also corroborated in several other prospective ABPM studies,[39,43,46,56,59–61] but it further substantiates that reduction of the asleep SBP mean by a hypertension treatment strategy defined by ingestion of the entire daily dose of one or more conventional BP-lowering medications at bedtime, especially when including an ARB, significantly and cost-effectively decreases (ie, chronoprevents) CVD risk both for patients of the general hypertension population[18] and those of greater vulnerability and enhanced CVD risk diagnosed with type 2 diabetes,[19,45] CKD,[20] and resistant hypertension[57] (Fig. 6). Of particular relevance to the usual readers of this journal is the finding of the MAPEC study of greater reduction of CHF risk by the bedtime chronotherapy than the customary on-awakening treatment regimen (HR = 0.25 [0.12–0.54], $P<.001$), with a rate of CHF during follow-up of 3.04% in the cohort of patients who routinely ingested all hypertension medications on awakening compared with only 0.75% in the cohort of

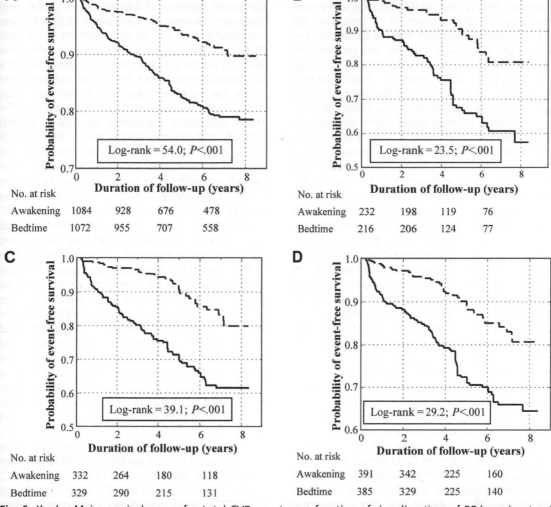

Fig. 6. Kaplan-Meier survival curves for total CVD events as a function of circadian time of BP-lowering treatment; that is, patients ingesting either all prescribed BP-lowering medications on awakening (*continuous black line*) or full daily dose of one or more of them at bedtime (*dashed blue line*), in the general hypertension population of the MAPEC study (*A*) and those additionally diagnosed on recruitment with type 2 diabetes (*B*) or CKD (*C*), or having resistant hypertension (*D*). Obvious is the markedly better reduction of CVD risk and prevention (ie, chronoprevention) of CVD events not only in the general population of patients with hypertension of the MAPEC study but, most importantly, in those with the compelling medical conditions conferring much greater vulnerability: those with type 2 diabetes, CKD, and resistant hypertension. (*Data from* Refs.[18–20,57])

patients who ingested one or more hypertension medications at bedtime.[18] Thus, several international medical and scientific societies[24,62,82–85] now acknowledge the clinical relevance of asleep BP as the prime target of therapy by recommending that physicians advise their hypertension patients to ingest one or more prescribed hypertension medications at bedtime. In so doing they directly endorse the importance of bedtime hypertension chronotherapy in the management of patients with high BP and, indirectly, the highly relevant and novel clinical concept of CVD chronoprevention.

SUMMARY

The diagnostic approaches and treatment strategies that now dominate clinical practice are founded on the incomplete biological concept of homeostasis, which leads practitioners to assume that clinical indicators of health and disease are invariable during the 24-hour period and other time domains. Therefore, OBPM, which are uniquely representative only of the particular time of day that a patient presents for examination, neither indicate the SBP and DBP at other times of the day and night nor in any way indicate the features of the 24-hour pattern that are most predictive of CVD risk. In addition, clinical practitioners either are unaware of or disregard the now well-established fact that the correlation between BP and CVD risk is far stronger for the ABPM-derived asleep SBP mean and sleep-time relative SBP decline than daytime OBPM.[39,42–46,52,53,56,57,59–61] From the substantial and indisputable evidence of the significantly better prognostic value of these ABPM-derived end points versus the unique single-time-of-day impression offered by OBPM, several international guidelines now propose as a requirement ambulatory BP measurements to confirm the OBPM-based diagnosis of hypertension.[25,86] The latest update of the guidelines for the clinical management of adult primary hypertension from the National Institute for Health and Clinical Excellence (NICE) recommend ABPM be conducted to corroborate the diagnosis of hypertension for all adults 18 years of age or older with increased OBPM.[86] However, the NICE guidelines specify that clinicians should rely on the average of at least 14 measurements taken during the person's usual waking hours to confirm a diagnosis of hypertension. The NICE guidelines, by explicitly recommending that clinical decisions be based solely on ABPM-derived daytime SBP/DBP means greater than or equal to 135/85 mm Hg (the established wake-time thresholds for adults,[23] regardless of sex and presence of the compelling clinical conditions of type 2 diabetes, CKD, and past history of CVD events associated with highest CVD risk),[24] thus disregard the most meaningful sleep-time data that are acquired by around-the-clock ABPM.[24] This unjustified recommendation of the NICE guidelines ignores the persuasive findings of the substantial number of investigations[39,42–46,52,53,56,57,59–61] that document that the sleep-time BP more strongly predicts future CVD events than does the wake-time ambulatory BP. The authors wish to call attention to the fact that the recommendations of the NICE guidelines preclude determination of the most relevant information provided by around-the-clock ABPM (ie, the asleep SBP/DBP means), and thus they disrespect the known high prevalence of sleep-time hypertension and associated increased CVD risk.[24,42,45,52,53] In addition, the NICE guidelines disregard the considerable prevalence and clinical implications of masked hypertension (ie, normal office BP but increased ambulatory BP),[44] and nondipping normotension, namely absence of sleep-time relative decline from the daytime BP mean level by 10% or more in individuals with otherwise normal ambulatory BP levels.[58]

The most recently issued guidelines of the European Society of Hypertension (ESH) and European Society of Cardiology (ESC) for the management of arterial hypertension state that, "it is now generally accepted that out-of-office BP is an important adjunct to conventional office BP measurement, but the latter currently remains the 'gold standard' for screening, diagnosis and management of hypertension."[23] These ESH/ESC guidelines provide a limited list of conditions "considered as clinical indications for out-of-office BP measurement for diagnostic purposes,"[23] specifically: suspected isolated-office and/or masked hypertension; considerable variability of OBPM during the same of between visits; autonomic, postural, postprandial, siesta, and medication-induced hypotension; increased OBPM or suspected preeclampsia in pregnant women; identification of true and false resistant hypertension; suspicion of nocturnal hypertension or absence of dipping; and assessment of BP variability.[23] As emphatically expressed in the ESH/ESC guidelines, out-of-office methods of ABPM and HBPM do not assess BP status equivalently: "since the two methods provide somehow different information on the subject's BP status and risk, they should thus be regarded as complementary, rather than competitive or alternative."[23] From the current evidence presented herein on the prognostic value of sleep-time BP, the ESH/ESC guidelines seem outdated and anchored in the past by advocating the supposedly time-honored value of OBPM.

The 2015 US Preventive Services Task Force (USPSTF) report[25] constitutes an important update as to the preferred means in primary care practice of making the differential diagnosis of hypertension versus normotension plus estimating patient CVD risk. The most important conclusions of this report are[25] (1) derived parameters from around-the-clock ABPM best predict long-term adverse CVD outcomes independently of daytime OBPM; and (2) around-the-clock ABPM, rather than traditional daytime OBPM, should now be considered the reference standard in primary care medicine to diagnose hypertension in adults 18 years of age or older. Thus, the report recommends application of ABPM to either corroborate or contradict single or repeated-interval daytime OBPM-diagnosed increased BP to avoid misdiagnosis and unnecessary treatment of persons who show increased OBPM but are proved to be normotensive by ABPM (commonly termed isolated-office hypertension, although the more accurate and preferred term is masked normotension).[24] From an exploratory meta-analysis of no apparent difference in

HR for CVD risk per increase of 10 mm Hg between the ABPM-derived nighttime, daytime, and 24-hour SBP means, the USPSTF report concludes that any one of these mean values might be used interchangeably to corroborate the diagnosis of hypertension in adults.[25] However, this conclusion is questionable because of large differences between the consulted studies as to how nighttime and daytime are defined, plus the absence of emphasis on the most clinically meaningful end point of the sleep-time BP to predict future CVD events.[63]

The findings of the MAPEC study that incorporated periodic systematic 48-hour ABPM evaluation of all participants during a median follow-up of 5.6 years constitute the first proof-of-concept evidence the progressive reduction of the asleep SBP mean and correction of the sleep-time relative SBP decline toward normal best attenuates the risk of CVD, stroke, and new-onset diabetes.[18–22,42,44,45,52,57,58,64,65] The results of the MAPEC study further substantiate that the clinical objectives of superior BP control plus greater CVD risk reduction can be accomplished easily without additional cost through a hypertension treatment strategy that entails ingestion of one or more conventional BP-lowering medications at bedtime in step with key physiologic, neuroendocrine, and other circadian rhythms that regulate the 24-hour BP pattern and its features. Thus, as discussed in detail herein, the bedtime chronotherapeutic hypertension strategy that targets two novel clinical treatment goals (normalization of the asleep SBP and sleep-time BP relative decline) is a much more effective and beneficial means of prevention (ie, chronoprevention) of CVD and other pathologic outcomes, particularly in individuals with high-risk CKD, type 2 diabetes, and resistant hypertension, as summarized in **Fig. 6**[18–20,57] and confirmed in upcoming publications by the Hygia outcomes project.[87]

REFERENCES

1. Albrecht U. Timing to perfection: the biology of central and peripheral circadian clocks. Neuron 2013; 74:246–60.

2. Reinberg A, Smolensky M. Biological rhythms and medicine. Berlin: Springer Verlag; 1983. p. 305.

3. Ticher A, Ashkenazi IE, Reinberg A. Preservation of the functional advantage of human time structure. FASEB J 1995;9:269–72.

4. Duffy JF, Czeisler CA. Effect of light on human circadian physiology. Sleep Med Clin 2009;4:165–77.

5. Smolensky MH, Sackett-Lundeen LL, Portaluppi F. Nocturnal night pollution and underexposure to daytime sunlight: complementary mechanisms of circadian disruption and related diseases. Chronobiol Int 2015;32:1029–48.

6. Hermida RC, Ayala DE, Portaluppi F. Circadian variation of blood pressure: the basis for the chronotherapy of hypertension. Adv Drug Deliv Rev 2007; 59:904–22.

7. Portaluppi F, Tiseo R, Smolensky MH, et al. Circadian rhythms and cardiovascular health. Sleep Med Rev 2012;16:151–66.

8. Fabbian F, Smolensky MH, Tiseo R, et al. Dipper and non-dipper blood pressure 24-hour patterns: circadian rhythm-dependent physiologic and pathophysiologic mechanisms. Chronobiol Int 2013;30:17–30.

9. Smolensky MH, Hermida RC, Portaluppi F. Circadian mechanisms of 24-hour blood pressure regulation and patterning. Sleep Med Rev 2017;33:4–16.

10. Hermida RC, Ayala DE, Calvo C, et al. Chronotherapy of hypertension: administration-time dependent effects of treatment on the circadian pattern of blood pressure. Adv Drug Deliv Rev 2007;59:923–39.

11. Smolensky MH, Hermida RC, Ayala DE, et al. Administration-time-dependent effect of blood pressure-lowering medications: basis for the chronotherapy of hypertension. Blood Press Monit 2010;15:173–80.

12. Hermida RC, Ayala DE, Fernández JR, et al. Circadian rhythms in blood pressure regulation and optimization of hypertension treatment with ACE inhibitor and ARB medications. Am J Hypertens 2011;24:383–91.

13. Hermida RC, Ayala DE, Fernández JR, et al. Administration-time-differences in effects of hypertension medications on ambulatory blood pressure regulation. Chronobiol Int 2013;30:280–314.

14. Hermida RC, Ayala DE, Smolensky MH, et al. Chronotherapy improves blood pressure control and reduces vascular risk in CKD. Nat Rev Nephrol 2013;9:358–68.

15. Hermida RC, Ayala DE, Smolensky MH, et al. Chronotherapeutics of conventional blood pressure-lowering medications: simple, low-cost means of improving management and treatment outcomes of hypertensive-related disorders. Curr Hypertens Rep 2014;16:412.

16. Smolensky MH, Hermida RC, Ayala DE, et al. Bedtime hypertension chronotherapy: concepts and patient outcomes. Curr Pharm Des 2015;21: 773–90.

17. Hermida RC, Ayala DE, Smolensky MH, et al. Chronotherapy with conventional blood pressure medications improves management of hypertension and reduces cardiovascular and stroke risks. Hypertens Res 2016;39:277–92.

18. Hermida RC, Ayala DE, Mojón A, et al. Influence of circadian time of hypertension treatment on cardiovascular risk: results of the MAPEC study. Chronobiol Int 2010;27:1629–51.

19. Hermida RC, Ayala DE, Mojón A, et al. Influence of time of day of blood pressure-lowering treatment on cardiovascular risk in hypertensive patients with type 2 diabetes. Diabetes Care 2011; 34:1270–6.

20. Hermida RC, Ayala DE, Mojón A, et al. Bedtime dosing of antihypertensive medications reduces cardiovascular risk in CKD. J Am Soc Nephrol 2011;22: 2313–21.

21. Hermida RC, Ayala DE, Mojón A, et al. Prognostic marker of type 2 diabetes and therapeutic target for prevention. Diabetologia 2016;59:244–54.

22. Hermida RC, Ayala DE, Mojón A, et al. Bedtime ingestion of hypertension medications reduces the risk of new-onset type 2 diabetes: a randomised controlled trial. Diabetologia 2016;59:255–65.

23. Mancia G, Fagard R, Narkiewicz K, et al. 2013 ESH/ESC guidelines for the management of arterial hypertension: the Task Force for the Management of Arterial Hypertension of the European Society of Hypertension (ESH) and of the European Society of Cardiology (ESC). J Hypertens 2013;31:1281–357.

24. Hermida RC, Smolensky MH, Ayala DE, et al. 2013 ambulatory blood pressure monitoring recommendations for the diagnosis of adult hypertension, assessment of cardiovascular and other hypertension-associated risk, and attainment of therapeutic goals. Joint recommendations from the International Society for Chronobiology (ISC), American Association of Medical Chronobiology and Chronotherapeutics (AAMCC), Spanish Society of Applied Chronobiology, Chronotherapy, and Vascular Risk (SECAC), Spanish Society of Atherosclerosis (SEA), and Romanian Society of Internal Medicine (RSIM). Chronobiol Int 2013;30:355–410.

25. Piper MA, Evans CV, Burda BU, et al. Diagnosis and predictive accuracy of blood pressure screening methods with consideration of rescreening intervals: a systematic review for the U.S. Preventive Services Task Force. Ann Intern Med 2015;162:192–204.

26. Hermida RC, Fernández JR, Ayala DE, et al. Circadian rhythm of double (rate-pressure) product in healthy normotensive young subjects. Chronobiol Int 2001;18:475–89.

27. Hermida RC, Ayala DE, Fernández JR, et al. Modeling the circadian variability of ambulatorily monitored blood pressure by multiple-component analysis. Chronobiol Int 2002;19:461–81.

28. Hermida RC, Calvo C, Ayala DE, et al. Relationship between physical activity and blood pressure in dipper and nondipper hypertensive patients. J Hypertens 2002;20:1097–104.

29. Lakatua DJ, Haus E, Halberg F, et al. Circadian characteristics of urinary epinephrine and norepinephrine from healthy young women in Japan and U.S.A. Chronobiol Int 1986;3:189–95.

30. Angeli A, Gatti G, Masera R. Chronobiology of the hypothalamic-pituitary-adrenal and renin-angiotensin-aldosterone systems. In: Touitou Y, Haus E, editors. Biologic rhythms in clinical and laboratory medicine. Berlin: Springer-Verlag; 1992. p. 292–314.

31. Gordon RD, Wolfe LK, Island DP, et al. A diurnal rhythm in plasma renin activity in man. J Clin Invest 1966;45:1587–92.

32. Portaluppi F, Trasforini G, Margutti A, et al. Circadian rhythm of calcitonin gene-related peptide in uncomplicated essential hypertension. J Hypertens 1992; 10:1227–34.

33. Sothern RB, Vesely DL, Kanabrocki EL, et al. Temporal (circadian) and functional relationship between atrial natriuretic peptides and blood pressure. Chronobiol Int 1995;12:106–20.

34. Kanabrocki EL, George M, Hermida RC, et al. Day-night variations in blood levels of nitric oxide, T-TFPI and E-selectin. Clin Appl Thromb Hemost 2001;7: 339–45.

35. Smolensky MH, Hermida RC, Castriotta RJ, et al. Role of sleep-wake cycle on blood pressure circadian rhythms and hypertension. Sleep Med 2007;8: 668–80.

36. Perloff D, Sokolow M, Cowan R. The prognostic value of ambulatory blood pressures. JAMA 1983; 249:2792–8.

37. Verdecchia P, Porcellati C, Schillaci G, et al. Ambulatory blood pressure: an independent predictor of prognosis in essential hypertension. Hypertension 1994;24:793–801.

38. Clement DL, De Buyzere ML, De Bacquer DA, et al. Prognostic value of ambulatory blood-pressure recordings in patients with treated hypertension. N Engl J Med 2003;348:2407–15.

39. Dolan E, Stanton A, Thijs L, et al. Superiority of ambulatory over clinic blood pressure measurement in predicting mortality: the Dublin Outcome Study. Hypertension 2005;46:156–61.

40. Eguchi K, Pickering TG, Hoshide S, et al. Ambulatory blood pressure is a better marker than clinic blood pressure in predicting cardiovascular events in patients with/without type 2 diabetes. Am J Hypertens 2008;21:443–50.

41. Salles GF, Cardoso CR, Muxfeldt ES. Prognostic influence of office and ambulatory blood pressures in resistant hypertension. Arch Intern Med 2008; 168:2340–6.

42. Hermida RC, Ayala DE, Mojón A, et al. Decreasing sleep-time blood pressure determined by ambulatory monitoring reduces cardiovascular risk. J Am Coll Cardiol 2011;58:1165–73.

43. Minutolo R, Agarwal R, Borrelli S, et al. Prognostic role of ambulatory blood pressure measurement in patients with nondialysis chronic kidney disease. Arch Intern Med 2011;171:1090–8.

44. Hermida RC, Ayala DE, Mojón A, et al. Sleep-time blood pressure and the prognostic value of isolated-office and masked hypertension. Am J Hypertens 2012;25:297–305.

45. Hermida RC, Ayala DE, Mojón A, et al. Sleep-time blood pressure as a therapeutic target for cardiovascular risk reduction in type 2 diabetes. Am J Hypertens 2012;25:325–34.

46. Roush GC, Fagard RH, Salles GF, et al. Prognostic impact from clinic, daytime, and nighttime systolic blood pressure in 9 cohorts on 13,844 patients with hypertension. J Hypertens 2014;32:2332–40.

47. Hermida RC, Ayala DE, Crespo JJ, et al. Influence of age and hypertension treatment-time on ambulatory blood pressure in hypertensive patients. Chronobiol Int 2013;30:176–91.

48. Ayala DE, Moyá A, Crespo JJ, et al. Circadian pattern of ambulatory blood pressure in hypertensive patients with and without type 2 diabetes. Chronobiol Int 2013;30:99–115.

49. Mojón A, Ayala DE, Piñeiro L, et al. Comparison of ambulatory blood pressure parameters of hypertensive patients with and without chronic kidney disease. Chronobiol Int 2013;30:145–58.

50. Ríos MT, Domínguez-Sardiña M, Ayala DE, et al. Prevalence and clinical characteristics of isolated-office and true resistant hypertension determined by ambulatory blood pressure monitoring. Chronobiol Int 2013;30:207–20.

51. Portaluppi F, Hermida RC. Circadian rhythms in cardiac arrhythmias and opportunities for their chronotherapy. Adv Drug Deliv Rev 2007;59:940–51.

52. Hermida RC, Ayala DE, Fernández JR, et al. Sleep-time blood pressure: prognostic value and relevance as a therapeutic target for cardiovascular risk reduction. Chronobiol Int 2013;30:68–86.

53. Hermida RC, Ayala DE, Mojón A, et al. Sleep-time ambulatory blood pressure as a novel therapeutic target for cardiovascular risk reduction. J Hum Hypertens 2014;28:567–74.

54. Ohkubo T, Hozawa A, Yamaguchi J, et al. Prognostic significance of the nocturnal decline in blood pressure in individuals with and without high 24-h blood pressure: the Ohasama study. J Hypertens 2002;20:2183–9.

55. Ingelsson E, Bjorklund-Bodegard K, Lind L, et al. Diurnal blood pressure pattern and risk of congestive heart failure. JAMA 2006;295:2859–66.

56. Boggia J, Li Y, Thijs L, et al. Prognostic accuracy of day versus night ambulatory blood pressure: a cohort study. Lancet 2007;370:1219–29.

57. Ayala DE, Hermida RC, Mojón A, et al. Cardiovascular risk of resistant hypertension: dependence on treatment-time regimen of blood pressure-lowering medications. Chronobiol Int 2013;30:340–52.

58. Hermida RC, Ayala DE, Mojón A, et al. Blunted sleep-time relative blood pressure decline increases cardiovascular risk independent of blood pressure level – The "normotensive non-dipper" paradox. Chronobiol Int 2013;30:87–98.

59. Ben-Dov IZ, Kark JD, Ben-Ishay D, et al. Predictors of all-cause mortality in clinical ambulatory monitoring. Unique aspects of blood pressure during sleep. Hypertension 2007;49:1235–41.

60. Fagard RH, Celis H, Thijs L, et al. Daytime and nighttime blood pressure as predictors of death and cause-specific cardiovascular events in hypertension. Hypertension 2008;51:55–61.

61. Fan HQ, Li Y, Thijs L, et al. Prognostic value of isolated nocturnal hypertension on ambulatory measurement in 8711 individuals from 10 populations. J Hypertens 2010;28:2036–45.

62. Hermida RC, Smolensky MH, Ayala DE, et al. Ambulatory blood pressure monitoring (ABPM) as the reference standard for diagnosis of hypertension and assessment of vascular risk in adults. Chronobiol Int 2015;32:1329–42.

63. Smolensky MH, Ayala DE, Hermida RC. Ambulatory blood pressure monitoring (ABPM) as THE reference standard to confirm diagnosis of hypertension in adults: recommendation of the 2015 U.S. Preventive Services Task Force (USPSTF). Chronobiol Int 2015;32:1320–2.

64. Hermida RC, Ayala DE, Mojón A, et al. Cardiovascular risk of essential hypertension: influence of class, number, and treatment-time regimen of hypertension medications. Chronobiol Int 2013;30:315–27.

65. Hermida RC, Ayala DE, Mojón A, et al. Role of time-of-day of hypertension treatment on the J-shaped relationship between blood pressure and cardiovascular risk. Chronobiol Int 2013;30:328–39.

66. Hermida RC, Ayala DE, Fontao MJ, et al. Ambulatory blood pressure monitoring: importance of sampling rate and duration – 48 versus 24 hours – on the accurate assessment of cardiovascular risk. Chronobiol Int 2013;30:55–67.

67. Hermida RC, Fernández JR, Mojón A, et al. Reproducibility of the hyperbaric index as a measure of blood pressure excess. Hypertension 2000;35:118–25.

68. Hermida RC, Mojón A, Fernández JR, et al. The tolerance-hyperbaric test: a chronobiologic approach for improved diagnosis of hypertension. Chronobiol Int 2002;19:1183–211.

69. Crespo C, Fernández JR, Aboy M, et al. Clinical application of a novel automatic algorithm for actigraphy-based activity and rest period identification to accurately determine awake and asleep ambulatory blood pressure parameters and cardiovascular risk. Chronobiol Int 2013;30:43–54.

70. Yusuf S, Sleight P, Pogue J, et al. Effects of an angiotensin-converting-enzyme inhibitor, ramipril, on cardiovascular events in high-risk patients: the Heart Outcomes Prevention Evaluation Study Investigators. N Engl J Med 2000;342:145–53.

71. Svensson P, de Faire U, Sleight P, et al. Comparative effects of ramipril on ambulatory and office blood pressures. A HOPE substudy. Hypertension 2001; 38:e28–32.

72. Hermida RC, Ayala DE. Chronotherapy with the angiotensin-converting enzyme inhibitor ramipril in essential hypertension: improved blood pressure control with bedtime dosing. Hypertension 2009; 54:40–6.

73. Hermida RC, Ayala DE, Fontao MJ, et al. Administration-time-dependent effects of spirapril on ambulatory blood pressure in uncomplicated essential hypertension. Chronobiol Int 2010;27:560–74.

74. Staessen JA, Fagard R, Thijs L, et al. Randomised double-blind comparison of placebo and active treatment for older patients with isolated systolic hypertension. Lancet 1997;350:757–64.

75. Liu L, Wang JG, Gong L, et al. Comparison of active treatment and placebo in older Chinese patients with isolated systolic hypertension. Systolic Hypertension in China (Syst-China) Collaborative Group. J Hypertens 1998;16:1823–9.

76. Hermida RC, Calvo C, Ayala DE, et al. Dose- and administration-time-dependent effects of nifedipine GITS on ambulatory blood pressure in hypertensive subjects. Chronobiol Int 2007;24:471–93.

77. Hermida RC, Ayala DE, Mojon A, et al. Chronotherapy with nifedipine GITS in hypertensive patients: improved efficacy and safety with bedtime dosing. Am J Hypertens 2008;21:948–54.

78. Black HR, Elliott WJ, Grandits G, et al. Principal results of the Controlled Onset Verapamil Investigation of Cardiovascular End Points (CONVINCE) trial. JAMA 2003;289:2073–82.

79. White WB, Black HR, Weber MA, et al. Comparison of effects of controlled-onset extended-release verapamil at bedtime and nifedipine gastrointestinal therapeutic system on arising on early morning blood pressure, heart rate, and the heart rate-blood pressure product. Am J Cardiol 1998;81: 424–31.

80. Roush GC, Fapohunda J, Kostis JB. Evening dosing of antihypertensive therapy to reduce cardiovascular events: a third type of evidence based on a systematic review and meta-analysis of randomized trials. J Clin Hypertens (Greenwich) 2014;16:561–8.

81. Law MR, Morris JK, Wald NJ. Use of blood pressure lowering drugs in the prevention of cardiovascular disease: meta-analysis of 147 randomised trials in the context of expectations from prospective epidemiological studies. BMJ 2009;338:b1665.

82. American Diabetes Association. Standards of medical care in diabetes – 2012. Diabetes Care 2012; 35(Suppl 1):S11–63.

83. Authors/Task Force Members, Rydén L, Grant PJ, et al. ESC guidelines on diabetes, pre-diabetes, and cardiovascular diseases developed in collaboration with the EASD: the Task Force on Diabetes, Pre-diabetes, and Cardiovascular Diseases of the European Society of Cardiology (ESC) and developed in collaboration with the European Association for the Study of Diabetes (EASD). Eur Heart J 2013; 34:3035–87.

84. Shimamoto K, Ando K, Fujita T, et al. The Japanese Society of Hypertension guidelines for the management of hypertension (JSH 2014). Hypertens Res 2014;37:253–90.

85. Chiang CE, Wang TD, Ueng KC, et al. 2015 guidelines of the Taiwan Society of Cardiology and the Taiwan Hypertension Society for the Management of Hypertension. J Chin Med Assoc 2015;78:1–47.

86. National Institute for Health and Clinical Excellence. Hypertension: the clinical management of primary hypertension in adults. NICE clinical guidelines 127: methods, evidence and recommendations. London: National Clinical Guidelines Centre; 2011. Available at: http://guidance.nice.org.uk/CG/Wave2/14.

87. Hermida RC. Sleep-time ambulatory blood pressure as a prognostic marker of vascular and other risks and therapeutic target for prevention by hypertension chronotherapy: rationale and design of the Hygia Project. Chronobiol Int 2016;33:906–36.

UNITED STATES POSTAL SERVICE®

Statement of Ownership, Management, and Circulation
(All Periodicals Publications Except Requester Publications)

1. Publication Title	2. Publication Number	3. Filing Date
HEART FAILURE CLINICS	025 – 055	6/18/2017

4. Issue Frequency	5. Number of Issues Published Annually	6. Annual Subscription Price
JAN, APR, JUL, OCT	4	$247.00

7. Complete Mailing Address of Known Office of Publication (Not printer) (Street, city, county, state, and ZIP+4®)

ELSEVIER INC.
230 Park Avenue, Suite 800
New York, NY 10169

Contact Person
STEPHEN R. BUSHING
Telephone (include area code)
215-239-3688

8. Complete Mailing Address of Headquarters or General Business Office of Publisher (Not printer)

ELSEVIER INC.
230 Park Avenue, Suite 800
New York, NY 10169

9. Full Names and Complete Mailing Addresses of Publisher, Editor, and Managing Editor (Do not leave blank)

Publisher (Name and complete mailing address)

ADRIANNE BRIGIDO, ELSEVIER INC.
1600 JOHN F KENNEDY BLVD. SUITE 1800
PHILADELPHIA, PA 19103-2899

Editor (Name and complete mailing address)

STACY EASTMAN, ELSEVIER INC.
1600 JOHN F KENNEDY BLVD. SUITE 1800
PHILADELPHIA, PA 19103-2899

Managing Editor (Name and complete mailing address)

PATRICK MANLEY, ELSEVIER INC.
1600 JOHN F KENNEDY BLVD. SUITE 1800
PHILADELPHIA, PA 19103-2899

10. Owner (Do not leave blank. If the publication is owned by a corporation, give the name and address of the corporation immediately followed by the names and addresses of all stockholders owning or holding 1 percent or more of the total amount of stock. If not owned by a corporation, give the names and addresses of the individual owners. If owned by a partnership or other unincorporated firm, give its name and address as well as those of each individual owner. If the publication is published by a nonprofit organization, give its name and address.)

Full Name	Complete Mailing Address
WHOLLY OWNED SUBSIDIARY OF REED/ELSEVIER, US HOLDINGS	1600 JOHN F KENNEDY BLVD. SUITE 1800 PHILADELPHIA, PA 19103-2899

11. Known Bondholders, Mortgagees, and Other Security Holders Owning or Holding 1 Percent or More of Total Amount of Bonds, Mortgages, or Other Securities. If none, check box ☑ None

Full Name	Complete Mailing Address
N/A	

12. Tax Status (For completion by nonprofit organizations authorized to mail at nonprofit rates) (Check one)
The purpose, function, and nonprofit status of this organization and the exempt status for federal income tax purposes:
☑ Has Not Changed During Preceding 12 Months
☐ Has Changed During Preceding 12 Months (Publisher must submit explanation of change with this statement)

13. Publication Title	14. Issue Date for Circulation Data Below
HEART FAILURE CLINICS	JULY 2017

15. Extent and Nature of Circulation			Average No. Copies Each Issue During Preceding 12 Months	No. Copies of Single Issue Published Nearest to Filing Date
a. Total Number of Copies (Net press run)			117	89
b. Paid Circulation (By Mail and Outside the Mail)	(1)	Mailed Outside-County Paid Subscriptions Stated on PS Form 3541 (include paid distribution above nominal rate, advertiser's proof copies, and exchange copies)	23	26
	(2)	Mailed In-County Paid Subscriptions Stated on PS Form 3541 (include paid distribution above nominal rate, advertiser's proof copies, and exchange copies)	0	0
	(3)	Paid Distribution Outside the Mails Including Sales Through Dealers and Carriers, Street Vendors, Counter Sales, and Other Paid Distribution Outside USPS®	16	17
	(4)	Paid Distribution by Other Classes of Mail Through the USPS (e.g., First-Class Mail®)	0	0
c. Total Paid Distribution (Sum of 15b (1), (2), (3), and (4))			39	43
d. Free or Nominal Rate Distribution (By Mail and Outside the Mail)	(1)	Free or Nominal Rate Outside-County Copies included on PS Form 3541	34	46
	(2)	Free or Nominal Rate In-County Copies Included on PS Form 3541	0	0
	(3)	Free or Nominal Rate Copies Mailed at Other Classes Through the USPS (e.g., First-Class Mail)	0	0
	(4)	Free or Nominal Rate Distribution Outside the Mail (Carriers or other means)	0	0
e. Total Free or Nominal Rate Distribution (Sum of 15d (1), (2), (3) and (4))			34	46
f. Total Distribution (Sum of 15c and 15e)			73	89
g. Copies not Distributed (See Instructions to Publishers #4 (page #3))			44	0
h. Total (Sum of 15f and g)			117	89
i. Percent Paid (15c divided by 15f times 100)			53.42%	48.31%

* If you are claiming electronic copies, go to line 16 on page 3. If you are not claiming electronic copies, skip to line 17 on page 3.

16. Electronic Copy Circulation	Average No. Copies Each Issue During Preceding 12 Months	No. Copies of Single Issue Published Nearest to Filing Date
a. Paid Electronic Copies	0	0
b. Total Paid Print Copies (Line 15c) + Paid Electronic Copies (Line 16a)	39	43
c. Total Print Distribution (Line 15f) + Paid Electronic Copies (Line 16a)	73	89
d. Percent Paid (Both Print & Electronic Copies) (16b divided by 16c × 100)	53.42%	48.31%

☑ I certify that 50% of all my distributed copies (electronic and print) are paid above a nominal price.

17. Publication of Statement of Ownership
☑ If the publication is a general publication, publication of this statement is required. Will be printed   ☐ Publication not required.
in the _____ OCTOBER 2017 _____ issue of this publication.

18. Signature and Title of Editor, Publisher, Business Manager, or Owner _____ Date 6/18/2017

STEPHEN R. BUSHING - INVENTORY DISTRIBUTION CONTROL MANAGER

I certify that all information furnished on this form is true and complete. I understand that anyone who furnishes false or misleading information on this form or who omits material or information requested on the form may be subject to criminal sanctions (including fines and imprisonment) and/or civil sanctions (including civil penalties).

PS Form **3526**, July 2014 (Page 3 of 4)

PS Form **3526**, July 2014 (Page 1 of 4 (see instructions page 4))   PSN: 7530-01-000-9931   PRIVACY NOTICE: See our privacy policy on www.usps.com.

Moving?

Make sure your subscription moves with you!

To notify us of your new address, find your **Clinics Account Number** (located on your mailing label above your name), and contact customer service at:

Email: journalscustomerservice-usa@elsevier.com

800-654-2452 (subscribers in the U.S. & Canada)
314-447-8871 (subscribers outside of the U.S. & Canada)

Fax number: 314-447-8029

Elsevier Health Sciences Division
Subscription Customer Service
3251 Riverport Lane
Maryland Heights, MO 63043

*To ensure uninterrupted delivery of your subscription, please notify us at least 4 weeks in advance of move.

Printed and bound by CPI Group (UK) Ltd, Croydon, CR0 4YY

03/10/2024

01040298-0010